Detection Systems in Lung Cancer and Imaging, Volume 1

Detection Systems in Lung Cancer and Imaging, Volume 1

Edited by
Ayman El-Baz
University of Louisville, Louisville, Kentucky, USA and
University of Louisville at AlAlamein International University (UofL-AIU),
New Alamein City, Egypt

Jasjit S Suri
AtheroPoint LLC, Roseville, CA, USA

IOP Publishing, Bristol, UK

ISBN 978-0-7503-3355-9 (ebook)
ISBN 978-0-7503-3353-5 (print)
ISBN 978-0-7503-3356-6 (myPrint)
ISBN 978-0-7503-3354-2 (mobi)

DOI 10.1088/978-0-7503-3355-9

Version: 20220101

IOP ebooks

British Library Cataloguing-in-Publication Data: A catalogue record for this book is available from the British Library.

Published by IOP Publishing, wholly owned by The Institute of Physics, London

IOP Publishing, Temple Circus, Temple Way, Bristol, BS1 6HG, UK

US Office: IOP Publishing, Inc., 190 North Independence Mall West, Suite 601, Philadelphia, PA 19106, USA

With love and affection to my mother and father, whose loving spirit sustains me still

—Ayman El-Baz

To my late loving parents, immediate family, and children

—Jasjit S Suri

Contents

Preface

The book covers the state-of-the-art techniques for the early detection of lung cancer, focusing on non-invasive approaches. Lung cancer is the second most common cancer in men and women; it comes after prostate cancer in men and after breast cancer in women. It is considered the leading cause of cancer-related deaths among both genders in the United States; however, the early detection of lung cancer increases the survival rate among patients. This book discusses the development of accurate and reliable techniques for the early detection of lung cancer. Among the topics discussed in the book are lung cancer classification using wavelet recurrent neural network; diffusion-weighted magnetic resonance imaging (DWI) for lung cancer; handcrafted features; radiation therapy in lung cancer treatment; visual sensing technology in lung cancer screening; automatic lung segmentation; molecular imaging; computed tomography ventilation imaging; and heat shock proteins.

In summary, the main aim of this book is to help advance scientific research within the broad field of the early detection of lung cancer. The book focuses on major trends and challenges in this area, and it presents work aimed at identifyng new techniques and their use in biomedical image analysis.

Ayman El-Baz
Jasjit S Suri

Acknowledgement

The completion of this book could not have been possible without the participation and assistance of so many people whose names cannot all be enumerated. Their contributions are sincerely appreciated and gratefully acknowledged. However, the editors would like to express their deep appreciation and indebtedness particularly to Dr Ali H Mahmoud and Kamal Hammouda for their endless support.

Ayman El-Baz
Jasjit S Suri

Editor biographies

Ayman El-Baz

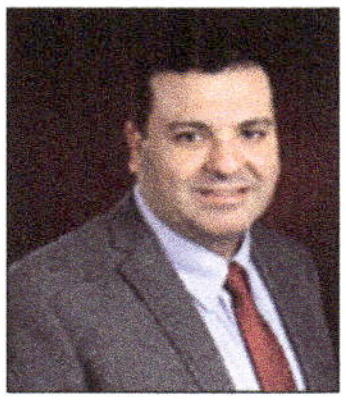

Ayman El-Baz is a Distinguished Professor at University of Louisville, Kentucky, United States and University of Louisville at AlAlamein International University (UofL-AIU), New Alamein City, Egypt. Dr El-Baz earned his BSc and MSc degrees in electrical engineering in 1997 and 2001, respectively. He earned his PhD in electrical engineering from the University of Louisville in 2006. Dr El-Baz was named as a Fellow for Coulter, AIMBE and NAI for his contributions to the field of biomedical translational research. Dr El-Baz has almost two decades of hands-on experience in the fields of bio-imaging modeling and non-invasive computer-assisted diagnosis systems. He has authored or coauthored more than 500 technical articles (182 journals, 44 books, 95 book chapters, 253 refereed-conference papers, 215 abstracts, and 38 US patents and Disclosures).

Jasjit S Suri

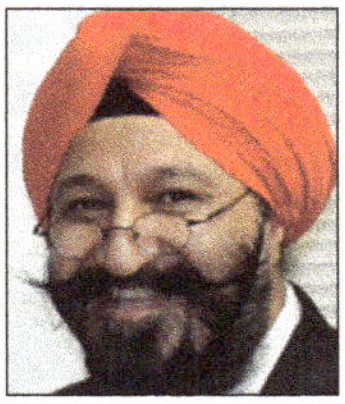

Jasjit S Suri, PhD, MBA is a Fellow of IEEE, AIMBE, SVM, AIUM, and APVS. He is currently the Chairman of AtheroPoint, Roseville, CA, USA, dedicated to imaging technologies for cardiovascular and stroke. He has nearly ~22,000 citations, coauthored 50 books, and has an H-index of 72.

List of contributors

Abdurakhman
Mathematics Department, Universitas Gadjah Mada, Yogyakarta, Indonesia

Kshitish Acharya
Institute of Bioinformatics and Applied Biotechnology (IBAB), Phase I, Electronic City, Bengaluru (Bangalore) - 560 100, Karnataka, India (www.ibab.ac.in)
and
Founder Director, Shodhaka Life Sciences Pvt. Ltd., Electronic city, Phase I, Bengaluru (Bangalore) - 560100, Karnataka, India (www.shodhaka.net)
and
Founder, Biological Data Analysers' Association (http://startbioinfo.org/BdataA)

Guilherme Aresta
INESC TEC, Porto, Portugal

Özlem Çoban
Department of Pharmaceutical Technology, Faculty of Pharmacy, Karadeniz Technical University, Trabzon, Turkey
and
Drug and Pharmaceutical Technology Application and Research Center, Karadeniz Technical University, Trabzon, Turkey

Carlos Ferreira
INESC TEC, Porto, Portugal

Adria Hasan
Molecular Cell Biology Laboratory, Integral Information and Research Centre-4 (IIRC-4), and Department of Bioengineering, Faculty of Engineering, Integral University, Kursi Road, Lucknow 226026, India
and
Department of Bioengineering, Faculty of Engineering, Integral University, Kursi Road, Lucknow, 226026, India

Seifedine Kadry
Department of Mathematics and Computer Science, Faculty of Science, Lebanon

Puja Khaitan
Medstar Washington Hospital Center, Washington, DC, USA

Rongpeng Li
Jiangsu Normal University, Xuzhou, China

Jonathan Lischalk
NYU Langone, New York, USA

Mary McGunigal
Medstar Georgetown University Hospital, Washington, DC, USA

Snober S Mir
Molecular Cell Biology Laboratory, Integral Information and Research Centre-4 (IIRC-4), and Department of Bioengineering, Faculty of Engineering, Integral University, Kursi Road, Lucknow 226026, India
and
Department of Bioengineering, Faculty of Engineering, Integral University, Kursi Road, Lucknow, 226026, India

Devi Nurtiyasari
Mathematics Education Study Program, Universitas Islam Negeri Sunan Kalijaga, Yogyakarta, Indonesia

Sana Parveen
Molecular Cell Biology Laboratory, Integral Information and Research Centre-4 (IIRC-4), and Department of Bioengineering, Faculty of Engineering, Integral University, Kursi Road, Lucknow 226026, India
and
Department of Biosciences, Faculty of Science, Integral University, Kursi Road, Lucknow, 226026, India

João Pedrosa
INESC TEC, Porto, Portugal

Venkatesan Rajinikanth
Department of Electronics and Instrumentation Engineering, OMR, Chennai 600119, TN, India

Pamela Randolph-Jackson
Medstar Washington Hospital Center, Washington, DC, USA

Suroor Fatima Rizvi
Molecular Cell Biology Laboratory, Integral Information and Research Centre-4 (IIRC-4), and Department of Bioengineering, Faculty of Engineering, Integral University, Kursi Road, Lucknow 226026, India
and
Department of Bioengineering, Faculty of Engineering, Integral University, Kursi Road, Lucknow, 226026, India

Dedi Rosadi
Mathematics Department, Universitas Gadjah Mada, Yogyakarta, Indonesia

Bilal A Tahir
Department of Oncology and Metabolism, The University of Sheffield, Sheffield, UK

Hidetaka Uramoto
Department of Thoracic Surgery, Kanazawa Medical University, Uchinada, Japan

Katsuo Usuda
Department of Thoracic Surgery, Kanazawa Medical University, Uchinada, Japan

Yonghong Xu
Jiangsu Normal University, Xuzhou, China

Nana Xu
Xuzhou Medical University, Xuzhou, China

Yeşim Kaya Yaşar
Department of Pharmaceutical Technology, Faculty of Pharmacy, Karadeniz Technical University, Trabzon, Turkey
and
Drug and Pharmaceutical Technology Application and Research Center, Karadeniz Technical University, Trabzon, Turkey

IOP Publishing

Detection Systems in Lung Cancer and Imaging, Volume 1

Ayman El-Baz and Jasjit S Suri

Chapter 1

Lung cancer classification using wavelet recurrent neural network

Devi Nurtiyasari, Dedi Rosadi and Abdurakhman

1.1 Introduction

Cancer is one of the leading causes of death in the world [1]. One of the most common types is lung cancer which has the highest mortality rate among all types of cancer [2]. Early detection may increase the survival rate of patients significantly. An early detection method to find out if someone has lung cancer is a lung radiology test (lung image). This image provides information on whether the lung is normal or not. A normal lung will show no nodules in the image, whereas an abnormal lung will show some nodules in the image. However, these nodules do not always indicate lung cancer since they can be caused by other diseases such as pneumonia or tuberculosis [3]. Nodules detected in the lung can be classified into two categories, namely non-cancerous nodules (benign) and cancerous nodules (malignant).

Therefore, to be able to classify the nodules for early detection of lung cancer based on the lung image, we need classification methods. The neural network model has been developed by researchers to classify lung cancer based on lung image. The recurrent neural network is one type of neural network model that has a feedback link on the network. As an image contains noise, the noise needs to be removed from the original image before applying the neural network network model for the classification process. This is known as the image denoising process. This process aims to get an image with better/higher quality. One of the methods of image denoising is using wavelet. The model that combines wavelet and recurrent neural network is called wavelet recurrent neural network (WRNN) [4].

Most of the models for lung cancer classification based on lung cancer images are various types of neural network model with binarization image pre-processing. The previous research for lung cancer classification has been done using the neural

doi:10.1088/978-0-7503-3355-9ch1

network model and it provides an accuracy of 80% [5]. Further research has been done using recurrent neural network model and it provides result with accuracy of 81.33% [6]. This research is not concerned with the image characteristics. Therefore, in this chapter, we will use WRNN to classify lung cancer based on lung images. Wavelet is concerned with the image characteristics and is used to remove the noise from the original image, while recurrent neural network is used for the classification process. As it is an elaborated model, it is expected to produce better/higher accuracy.

1.2 Lung cancer and lung image

1.2.1 Lung cancer

Cancer is a leading cause of death worldwide. According to the report, there were an estimated 9.6 million deaths in 2018 caused by cancer [1]. Globally, 1 in 6 deaths is caused by cancer. Lung cancer is the most common cancer and is responsible for 2.09 million cases. Moreover lung cancer is also the most common cause of cancer death with 1.76 million deaths [2].

Smoking is not the only cause of lung cancer. However, smoking is a significant factor that causes lung cancer. It is responsible for about 22% of deaths from lung cancer [1]. Active smokers are the most vulnerable group to lung cancer. Passive smokers also have a risk of lung cancer. Cigarettes and cigarette smoke contain more than 4000 chemicals and more than 60 toxic and carcinogenic substances. In the initial stages, the toxic substances do not affect the function of the lung organs, but the longer a person smokes, the damage to lung tissue will increase. This damage will cause cells to react abnormally and uncontrollably until cancer cells finally appear.

Early detection may increase the survival rate of patients significantly. Early detection that can be used to establish whether someone has lung cancer can be done through lung radiology tests (images of the lungs), called chest x-ray radiography. These images provide information on whether the lungs are normal or not. Normal lungs will show no nodules in the image, whereas abnormal lungs will show some nodules in the lung images. However, these nodules are not always indications of lung cancer since they can be caused by other diseases such as pneumonia or tuberculosis [3]. Nodules detected in the lungs can be classified into two categories, namely non-cancerous nodules (benign) and cancerous nodules (malignant).

1.2.2 Lung image

The image is a matrix of the pixel. It is arranged in rows and columns. The pixel describes the row and column location. It also has intensity symbolized as $p(x,y)$, where x is the row location and y is the column location of the pixel. Based on its intensity, the image can be categorized into three types, namely RGB, grayscale, and binary.

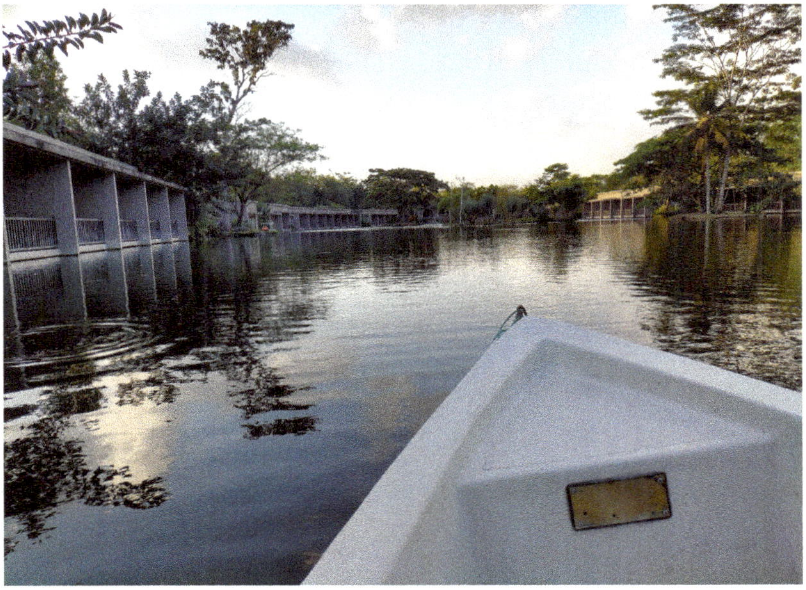

Figure 1.1. RGB image.

1.2.2.1 RGB image

RGB (red, green, blue) are the basic colors accepted by human eyes. Each pixel in the RGB image represents three basic colors. Each base color has intensity with a minimum value of 0 and a maximum value of 255. Mathematically, the intensity of each basic color of an RGB image is:

$$0 \leqslant p(x, y) \leqslant 255 \tag{1.1}$$

Figure 1.1 is an example of an RGB image. This image can be defined in a matrix sized 8×8 which contains its pixel. The red color matrix of figure 1.1 is as follows:

$$\begin{matrix} 177 & 224 & 172 & 205 & 202 & 205 & 197 & 161 \\ 87 & 113 & 173 & 239 & 231 & 241 & 181 & 113 \\ 47 & 41 & 72 & 118 & 140 & 144 & 95 & 68 \\ 68 & 54 & 55 & 92 & 129 & 154 & 98 & 72 \\ 42 & 50 & 87 & 165 & 149 & 157 & 132 & 113 \\ 104 & 162 & 100 & 102 & 129 & 139 & 143 & 136 \\ 68 & 125 & 66 & 83 & 139 & 120 & 110 & 114 \\ 72 & 58 & 46 & 128 & 123 & 106 & 110 & 110 \end{matrix}$$

The green color matrix of figure 1.1 is as follows:

176	226	176	212	210	215	199	145
94	120	177	244	238	240	173	104
55	53	84	125	141	138	86	64
80	70	70	98	126	139	88	68
53	58	93	169	159	163	128	100
102	151	108	112	141	153	153	141
68	125	91	101	150	129	114	122
94	84	70	137	133	116	115	115

The blue color matrix of figure 1.1 is as follows:

173	228	182	223	222	230	199	123
87	120	171	246	244	238	150	62
61	58	76	115	123	110	54	31
86	75	63	92	113	118	59	29
44	48	85	169	167	171	121	71
89	135	112	120	153	171	170	146
61	122	111	116	162	137	115	135
103	97	80	146	143	124	120	124

1.2.2.2 *Grayscale image*

A grayscale image has only one intensity value for each pixel. It determines that red = green = blue. Each pixel of the grayscale image is a gray shadow that has an intensity value of 0 (black) to 255 (white). Mathematically, the intensity of the grayscale image can be written as follows:

$$0 \leqslant p(x, y) \leqslant 255 \tag{1.2}$$

Figure 1.2 is lung image as one of the example of grayscale image lung image [7]. The graysacle matrix of figure 1.2 is as follows:

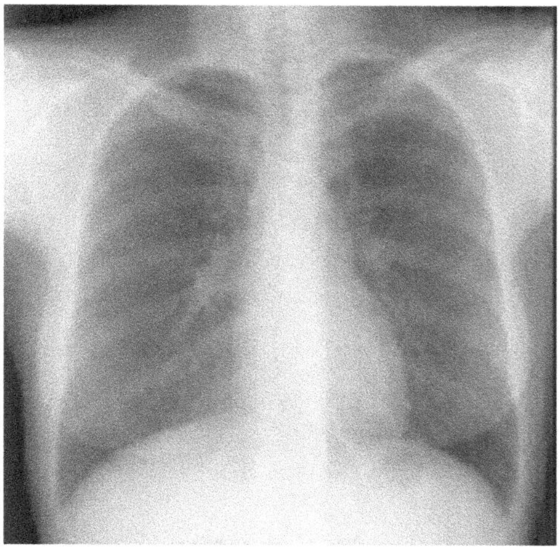

Figure 1.2. Grayscale image. Credit: Japanese Society of Radiological Technology.

124	127	140	182	183	143	148	134
207	196	151	160	182	140	177	190
207	177	117	160	187	111	147	178
178	170	118	169	201	124	141	153
154	163	126	181	218	150	137	149
139	160	130	184	223	170	133	141
111	152	176	208	220	179	132	109
96	195	222	228	229	219	197	110

1.2.2.3 Binary image

A binary image only contains two colors, that is black (0) and white (1). Mathematically, the intensity of a binary image can be defined as follows.

$$p(x, y) = \begin{cases} 0, \text{ black} \\ 1, \text{ white} \end{cases} \tag{1.3}$$

If we transform figure 1.2 to a binary image, the image will be as figure 1.3. The matrix of figure 1.3 is as follows:

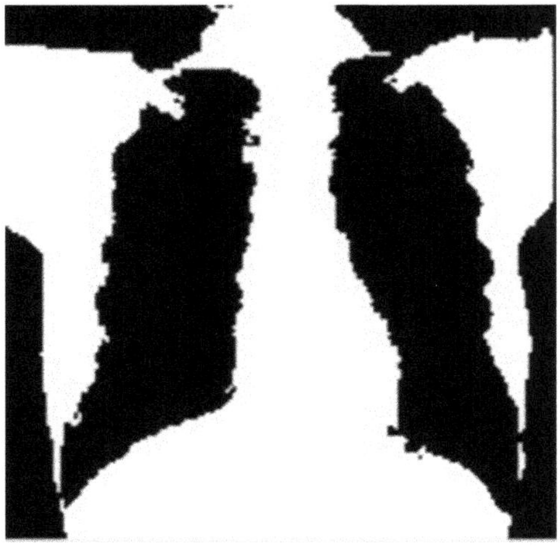

Figure 1.3. Binary image.

1	1	1	1	1	1	1	1
1	1	1	1	1	1	1	1
1	1	0	1	1	0	1	1
1	1	0	1	1	0	1	1
1	1	1	1	1	1	1	1
1	1	1	1	1	1	1	1
0	1	1	1	1	1	0	0
0	1	1	1	1	1	1	0

1.2.3 Image processing

Image processing applies to visually analyzing the lung image. This is a method for performing several operations on an image. Image processing aims to extract useful information from an image. Some extraction features to signify the lung classification can be extracted using several image processing techniques, such as an enhancement method to get a better image quality. Enhancements are applied to reduce or eliminate noise.

Noise is random speckles on the surface of the image, it is not part of the image. One of the most common noise models is additive noise. This noise adds uniformly in the field of imagery. Additive noise is formulated as follows:

$$p(x, y) = p_a(x, y) + p_n(x, y) \tag{1.4}$$

where $p(x,y)$ is the pixel value the original image, $p_a(x, y)$ is the pixel value of the denoised image, and $p_n(x, y)$ is the pixel value of the noise.

Removing noise from an image is called as the denoising step/pre-processing process before the image processing. One technique of the denoising step is to use the wavelet transforms. Wavelet will be discussed in the next section.

After the denoised image is obtained, the next step is to get feature extraction by applying the gray level co-occurrence matrix (GLCM). This is a second-order statistical method which is different from first-order statistical methods. Second-order statistical methods involve environmental values with the consideration that the input is in the form of a matrix. In the next section, we will discuss the GLCM to obtain some feature extractions.

1.3 Classification process

1.3.1 Classification

Classification is defined as a grouping process based on the characteristics of similarity and difference. This can be used when the information about how the data is grouped has been predetermined. The training process is carried out with training data that has been labeled into groups, while the testing process will classify the testing data into the existing groups. Classification is a type of supervised learning. Supervised learning is a machine learning task to learn functions that map input to output based on examples of input–output pairs [8].

Sometimes there is a misinterpretation between classifications and clustering. Both classification and clustering are used to categorize objects into one or several classes based on features/characteristics. They appear to be a similar process, but in this case clustering is used when it is not known how the data should be grouped. The number of groups in the clustering process is self-assumed by the model without predetermination. The output of the clustering process is grouped data. The differences of classification and clustering are summarized in table 1.1.

Based on the summarization table 1.1, classification is type of supervised learning. There is an output target in classification, while clustering is a type of unsupervised learning. There is no output target in clustering. Classification is more complex than clustering since there are many levels in the classification process, whereas the clustering process is only a grouping process based on similarities of the given data.

Table 1.1. Classification and clustering.

Classification	Clustering
Supervised learning	Unsupervised learning
Infinite set of input data	Finite set of data
Based on training data	Based on prior knowledge
Output target	No output target
Used to classify future observations	Used to understand the data
Goal: assigning new input to a class	Goal: finding similarities within given data

Examples of classification methods are logistic regression, Naive Bayes classifier, support vector machines, neural networks, etc. Examples of clustering methods are the *k*-means clustering algorithm, the fuzzy *c*-means clustering algorithm, the Gaussian clustering algorithm, etc. In the next section we will discuss classification using neural networks.

1.3.2 Features extraction

Image extraction is a technique for collecting features from an image. The GLCM method is one of the methods that can be used for image extraction. This type of image extractions results in 14 features, i.e., energy, contrast, correlation, the sum of square variance, Inverse Difference Moment (IDM), sum average, sum entropy, sum variance, entropy, difference variance, difference entropy, maximum probability, homogeneity, and dissimilarity [9]. All of the features extraction formulated as following detailed:

1. Energy: energy is the sum of square elements in GLCM. If the energy value equals 1 then the image is a constants image. The equation of energy is:

$$\text{Energy} = \sum_x \sum_y \left(\frac{p(x, y)}{R} \right)^2 \tag{1.5}$$

   with $p(x,y)$ = pixel value row- x and column- y, $R = \sum p(x, y)$. R is a constant of normalization such that the normalized pixel value satisfies the mass probability function characteristics, that is $0 \leqslant \frac{p(x, y)}{R} \leqslant 1$ and $\sum \frac{p(x, y)}{R} = 1$.

2. Contrast: contrast is the measure of contrast intensity between one pixel and another pixel. It is formulated as follows.

$$\text{Contrast} = \sum_x \sum_y \frac{p(x, y)}{R} (x - y)^2 \tag{1.6}$$

3. Correlation: correlation is used to measure the linear level dependence of gray (gray level) between pixels in one position to another position. The equation of correlation is formulated as follows:

$$\text{Correlation} = \sum_x \sum_y \frac{\dfrac{xyp(x, y)}{R} - \mu_x \mu_y}{\sigma_x \sigma_y} \tag{1.7}$$

   with $\mu_x = \sum_x \sum_y xp(x, y)$, $\mu_y = \sum_x \sum_y yp(x, y)$, $\sigma_x = \sum_x \sum_y (x - \mu_x)^2 p(x, y)$, and $\sigma_y = \sum_x \sum_y (x - \mu_y)^2 p(x, y)$.

4. Sum of square variance: the equation of sum of square variance is:

$$\text{Sum of Square Variance} = \sum_x \sum_y \frac{p(x, y)}{R}(x - \mu)^2 \tag{1.8}$$

with $\mu = \frac{\sum_x \sum_y p(x, y)}{xy}$.

5. Inverse different moment: inverse different moment is a measure of local homogeneity. It is formulated as follows.

$$\text{Inverse Different Moment} = \sum_x \sum_y \frac{\frac{p(x, y)}{R}}{1 + (x - y)^2} \tag{1.9}$$

6. Sum average: sum average is formulated as follows.

$$\text{Sum Avearge} = -\sum_k k p_{x+y}(k) \tag{1.10}$$

with $p_{x+y}(k) = \sum_{x=1}^{N_g} \sum_{y=1}^{N_g} \frac{p(x, y)}{R}; x + y = k; k = 2, 3, \ldots, 2N_g$ and N_g is the biggest dimension of the image row and column.

7. Sum entropy: sum entropy is formulated as follows.

$$\text{Sum Entropy} = -\sum_k p_{x+y}(k) \log p_{x+y}(k) \tag{1.11}$$

8. Sum variance: sum variance shows how many gray levels vary from the average value. The equation of sum variance is as follows.

$$\text{Sum Variance} = \sum_k (i - SE)^2 p_{x+y}(k) \tag{1.12}$$

9. Entropy: the equation of entropy is:

$$\text{Entropy} = -\sum_x \sum_y \frac{p(x, y)}{R} \log p(x, y) \tag{1.13}$$

10. Difference variance: difference variance is formulated as follows.

$$\text{Different Variance} = \text{variance of } p_{x-y}(k) \tag{1.14}$$

with $p_{x-y(\mathrm{k})} = \sum_{x=1}^{N_g} \sum_{y=1}^{N_g} \frac{p(x, y)}{R}, \mid x - y \mid = k$ and $k = 0, 1, 2, \ldots, (N_g - 1)$.

11. Difference entropy: difference entropy is formulated as follows.

$$\text{Different Entropy} = -\sum_k p_{x+y}(k) \log p_{x+y}(k) \tag{1.15}$$

12. Maximum probability: the equation of maximum probability is:

$$\text{Maximum Probability} = \max_{x,y}\left\{\frac{p(x, y)}{R}\right\} \tag{1.16}$$

13. Homogeneity: homogeneity is a measure of the closeness of distribution of elements in the GLCM to the diagonal of the GLCM. It is formulated as follows:

$$\text{Homogeneity} = \sum_x\sum_y\frac{\frac{p(x, y)}{R}}{1 + |x - y|} \tag{1.17}$$

14. Dissimilarity shows the difference of each pixel. It is formulated as follows. Dissimilarity:

$$\text{Dissimilarity} = \sum_x\sum_y\frac{p(x, y)}{R}|x - y| \tag{1.18}$$

Here is an example of feature extraction's manual calculation. Let us do features extraction of figure 1.3, then the energy and dissimilarity value are calculated as follow:

$$R = \sum p(x, y) = p(1, 1) + p(1, 2) + \ldots + p(8, 7) + p(8, 8) = 1 + 1 + \ldots$$
$$+1 + 0 = 55$$

$$\text{Energy} = \sum_x\sum_y p(x, y)^2 = \frac{p(1, 1)^2}{R} + \ldots + \frac{p(8, 7)^2}{R} + \frac{p(8, 8)^2}{R} = \frac{1}{55}^2 + \ldots$$
$$+\frac{1}{55}^2 + \frac{0}{55}^2 = 0.018182$$

$$\text{Dissimilarity} = \sum_x\sum_y\frac{p(x, y)}{R}|x - y| = \frac{p(1, 1)^2}{R}|1 - 1| + \frac{p(1, 2)^2}{R}|1 - 2| + \ldots$$
$$+\frac{p(8, 7)^2}{R}|8 - 1| + \frac{p(8, 8)^2}{R}|8 - 8| = \frac{1}{55}^2 . 0 + \frac{1}{55}^2 . 1 + \ldots$$
$$+\frac{1}{55}^2 . 1 + \frac{0}{55}^2 . 0 = 0.05124$$

From the calculation above, we can conclude that figure 1.3 has an energy value 0.018 182 and a dissimilarity value 0.051 24.

1.3.3 Wavelet

Wavelet is an analytical tool commonly used to present data or functions operators into different frequency components, and then review each component with a resolution according to its scale [10]. Wavelet is a small wave that has its energy concentrated in time to give a tool for the analysis of transient, non-stationary, or time-varying phenomena [11]. Wavelet can concentrate image energy in some coefficients. The coefficients separate into two categories: coefficients with high energy and coefficients with low energy. The coefficients with low energy can be removed since they do not give significant information.

Wavelet has a gender, i.e., the father wavelet φ and the mother wavelet ψ [12]. The integral of the father wavelet equals 1 and the integral of the mother wavelet equals 0. They are mathematically defined as follows.

$$\int \varphi(t)dt = 1 \text{ and } \int \psi(t)dt = 0 \tag{1.19}$$

The father wavelet is used to represent the smooth and low-frequency part of the signal and the mother wavelet is used to represent the detailed and high-frequency part of the signal.

1.3.3.1 Haar wavelet

Haar Wavelet is the base of the other wavelet types (figure 1.4). The mother wavelet function is defined as follows:

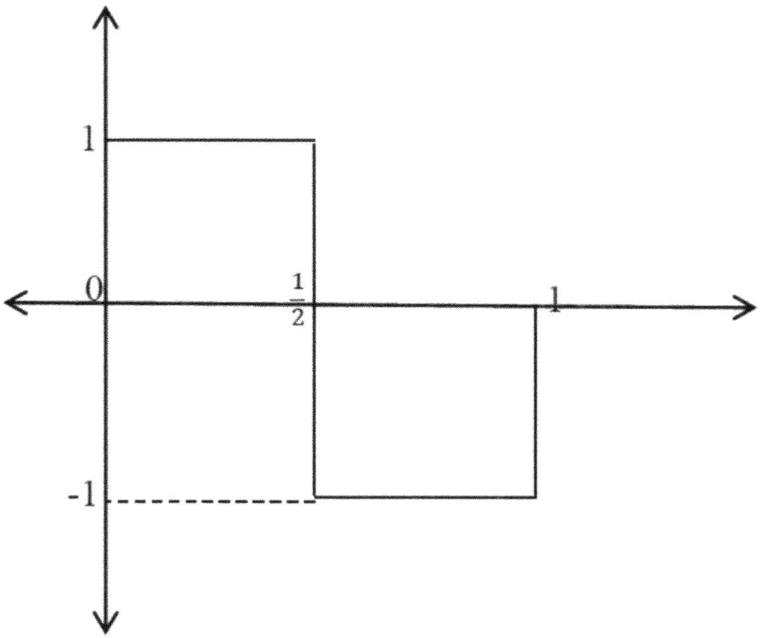

Figure 1.4. Haar wavelet.

$$\psi_{j,k}(x) = \begin{cases} 1, & x \epsilon \left[0, \frac{1}{2}\right) \\ -1, & x \epsilon \left[\frac{1}{2}, 1\right) \\ 0, & others \end{cases} \tag{1.20}$$

While the father wavelet function is defined as follows.

$$\varphi_{j,k}(x) = \begin{cases} 1, & x \epsilon [0, 1) \\ 0, & others \end{cases} \tag{1.21}$$

Given a signal that is defined by $f = (f_1, f_2, f_3, \dots, f_N)$, where $N = 2^J$ and J is a positive integer, so the first level of Haar transformation decomposed the signal f becoming two sub-signal a^1 and d^1, where the length of each sub-signal is half the length of signal f. Sub-signal $a^1 = (a_1, a_2, a_3, \dots a_{\frac{N}{2}})$ is the trend component of Haar transformation and the sub-signal $d^1 = (d_1, d_2, d_3, \dots d_{\frac{N}{2}})$ is the fluctuation component of the Haar transformation. Scaling signal V_m^1 of the first level of Haar wavelet is $V_1^1 = (\alpha_1, \alpha_2, 0, 0, \dots, 0, 0)$, $V_2^1 = (0, 0, \alpha_1, \alpha_2, 0, 0, \dots, 0, 0), \dots,$ $V_{N/2}^1 = (0, 0, \dots, 0, 0, \alpha_1, \alpha_2)$, where $\alpha_1 = \alpha_2 = \frac{1}{\sqrt{2}}$, while the wavelet signal W_m^1 of the first level of Haar wavelet is $V_1^1 = (\beta_1, \beta_2, 0, 0, \dots, 0, 0)$, $V_2^1 = (0, 0, \beta_1, \beta_2, 0, 0, \dots, 0, 0)$, $\dots,$ $V_{N/2}^1 = (0, 0, \dots, 0, 0, \beta_1, \beta_2)$, where $\beta_1 = \frac{1}{\sqrt{2}}$ and $\beta_2 = -\frac{1}{\sqrt{2}}$. Then the sub-signal of the Haar transformation can be written as follows:

$$a_m = f.\ V_m^1 \text{ and } d_m = f.\ W_m^1 \tag{1.22}$$

where $m = 1, 2, 3, \dots, \frac{N}{2}$. The wavelet decomposition of each level is as follows.

$$f \xrightarrow{H_1} (a^1 | d^1) \tag{1.23}$$

Then, analogously with the pyramid algorithm, the next level of Haar transformation is as follows:

$$f \xrightarrow{H_2} (a^2 \mid d^2 \mid d^1) \tag{1.24}$$

where a^2 and d^2 are calculated from

$$a^1 \xrightarrow{H_1} (a^2 \mid d^2) \tag{1.25}$$

1.3.3.2 Daubhecies wavelet

Daubhecies wavelet is a kind of wavelet which was recognized by Ingrid Daubchecies. There are many kinds of Daubhecies wavelet. In this research, the type of Daubhecies wavelet used is Daubh4. The concept of the Daubh4 wavelet is similar to the Haar wavelet, the difference is the scaling signal V_m^1 and the wavelet function W^1_m. Scaling signal V^1_m of the first level of Daubh4 wavelet is $V^1_1 = (\alpha_1, \alpha_2, \alpha_3, \alpha_4, \dots, 0, 0)$, $V^1_2 = (0, 0, 0, 0, \alpha_1, \alpha_2, \alpha_3, \alpha_4, \dots, 0, 0)$, …, $V^1_{N/2} = (0, 0, \dots, 0, 0, \alpha_1, \alpha_2, \alpha_3, \alpha_4)$, where $\alpha_1 = \frac{1+\sqrt{3}}{4\sqrt{2}}$, $\alpha_2 = \frac{3+\sqrt{3}}{4\sqrt{2}}$, $\alpha_3 = \frac{3-\sqrt{3}}{4\sqrt{2}}$, and $\alpha_4 = \frac{1-\sqrt{3}}{4\sqrt{2}}$. While the wavelet signal W^1_m of the first level of Daubh4 wavelet is $W^1_1 = (\beta_1, \beta_2, \beta_3, \beta_4, \dots, 0, 0)$, $W^1_2 = (0, 0, 0, 0, \beta_1, \beta_2, \beta_3, \beta_4, \dots, 0, 0)$, …, $W^1_{N/2} = (0, 0, \dots, 0, 0, \beta_1, \beta_2, \beta_3, \beta_4)$, where $\beta_1 = \frac{1-\sqrt{3}}{4\sqrt{2}}$, $\beta_2 = \frac{\sqrt{3}-3}{4\sqrt{2}}$, $\beta_3 = \frac{3+\sqrt{3}}{4\sqrt{2}}$, and $\beta_4 = \frac{-1-\sqrt{3}}{4\sqrt{2}}$. The decomposition of the first level of Daubh4 wavelet is as follows.

$$f \xrightarrow{D_1} (a^1 \mid d^1) \tag{1.26}$$

Then, analogously with the pyramid algorithm, the next level of Daubh4 transformation is as follows:

$$f \xrightarrow{D_2} (a^2 \mid d^2 \mid d^1) \tag{1.27}$$

where a^2 and d^2 are calculated from

$$a^1 \xrightarrow{D_1} (a^2 \mid d^2) \tag{1.28}$$

Here is an example of manual calculation, given a signal $f = (f_1, f_2, f_3, f_4, f_5, f_6, f_7, f_8) = (2, 1, 3, -1, 2, 4, 3, 4)$, then the signal f can be transformed as $j = 1, \dots, ((\log_2 8) - 1 = 2)$. The Haar level 1 transformation is as follows.

$$a^1_1 = \frac{f_1 + f_2}{\sqrt{2}} = \frac{2+1}{\sqrt{2}} = \frac{3}{\sqrt{2}}$$

$$a^1_2 = \frac{f_3 + f_4}{\sqrt{2}} = \frac{3+(-1)}{\sqrt{2}} = \frac{2}{\sqrt{2}}$$

$$a^1_3 = \frac{f_5 + f_6}{\sqrt{2}} = \frac{2+4}{\sqrt{2}} = \frac{6}{\sqrt{2}}$$

$$a^1_4 = \frac{f_7 + f_8}{\sqrt{2}} = \frac{3+4}{\sqrt{2}} = \frac{7}{\sqrt{2}}$$

and

$$d^1_1 = \frac{f_2 - f_1}{\sqrt{2}} = \frac{1-2}{\sqrt{2}} = -\frac{1}{\sqrt{2}}$$

$$d^1_2 = \frac{f_4 - f_3}{\sqrt{2}} = \frac{-1-3}{\sqrt{2}} = -\frac{4}{\sqrt{2}}$$

$$d_3^1 = \frac{f_6 - f_5}{\sqrt{2}} = \frac{4 - 2}{\sqrt{2}} = \frac{2}{\sqrt{2}}$$

$$d_4^1 = \frac{f_8 - f_7}{\sqrt{2}} = \frac{4 - 3}{\sqrt{2}} = \frac{1}{\sqrt{2}}$$

It can be written as follows.

$$f \xrightarrow{H_1} (a_1^1, a_2^1, a_3^1, a_4^1 | d_1^1, d_2^1, d_3^1, d_4^1)$$

$$f \xrightarrow{H_1} \left(\frac{3}{\sqrt{2}}, \frac{2}{\sqrt{2}}, \frac{6}{\sqrt{2}}, \frac{7}{\sqrt{2}} \middle| -\frac{1}{\sqrt{2}}, -\frac{4}{\sqrt{2}}, \frac{2}{\sqrt{2}}, \frac{1}{\sqrt{2}} \right)$$

Haar level 2 transformation is as follows.

$$a_1^2 = \frac{a_1^1 + a_2^1}{\sqrt{2}} = \frac{\frac{3}{\sqrt{2}} + \frac{2}{\sqrt{2}}}{\sqrt{2}} = \frac{5}{2}$$

$$a_2^2 = \frac{a_3^1 + a_4^1}{\sqrt{2}} = \frac{\frac{6}{\sqrt{2}} + \frac{7}{\sqrt{2}}}{\sqrt{2}} = \frac{13}{2}$$

$$d_1^2 = \frac{a_2^1 - a_1^1}{\sqrt{2}} = \frac{\frac{2}{\sqrt{2}} - \frac{3}{\sqrt{2}}}{\sqrt{2}} = \frac{-1}{2}$$

$$d_2^2 = \frac{a_2^1 - a_1^1}{\sqrt{2}} = \frac{\frac{7}{\sqrt{2}} - \frac{6}{\sqrt{2}}}{\sqrt{2}} = \frac{1}{2}$$

It is also can be written as follows.

$$f \xrightarrow{H_2} (a_1^2, a_2^2 \mid d_1^2, d_2^2 | d_1^1, d_2^1, d_3^1, d_4^1)$$

$$f \xrightarrow{H_2} \left(\frac{5}{2}, \frac{11}{2} \middle| -\frac{1}{2}, \frac{1}{2} \middle| -\frac{1}{\sqrt{2}}, -\frac{4}{\sqrt{2}}, \frac{2}{\sqrt{2}}, \frac{1}{\sqrt{2}} \right)$$

Furthermore, the first average signal and the first fluctuation signal are:

$$A^1 = \left(\frac{a_1^1}{\sqrt{2}}, \frac{a_1^1}{\sqrt{2}}, \ldots, \frac{a_4^1}{\sqrt{2}}, \frac{a_4^1}{\sqrt{2}} \right) = (1.5,\ 1.5,\ 1,\ 1,\ 3,\ 3,\ 3.5,\ 3.5)$$

$$D^1 = \left(\frac{d_1^1}{\sqrt{2}}, -\frac{d_1^1}{\sqrt{2}}, \ldots, \frac{d_{N/2}^1}{\sqrt{2}}, -\frac{d_{N/2}^1}{\sqrt{2}} \right) = (0.5,\ -0.5,\ 2,\ -2,\ -1,\ 1,\ -0.5,\ 0.5)$$

Then the signal $f = A^1 + D^1 = (2, 1, 3, -1, 2, 4, 3, 4)$. In the same way, the second average signal and the second fluctuation signal are:

$$A^2 = (1.25,\ 1.25,\ 1.25,\ 1.25,\ 3.25,\ 3.25,\ 3.25,\ 3.25)$$

$$D^2 = (0.25,\ 0.25,\ -0.25,\ -0.25,\ -0.25,\ -0.25,\ 0.25,\ 0.25)$$

Then we get $A^1 = (1.5,\ 1.5,\ 1,\ 1,\ 3,\ 3,\ 3.5,\ 3.5)$ and $f = A^2 + D^2 + D^1 = (2, 1, 3, -1, 2, 4, 3, 4)$.

1.3.3.3 Image denoising with wavelet

Wavelet 2D is used for image denoising. The algorithm used for image denoising is the tree-adapted wavelet shrinkage (TAWS) algorithm. The TAWS algorithm is a simple, but highly effective, wavelet-based image denoising algorithm [13]. The wavelet transformation for an image can be calculated for an image with odd numbers of rows and columns. Consider an image f,

$$f = \begin{pmatrix} f_{1,M} & f_{2,M} & \cdots & f_{N,M} \\ \vdots & \vdots & \ddots & \vdots \\ f_{1,2} & f_{2,2} & \cdots & f_{N,2} \\ f_{1,1} & f_{2,2} & \cdots & f_{N,1} \end{pmatrix} \tag{1.29}$$

The first level of wavelet transformation is started by calculating the 1D wavelet transform (first level) on each row of f, so that it produces a new image. On the new image obtained from step 1, calculate the same 1D wavelet transforms on each of its columns. The wavelet transformation of an image f can be symbolized as follows:

$$f \longmapsto \begin{pmatrix} h^1 & d^1 \\ a^1 & v^1 \end{pmatrix} \tag{1.30}$$

where the sub-images h^1, d^1, a^1, and v^1 each of them has $M/2$ rows and $N/2$ columns. The sub-image a^1 is trends along rows of f followed by computing trends along with columns. The sub-image d^1 is created from the fluctuations along both rows and columns. The sub-image h^1 is created by computing trends along the image f followed by computing the fluctuations along with columns. The sub-image v^1 is the reverse of the sub-image h^1. The next step is thresholding with the formula as follows.

$$f_t(x, y) = \begin{cases} |f(x, y)| - T_B, & \text{if } \ |f(x, y)| \geqslant T_B \\ 0, & \text{if } \ |f(x, y)| < T_B \end{cases} \tag{1.31}$$

where $T_B = \sigma\sqrt{2logM}$, σ is the standard deviation of the noise, and M is the maximum dimension of the rows and column of the image. Then the last step is calculating the inverse of the wavelet transformation. Then, analogously with the pyramid algorithm, the next level of the transformation is as follows:

$$f \longmapsto \begin{pmatrix} h^1 & d^1 \\ h^2\, d^2 & v^1 \\ a^2\, v^2 & \end{pmatrix} \tag{1.32}$$

where h^2, d^2, a^2, and v^2 are calculated from

$$a^1 \longmapsto \begin{pmatrix} h^2 & d^2 \\ a^2 & v^2 \end{pmatrix} \tag{1.33}$$

1.3.4 Machine learning

Artificial intelligence (AI) has been discussed by scientists worldwide for decades. The main idea of AI initially suggests that machines ccould think like humans. AI is a simulation of human intelligence (HI) processed using a machine or computer. AI develops a computer system to do a task that involves a thought process like the human brain. In human intelligence, the cognitive process is complex, the decisions and thought processes are influenced by subjective factors. The decisions in AI are objective as they are not influenced by any motivation or emotions.

Machine learning is approach learning using mathematics equations linearly to make the decision. Machine learning is an AI. It describes an AI system that is taught to learn and make decisions by examining large amounts of input data. It makes calculated predictions based on analyzing the input information and performs tasks that are considered to require human intelligence. In the machine learning approach, the computer does not rely on the rules programmed by humans. It looks for certain patterns appearing in the data. These patterns are learned by the computer/machine and become a reference when the system is used.

Machine learning imitates human intelligence to make decision by providing the systems with the ability to automatically learn and improve from experience. Machine learning has the ability to generalize decisions using training processes. The training process is a repeated process of a dataset which contains input and target information. There are some machine learning alghorithms such as neural networks, perceptron, learning vector quantization, recurrent neural network, etc.

1.3.5 Neural network

1.3.5.1 Activation function

Neural network (NN) is an algorithm that is inspired by the workings of neurons in the human brain that are interconnected through chemical reactions. Each neuron will flow information that is connected to each synapsis. NN is an architecture consisting of many neurons that work together to respond to the inputs. Neurons are information processing units that form the basis of NN operations. NN consists of three layers, i.e., the input layer, the hidden layer, and the output layer. The input layer receives inputs (problems) from the outside and the output layer provides answers to the problems received by the input layer. The input layer can be connected to the output layer via a hidden layer.

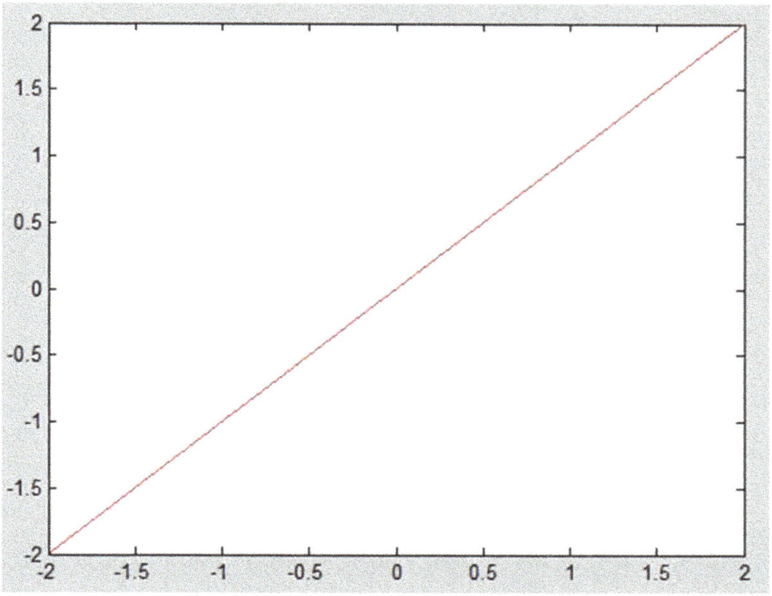

Figure 1.5. Linear function.

Each NN neuron is activated by an activation function. The activation function determines the output of a unit. It converts the input signal into an output signal which will be sent to another unit [14]. Activation functions that can be used as NN activators include linear functions, binary stepping functions, bipolar functions, binary sigmoid functions, and bipolar sigmoid function. The output value in the linear function is the same as the input value. The linear function (figure 1.5) is formulated as follows.

$$f(x) = x \tag{1.34}$$

The binary steps function is used to convert the input of a variable whose value is continuous to a binary output (0 and 1). The binary steps function (figure 1.6) is formulated as follows [15]:

$$f(x) = \begin{cases} 1, & x \geqslant 0 \\ 0, & \text{others} \end{cases} \tag{1.35}$$

The bipolar function is similar to the binary step function. The difference lies in the output value produced. The bipolar function produces an output value of 1 and −1. Bipolar functions, as shown in figure 1.7, are formulated as follows:

$$f(x) = \begin{cases} 1, & x \geqslant 0 \\ -1, & x < 0 \end{cases} \tag{1.36}$$

The binary sigmoid or log sig function has non-linear characteristics. It can be used to solve a complex problem with non-linear characteristics. The binary sigmoid

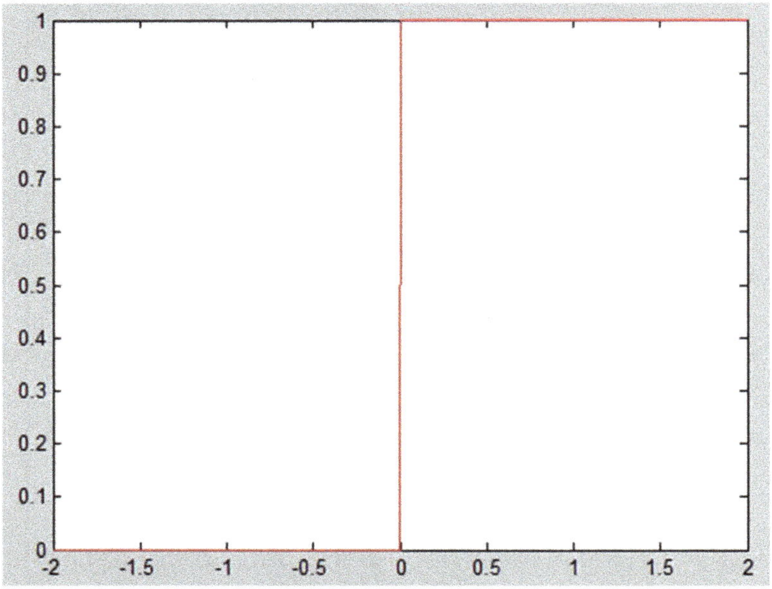

Figure 1.6. Binary step function.

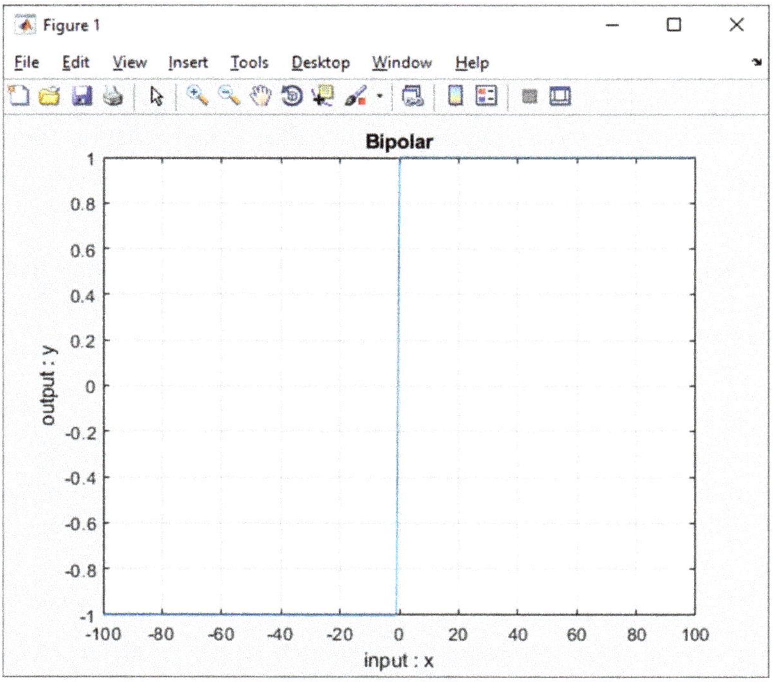

Figure 1.7. Bipolar function.

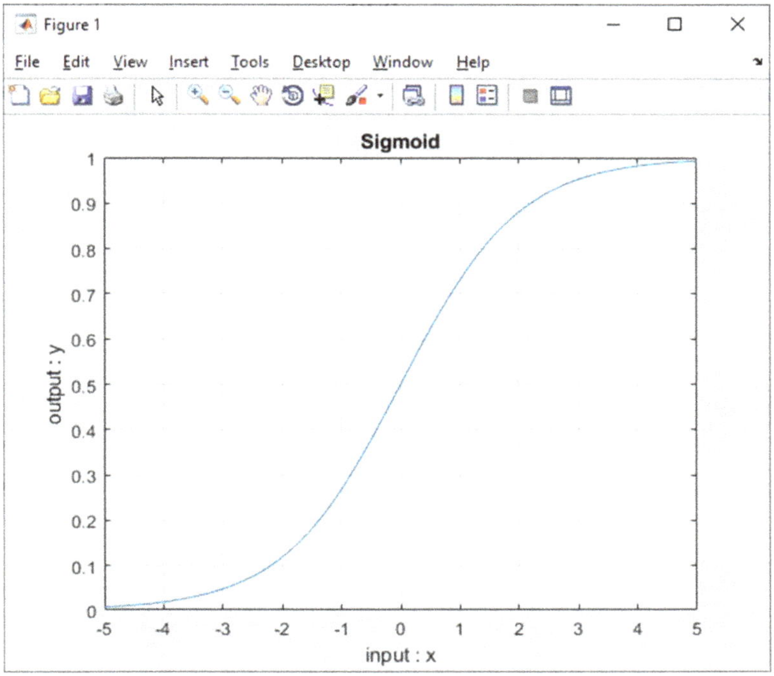

Figure 1.8. Binary sigmoid function.

function produces a value between 0 and 1 (figure 1.8). It is mathematically defined as follows.

$$f(x) = \frac{1}{1 + e^{-x}} \tag{1.37}$$

The bipolar or tansig sigmoid function is an activation function similar to the binary sigmoid function, the difference is in the range of output values. Bipolar sigmoid functions produce output values between −1 and 1 (figure 1.9). Bipolar sigmoid functions are formulated as follows.

$$f(x) = \frac{1 - e^{-x}}{1 + e^{-x}} \tag{1.38}$$

1.3.5.2 Architecture

Network architecture is an arrangement of neurons arranged in the NN layer. There are three types of NN architecture., i.e., NN with a single layer (single layered network), NN with multiple layers (multi-layer network), and NN with competitive layers. Single layer NN (figure 1.10) is the simplest type of NN architecture. NN with a single layer does not use a hidden layer. The input layer is directly connected to the output layer. NN with a single layer is an advanced feed network or feedforward [16]. Figure 1.10 shows that there are l neurons in the input layer

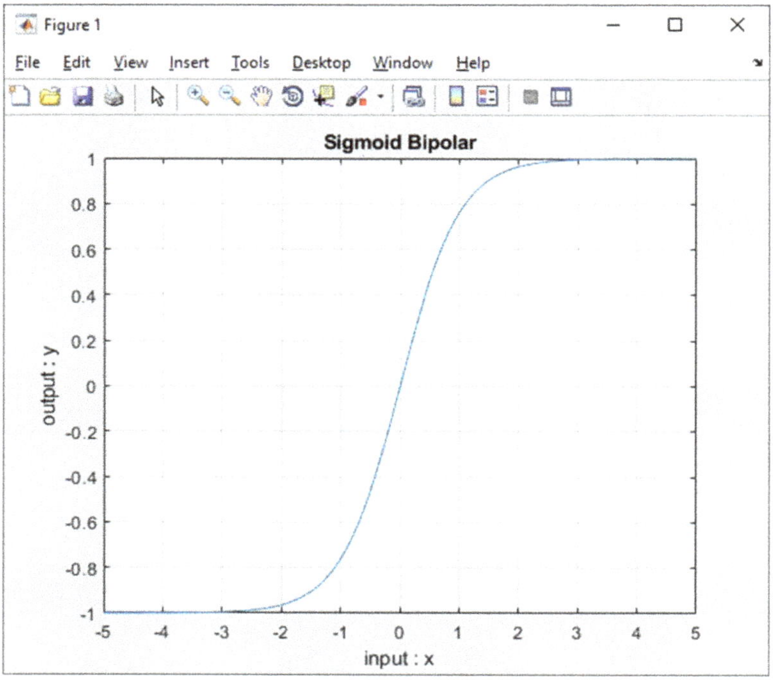

Figure 1.9. Bipolar sigmoid function.

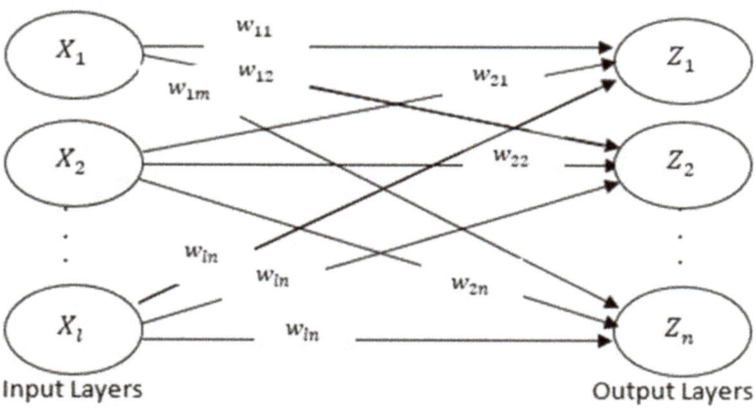

Figure 1.10. Single layered neural network.

and n neurons in the output layers, meanwhile w_{ik} is the weight connected input layer to the output layer with $i = 1, 2, \ldots, l$ and $k = 1, 2, \ldots, n$. The weighted input signal (z_in_k) to the neuron Z_k is the sum of the signal neuron weight $X_1, X_2, \ldots, X_l$, then:

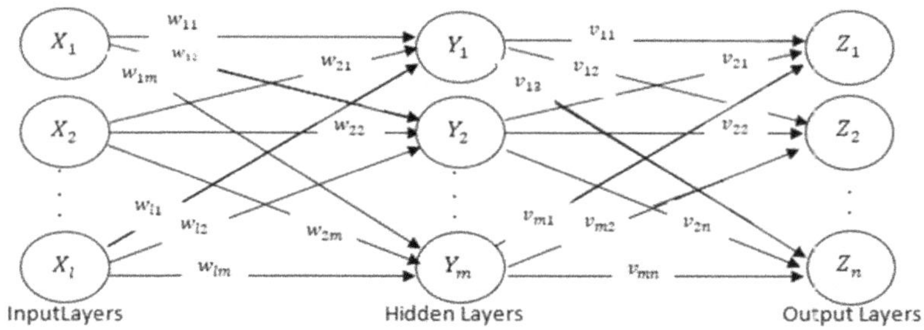

Figure 1.11. Multiple layered neural network.

$$z\_in_k = \sum_{i=1}^{l}\sum_{k=1}^{n} x_i w_{ik} \tag{1.39}$$

Activation z_k from neuron Z_k uses activation function f, then $z_k = f(z\_in_k)$.

If a single layer NN does not have a hidden layer then in NN with multiple layers there is at least one hidden layer (figure 1.11). Signals from the input layer on NN with multiple layers are transmitted to the output layer through one or more hidden layers. Figure 1.11 shows there are l neurons in the input layer, m neurons in the hidden layer, and n neurons in the output layer. The weight that connects the input layer to the hidden layer is w_{ik} with i=1,2,…,l and k=1,2,…,m. The weight that connects the hidden layer to the output layer is v_{kr} with k=1,2,…,m and r=1,2,…,n. The weighted input signal (y_in_k) to the neuron Y_k is the sum of neuron signal weight X_1, X_2, … , X_l then

$$y\_in_k = \sum_{i=1}^{l}\sum_{k=1}^{n} x_i w_{ik} \tag{1.40}$$

Activation y_k from neuron Y_k uses activation function f, then $y_k = f(y\_in_k)$. The weighted input signal (z_in_r) to the neuron Z_r is the sum of neuron signal weight Y_1, Y_2, … , Y_n then

$$z\_in_r = \sum_{k=1}^{m}\sum_{r=1}^{n} y_k v_{kr} \tag{1.41}$$

Activation z_r from neuron Z_r uses activation function f, then $z_r = f(z\_in_r)$.

The NN architecture with competitive layers is different from single layer NN or multiple layer NN. The neurons in the NN with the competitive layer can be interconnected. One of the examples of competitive layered NN is the recurrent neural network (RNN). It is a NN that has a feedback link. The layer on the RNN includes the input layer, the output layer, and the hidden layer as in the other networks, but in the RNN there is at least one feedback layer. RNN can be divided into two, i.e., the Elman RNN network and the Hopfield RNN network. The Elman RNN network has feedback from the hidden layer to the input layer while the Hopfield RNN network has feedback at each layer.

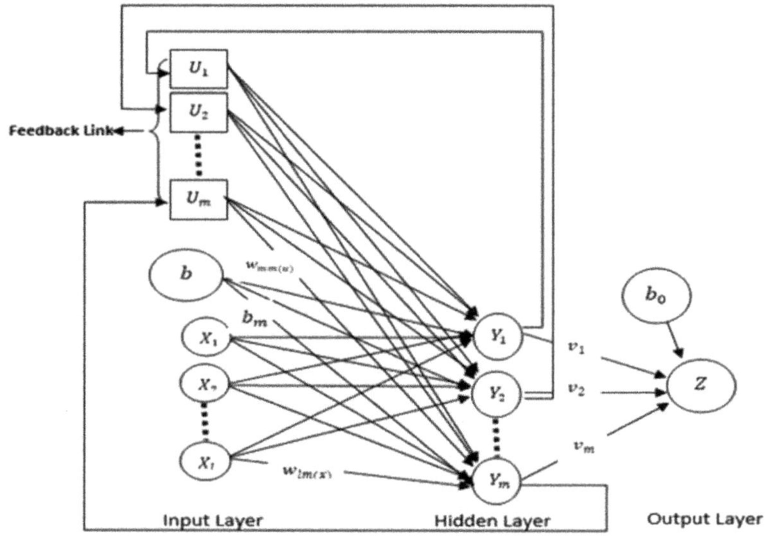

Figure 1.12. Recurrent neural network architecture. Copyright (2017) IEEE. Reprinted, with permission, from [4].

1.3.6 Recurrent neural network

RNN is a neural network with a feedback link. There are four layers in RNN: input layer, hidden layer, output layer, and feedback link. Activation function is used to connect one layer to another layer. The feedback link accommodates the network output to be re-input to the network. There are two RNN networks, namely the Hopfield network and the Elman network. The Hopfield network is a network single layer feedback with symmetrical weights introduced by John Hopfield in 1982. In this chapter, the researchers use RNN from the Elman Network which has a feedback link from the hidden layer to the input layer. The RNN architecture with the Elman Network is shown in figure 1.12.

1.3.7 Mean square error

Mean square error (MSE) measures the average of the errors of the network. It is the average squared difference between target and output of the network. The smaller the MSE value from which model is used for classification, the better the resulting classification. MSE is formulated as follows [17]:

$$\text{MSE} = \frac{1}{n}\sum_{t=1}^{n}(g_t - z_t)^2 \tag{1.42}$$

g_t is the target, z_t is the output, $t = 1,2,\ldots n$, and n = numbers of observed data.

1.3.8 Sensitivity, specificity, and accuracy

The possibilities that can happen in a diagnostic test are shown in table 1.2. There are four results for diagnostic tests. There are true positive (a) which means that sick

Table 1.2. Diagnostic test.

	True situation	
Measure	Performance indicator present	Performance indicator absent
Positive	True positive (a)	False positive (b)
Negative	False negative (c)	True negative (d)
Total	(a)+(c)	(b)+(d)

patients are correctly identified as sick, false positive (b) which means that healthy patients are incorrectly identified as sick, false negative (c) which means that sick patients arec incorrectly identified as healthy, and true negative (d) which means that healthy patients are correctly identified as healthy.

The sensitivity is the proportion ratio of true positive over the total number of true positive and false negative. It is mathematically calculated as follows:

$$\text{sensitivity} = \frac{a}{a + c} \tag{1.43}$$

The specificity is the proportion ratio of true negative over the total number of false positive and true negative. It is mathematically formulated as follows:

$$\text{specificity} = \frac{d}{b + d} \tag{1.44}$$

The accuracy is the proportion ratio of the total number of true positive and true negative over the whole total number of cases. It is measured by:

$$\text{accuracy} = \frac{a + d}{a + b + c + d} \tag{1.45}$$

1.4 Dataset

The Japanese Society of Radiology Technology (JSRT) released the Digital Image Database [7]. It is an open-access database of lung image radiology. This research uses JSRT dataset for as many as 100 lung images with details as follows:

1. the image format is *.jpg,
2. grayscale image,
3. the matrix of the image is 2048 × 2048.

The dataset is divided into three part (figure 1.13) and each image is named with prefix format as follows:

1. 35 normal lung images, named with the prefix a, such as a-1.jpg; a-2.jpg; a-3. jpg, etc

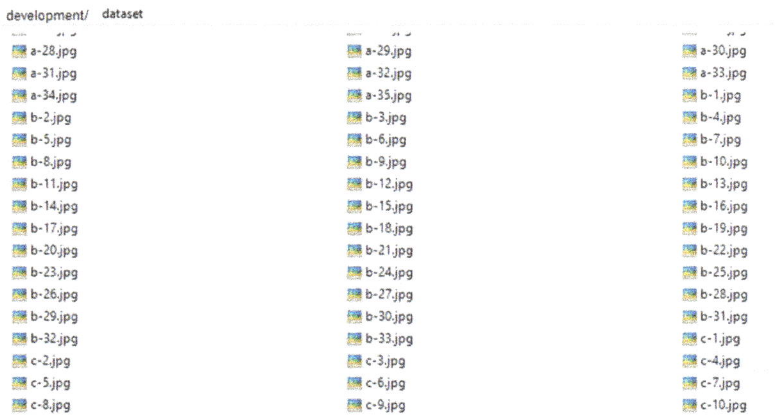

Figure 1.13. Dataset.

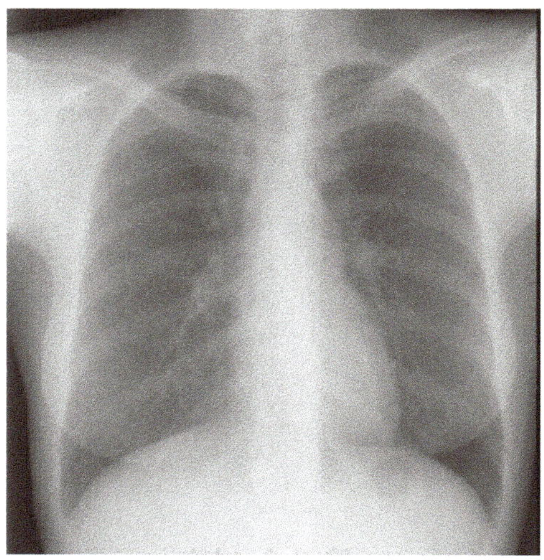

Figure 1.14. Normal lung image. Credit: Japanese Society of Radiological Technology.

2. 35 benign lung images, named with the prefix b, such as b-1.jpg; b-2.jpg; b-3. jpg, etc
3. 35 malignant lung images, named with the prefix c, such as c-1.jpg; c-2.jpg; c-3.jpg, etc

There were 100 lung images from the Japanese Society Radiology and Technology used in this paper (35 normal lung images, 33 benign lung images, and 32 malignant lung images). The images are grayscale images. Figures 1.14, 1.15, and 1.16 are the example of the normal lung image, benign lung image, and malignant lung image, respectively. The length of the matrix is 2048 that is 2^J where

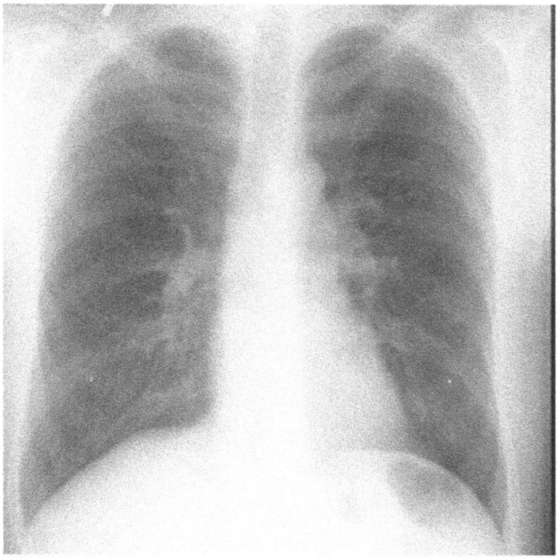

Figure 1.15. Benign lung image. Credit: Japanese Society of Radiological Technology.

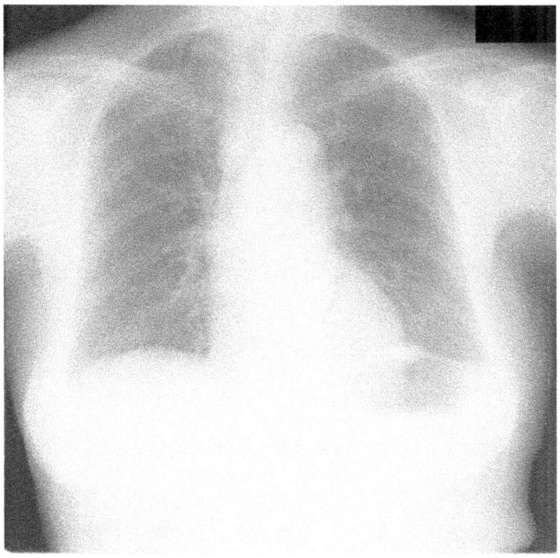

Figure 1.16. Malignant lung image. Credit: Japanese Society of Radiological Technology.

J=11. So that the image matrix can be decomposed with Haar Wavelet and Daubhecies Wavelet until level 10.

1.5 Modeling wavelet recurrent neural network for lung cancer nodule classification

1.5.1 Image denoising using wavelet

The denoised lung images with Haar Wavelet and Daubh4 Wavelet level 1 to level 10 were shown in figure 1.17 and 1.18. Figure 1.17 and 1.18 show denoised images

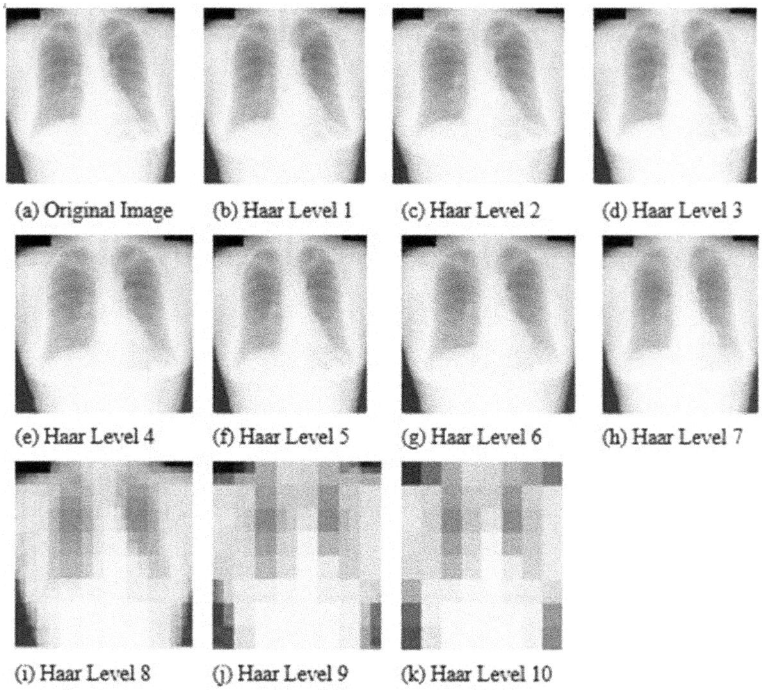

Figure 1.17. Denoising with Haar wavelet. Copyright (2017) IEEE. Reprinted, with permission, from [4].

were more obscure as the level increase. In this chapter we chose Haar Wavelet Level 4 for the denoising step and Daubh4 Wavelet Level 6. Another Haar Wavelet level and Daubh4 Wavelet level may be chosen for other research.

1.5.2 Wavelet recurrent neural network for lung cancer classification

WRNN modelling begins with the process of image denoising with the wavelet method. The denoised image is then extracted by the GLCM method. Feature extraction is used as the input variables in the classification process with RNN. The classification process uses the stage of the lung image as the target variable. Targets and outputs of the network are numerical data, namely 1 for normal lung images, 2 for benign lung images, and 3 for malignant lung images. In the classification process, there are three criteria, that is if the output value (z) is $1<y\leqslant 1,5$ then coded by 1 (the classification result is normal), if the output value (z) is $1,5<y\leqslant 2,5$, then coded by 2 (the classification result is benign), and if the output value (z) is $2,5<y<3$, then coded by 3 (the classification result is malignant). The next step is dividing the data. It was divided into training data (75 images of the lungs) and testing data (25 images of the lungs). The network used is RNN with backpropagation algorithm. The next procedure of choosing the best model is as follows.

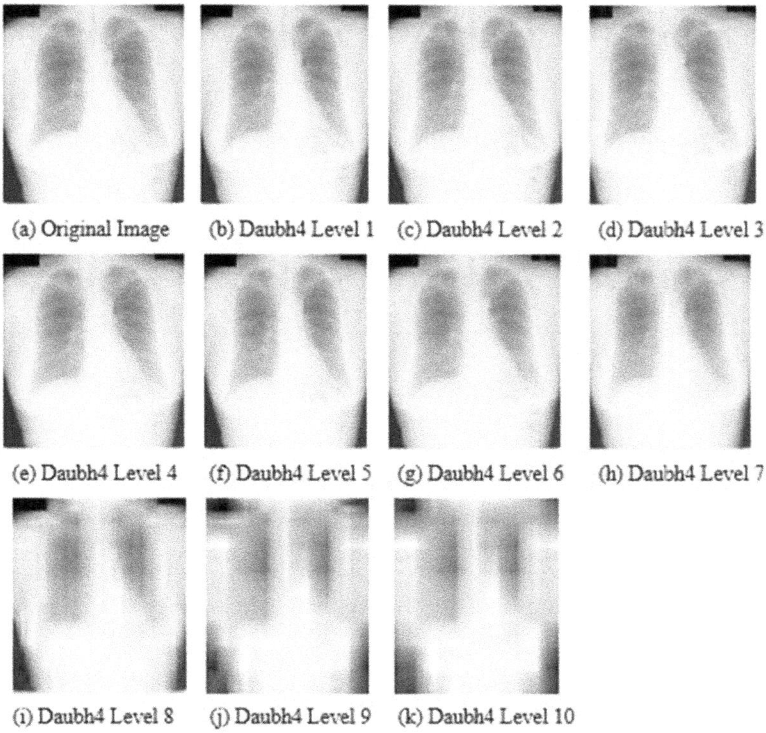

Figure 1.18. Denoising with Daubh4 wavelet.

Table 1.3. MSE for choosing the denoised image.

Extraction	Wavelet	MSE data training	MSE data testing
With binarization	Haar	0.483 27	0.638 45
	Daubh4	0.397 73	1.1982
Without binarization	Haar	0.467 22*	0.573 63*
	Daubh4	0.398 64*	0.412 26*

*Chosen model.

1. Choosing the denoised image: The denoised image can be directly extracted by the GLCM method. However, the denoised image can be transformed as a binary image before the extraction process. Table 1.3 describes the MSE of classification process with denoised image directly and binary image. Based on table 1.3, the best MSE is given by the extraction using Matlab software and without binarization process. Then the next step is using the 14 features extraction resulted from Matlab Software and without binarization process.

Table 1.4. MSE value for choosing how many neurons in the hidden layer.

Haar wavelet			Daubh4 wavelet		
Neuron	MSE data *training*	MSE data *testing*	Neuron	MSE data *training*	MSE data *testing*
1	0.467 22	0.573 63	1	0.398 64*	0.412 26*
2	0.415 38	0.512 01	2	0.315 49	0.484 66
3	0.382 06*	0.455 53*	3	0.357 19	0.477 06
4	0.345 26	0.584 08	4	0.315 85	0.523 37
5	0.292 48	0.696 55	5	0.308 12	1.5948

*Chosen model.

2. Choosing how many neurons in the hidden layer: Choosing how many neurons in the hidden layer is done by calculating the MSE value for the training data and testing the data as follows (table 1.4).

   Based on table 1.4, the RNN network with three neurons for the Haar Wavelet is better than the RNN network with other neurons in the hidden layer. Menawhile for the Daubh4 Wavelet, it is chosen by using only one hidden layer on the network.
3. Input Elimination: Table 1.5 is the MSE value for data training and data testing for the elimination input process.

   Based on table 1.5, 14 features are chosen as input variables for Haar wavelet and 13 Features (without X10) as input variables for the Daubh4 wavelet.

1.6 Results and discussion

The classification results using Haar WRNN and Daubh4 WRNN are shown in table 1.6 for training data and table 1.7 for testing data. Based on table 1.6 and table 1.7, the sensitivity, specificity, and accuracy of the model can be calculated (table 1.8 and table 1.9).

As shown in table 1.8 the accuracy when using Haar WRNN for training data is better than the accuracy when using Daubh4 WRNN for training data. The sensitivity, specificity, and accuracy using Haar WRNN for training data is respectively 93.75%, 66.67%, and 84%.

As shown in table 1.9 the accuracy using Haar WRNN for testing data is better than the accuracy using Daubh4 WRNN for tresting data. The sensitivity, specificity, and accuracy using Haar WRNN for testing data is respectively 88.24%, 62.5%, and 84%.

The highest accuracy value is given by WRNN model with Haar Wavelet that is 84% for tarining and testing data. However this model is not optimal to use as an indicator when the result is negative (normal lung) and when the result is positive (lung cancer). The accuracy of WRNN model was better than the previous research using NN [5] and RNN [6] which have accuracy respectively 80% and 81.33%.

Table 1.5. MSE value for input elimination.

Haar wavelet			
Elimination	Input (features)	MSE training	MSE testing
	14	0.382 06*	0.455 53*
X_8	13	0.369 33	0.572 39
$\boldsymbol{X_9}$	13	0.357 07	0.438 78
X_3	13	0.469 62	0.912 22
X_5	13	0.4859	0.605 63
X_{13}	13	0.374 78	0.6787
Daubh4 wavelet			
Elimination	Input(features)	MSE training	MSE testing
–	14	0.398 64	0.412 26*
X_{10}	13	0.394 94*	0.411 05*
X_9	13	0.398 98	0.411 54
X_3	13	0.458 64	0.641 94
X_5	13	0.423 06	0.537 84
X_{13}	13	0.442 13	0.7417
X_9, X_8	12	0.401 71	0.8217
X_9, X_3	12	0.458 35	0.838 02
X_9, X_5	12	0.371 95	0.603 21
X_9, X_{13}	12	0.475 99	0.486 46

*Chosen model.

Table 1.6. Diagnostic test for training data.

	TP	FP	FN	TN
Haar WRNN	45	9	3	18
Daubh4 WRNN	46	14	2	13

Table 1.7. Diagnostic test for testing data.

	TP	FP	FN	TN
Haar WRNN	15	2	2	6
Daubh4 WRNN	14	3	3	5

Table 1.8. Sensitivity, specificity, and accuracy for training data.

	Sensitivity	Specificity	Accuracy
Haar WRNN	93.75%	66.67%	84%
Daubh4 WRNN	95.83%	48.15%	78.67%

Table 1.9. Sensitivity, specificity, and accuracy for testing data.

	Sensitivity	Specificity	Accuracy
Haar WRNN	88.24%	74%	84%
Daubh4 WRNN	82.35%	62.5%	76%

1.7 Conclusion

The best WRNN model for lung classification was WRNN with three hidden layers and 14 features extraction as the input variables. The results it provided of sensitivity, specificity, and accuracy were respectively 93.75%, 66.67%, and 84% for training data and 88.24%, 75%, and 84% for testing data. The accuracy of WRNN model was better than the previous research using NN [5] and RNN [6] which have accuracy respectively 80% and 81.33%. Elaboration using other wavelet models such as Daubhecies, Symlet, or Coiflet can be done to denoise images. Meanwhile other image extractions and other neural networks such as Hopfield network and the convolutional neural network can be developed to get better accuracy in terms of lung cancer classification.

References

[1] World Health Organizations 2018 https://who.int/news-room/fact-sheets/detail/cancer

[2] Int. Agency for Research on Cancer 2020 *World Cancer Report 2020* ed C P Wild, E Weiderpass and B W Stewart (Lyon: World Health Organization)

[3] Udhesani K A G, Meegama R G N and Fernando T G I 2011 Statistical feature-based neural network approach for the detection of lung cancer *Int. J. Image Process.* **vol.5** 425–34

[4] Nurtiyasari D, Rosadi D and Abdurakhman 2017 The application of wavelet recurrent neural network for lung cancer classification *2017 3rd Int. Conf. on Science and Technology - Computer (ICST), Yogyakarta* 127–30

[5] Miah M and Yousuf M A 2015 Detection of lung cancer from CT image using image processing and neural network *Int'l Conf. on Electrical Engineering and Information & Communication Technology* 1–6

[6] Nurtiyasari D 2014 The application of recurrent neural network model and recurrent neuro fuzzy model for lung cancer nodule classification *BSc Thesis* Yogyakarta State University

[7] Japanese Society of Radiology Technology 1997 Digital Image Database

[8] Russell S J and Norvig P 2010 *Artificial Intelligence: A Modern Approach* 3rd edn (Englewood Cliffs, NJ: Prentice-Hall)

[9] Harralick R M, Shanmugam K and Dinstein I 1973 Texture features for image classification *IEEE Trans. on System, Man and Cybernet.* **3** 610

[10] Daubechies I 1992 Ten lectures of wavelets *CBMS-NSF Regional Conf. Series in Applied Mathematics, vol. 61* (Philadelpia: Society for Industrial and Applied Mathematics (SIAM))

[11] Burrus C S *et al* 1998 *Introduction to Wavelets and Wavelet Transforms.* (Englewood Cliffs, NJ: Prentice-Hall)

[12] Bruce A and Gao H 1996 *Applied Wavelet Analysis with S-PLUS.* (New York: Springer)

[13] Walker J S 2008 *A Primer on Wavelets and their Scientific Applications.* (Boca Raton, FL: Chapman and Hall (CRC Press))

[14] Fausett L 1994 *Fundamentals of Neural Network-Architectures, Algorithms, and Applications.* (Englewood Cliffs, NJ: Prentice-Hall)

[15] Yeung D S *et al* 2010 *Sensitivity Analysis for Neural Network.* (Berlin: Springer)

[16] Haykin S 1999 *Neural Networks and Comprehensive Foundation.* (New York: Prentice-Hall)

[17] Hanke J E and Wichern D W 2005 *Bussiness Forecasting* 8th edn (Englewood Cliffs, NJ: Prentice-Hall)

IOP Publishing

Detection Systems in Lung Cancer and Imaging, Volume 1

Ayman El-Baz and Jasjit S Suri

Chapter 2

Diagnosis of diffusion-weighted magnetic resonance imaging (DWI) for lung cancer

Katsuo Usuda and Hidetaka Uramoto

2.1 Introduction

Diffusion-weighted magnetic resonance imaging (DWI) is able to record the random, translational motion, or the so-called Brownian movement of water molecules in human tissue and organs and give an accurate visual representation [1]. To detect the restricted diffusion of water molecules in the body, the magnetic resonance imaging (MRI)'s DWI function has been used recently. One of the main uses of DWI has been for the diagnosis of acute ischemic stroke by imaging the brain, while also being used for the diagnosis of intracranial tumors and demyelinating diseases [2]. A tumor that is malignant has a lower apparent diffusion coefficient (ADC) value which ordinarily inhibits diffusion of the water molecule in DWI images compared to a benign lesion.

Over the last 30 years, MRI in lung cancer staging has been performed in a limited way in vessel invasion, mediastinum invasion or chest wall invasion of lung cancer due to the research conducted by Webb *et al* [3]. From the report in 1991, the Radiologic Diagnostic Oncology Group stated that the diagnostic ability of MRI was the same as CT concerning T factors or N factors except in mediastinum invasion or chest wall invasion of lung cancer. MRI has developed considerably since the technology was first introduced. The practice guidelines of the Japanese lung cancer society in 2018 [4] reported that MRI was recommended partly for the diagnosis of lung cancer. In Toronto in 2008, the recommendation of the usage of DWI was already discussed during the International Society for Magnetic Resonance in Medicine meeting [5]. Concerns about the lack of understanding of DWI were documented in the meeting report [5].

2.2 Diagnosis of lung cancer and the pulmonary nodules and masses (figures 2.1–2.6, table 2.1)

There are three papers of meta-analyses of DWI for differential diagnosis of pulmonary nodules and masses (PNMs) [6–8] and all of the meta-analyses was

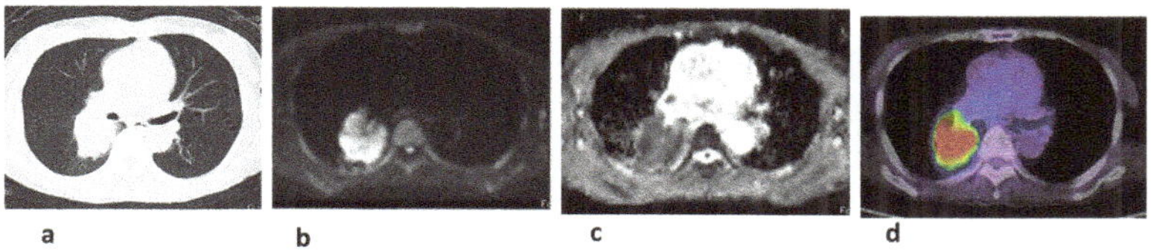

Figure 2.1. Case 1 Adenocarcinoma (acinar adenocarcinoma). (a) CT, (b) DWI, (c) ADC map, ADC 1.16×10^{-3} mm^2 s^{-1}, (d) FDG-PET/CT, SUV max 7.7.

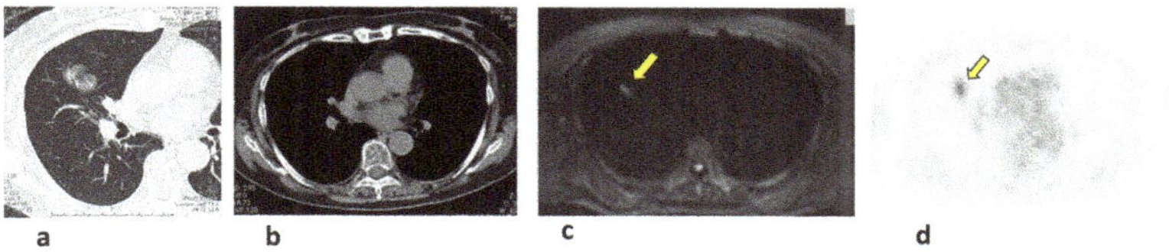

Figure 2.2. Case 2 Adenocarcinoma (lepidic adenocarcinoma) (a, b) CT, (c) DWI, ADC 1.364×10^{-3} mm^2 s^{-1}, (d) FDG-PET/CT, SUV max, 2.80.

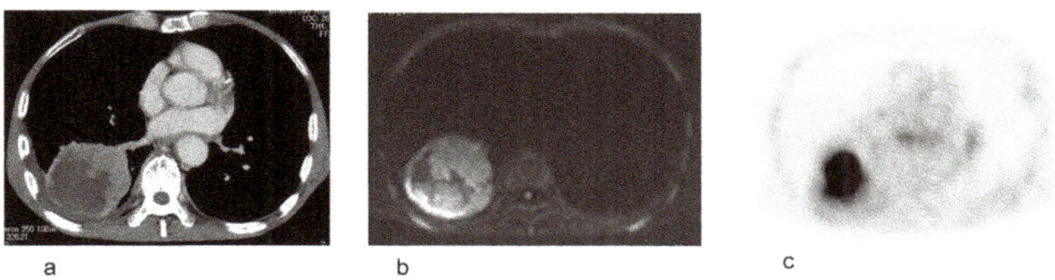

Figure 2.3. Case 3. Squamous cell carcinoma. (a) CT, (b) DWI, (c) FDG-PET/CT. This squamous cell carcinoma had central necrosis. Its ADC value was 1.11×10^{-3} mm^2 s^{-1}, and its SUV max was 24.7.

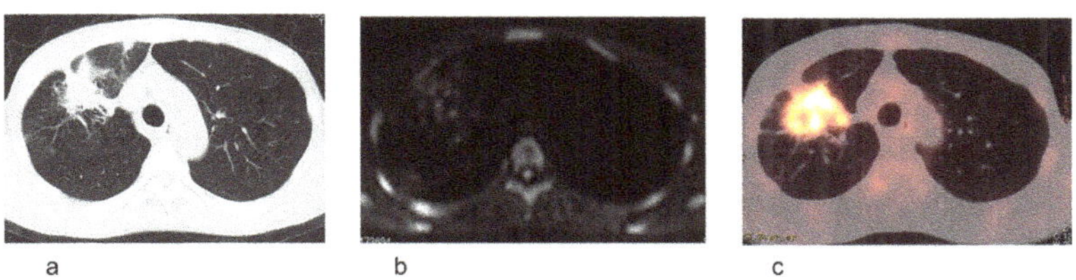

Figure 2.4. Case 4. Pulmonary abscess. (a) CT, (b) DWI, ADC 1.91×10^{-3} mm^2 s^{-1}, (c) FDG-PET/CT, SUV max 9.0.

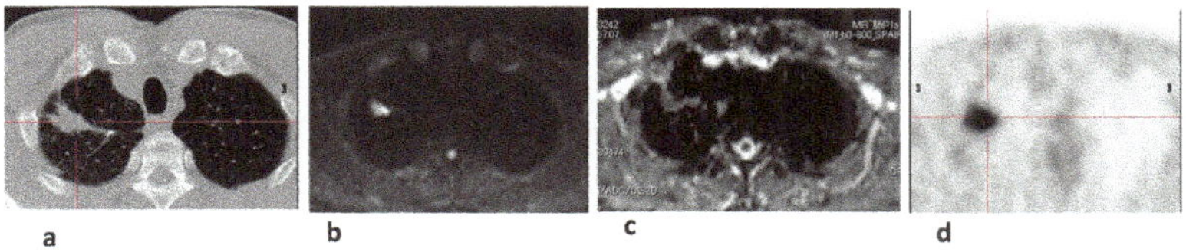

Figure 2.5. Case 5. Pulmonary tuberculosis. (a) CT, (b) DWI, (c) ADC map, ADC 1.13×10^{-3} mm^2 s^{-1}, (d) FDG-PET/CT, SUV max 3.60.

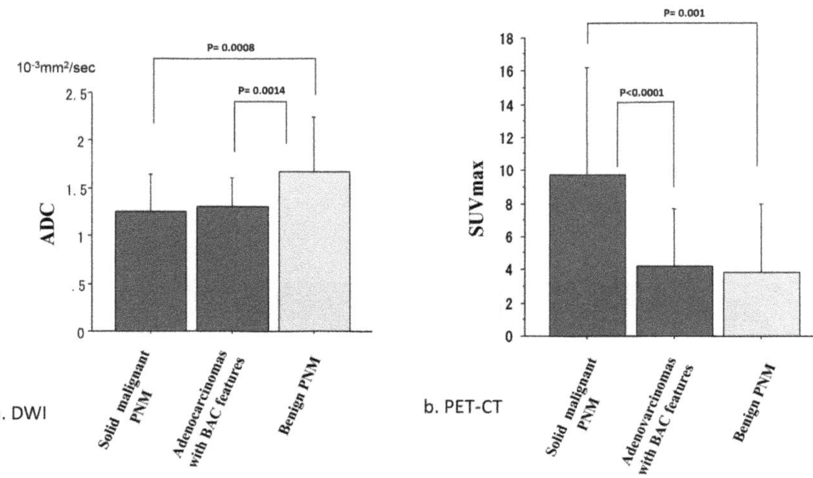

Figure 2.6. (a) Differences in ADC values in pulmonary nodules and masses (PNM). The ADC value (1.30 $\pm 0.30 \times 10^{-3}$ mm^2 s^{-1}) of the 65 adenocarciniomas with BAC features was significantly lower than that (1.66 $\pm 0.58 \times 10^{-3}$ mm^2 s^{-1}) of the 29 benign PNM (P=0.014). The ADC value ($1.25 \pm 0.39 \times 10^{-3}$ mm^2 s^{-1}) of the 95 solid malignant PNM was significantly lower than that of the 29 benign PNM (P=0.0008). (b) Differences in SUV max in PNM. The SUV max (4.18 ± 3.55) of adenocarciniomas with BAC features was significantly lower than that (9.72 ± 6.46) of the 95 solid malignant PNMs ($P<0.0001$), but similar to that (3.89 ± 4.05) of the 29 benign PNMs (P=0.779). Reprinted from [20] Copyright Asian Pacific Journal of Cancer Prevention.

Table 2.1. Assessment of DWI and FDG-PET in malignant and benign pulmonary nodules and masses (PNMs). Reprinted from [20] Copyright Asian Pacific Journal of Cancer Prevention.

		DWI				FDG-PET				
		TP	FN	TN	FP	TP	FN	TN	FP	Total
Malignant	Lung cancer	115	28			99	44			143
	Metastatic lung tumor	13	4			13	4			17
Benign	Chronic pneumonia			7	3			6	4	10
	Nontuberculous mycobacteria			2	2			2	2	4
	Hamartoma			4	0			4	0	4
	Pulmonary tuberculosis			0	3			3	0	3
	Granuloma			2	0			2	0	2
	Sarcoidosis			2	0			0	2	2
	Lung abscess			2	0			0	2	2
	Pulmonary scar			0	2			2	0	2
	Total	128	32	19	10	112	48	19	10	189

TP = true-positive, FN = false-negative, TN = true-negative, FP = false-positive

The sensitivity [80.0% (128/160)] of DWI was significantly higher than that [70.0% (112/160)] of FDG-PET for the malignant PNMs (p=0.0389). The specificity [65.5% (19/29)] of DWI was equal to that [65.5% (19/29)] of FDG-PET for the benign PNMs (p=0.80). The accuracy [77.8% (147/189)] of DWI was not significantly higher than that [69.3% (131/189)] of FDG-PET for all PNMs (p=0.0621).

reported that DWI could differentiate malignancy from benignity for PNMs (figure 2.1: acinar adenocarcinoma, figure 2.2: lepidic adenocarcinoma, figure 2.3: squamous cell carcinoma, figure 2.4: pulmonary abscess, figure 2.5: pulmonary tuberculosis, figure 2.6: differences in ADC values in PNMs.) For differentiating between malignancy and benignity in a tumor of the lungs [6, 9–11], the mediastinum [12], the thorax[13], the prostate [14], the breast [15], and the liver [16] DWI has been very useful. However, the use of DWI has been primarily regulated to the lungs but is recently showing its efficacy in the diagnosis and treatment of other organs.

In terms of diagnosing malignancy as well as diagnostic performance DWI was reported to be similar to that of 18-fluoro-2-deoxy-glucose positron emission tomography–computed tomography (FDG-PET/CT) [17], or to be more accurate and reliable than FDG-PET/CT [18].

FDG-PET/CT is well recognized as being able to predict how aggressive a tumor will be by standardized uptake value (SUV). That being said the ADC value and imaging pattern on DWI are also considered to correlate with FDG accumulation and tumor aggressiveness [9]. Nomori *et al* [19] in his research on primary lung cancer, classified the imaging pattern using DWI into three categories, i.e., faint-homogenous, dark-homogenous, and heterogeneous patterns. The report mentioned that DWI showed not only histological heterogeneity but also histological invasiveness, such as lymphatic, vascular, and pleural invasion. In FDG-PET/CT, a solid lung cancer shows positive FDG accumulation, but, well-differentiated adenocarcinoma and small-sized lung cancer with a little metabolic activity show little FDG accumulation, and are usually diagnosed as negative. ADC value of adenocarcinoma with bronchioloalveolar carcinoma features resembles to that of solid lung cancer, but SUVmax of adenocarcinoma with bronchioloalveolar carcinoma features looks like that of benign pulmonary lesions, which is the reason that some lung cancers are easy to be false-negative in FDG-PET/CT [20].

Two articles were published concerning comparison of diagnostic capability between DWI and FDG-PET/CT for PNMs [9, 20]. The sensitivity and the accuracy of DWI were remarkably better than those of FDG-PET/CT for PNMs [9]. For PNMs, the sensitivity (80.0%) of DWI was remarkably better than that(70.0%) of FDG-PET/CT (table 2.1) [20]. The specificity (65.5%) of DWI was as same as that (65.5%) of FDG-PET/CT, and the accuracy (77.8%) of DWI was not remarkably better than that(69.3%) of FDG-PET/CT (table 2.1) [20].

2.3 Diagnostic capability of nodal involvement in lung cancer (figures 2.7–2.9)

As non-invasive examinations CT and FDG-PET/CT are not only performed for the evaluation and staging of lung cancer but also to evaluate nodal involvement.

The limitations of FDG-PET/CT not being able to precisely stage some cases of lung cancer are well documented. Even though there are some instances with FDG-PET/CT showing false positives in the testing of lymph nodes for lung cancer, it is still superior to CT in the evaluation of lypmph nodes for lung cancer [21].

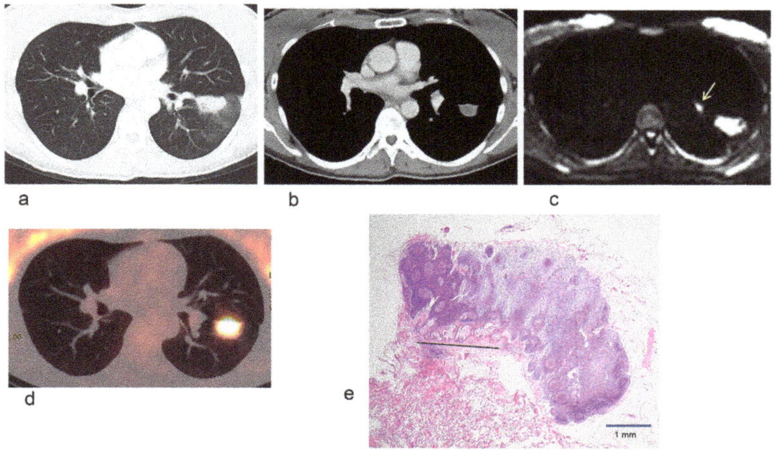

Figure 2.7. Case 6. Chest CT (a, b), DWI (c) and FDG-PET/CT (d) of a patient with adenocarcinoma. DWI and FDG-PET/CT identified the malignant lesion clearly. ADC value of the lung cancer was 1.239×10^{-3} $mm^2\ s^{-1}$, and its SUVmax was 11.3. A metastatic lesion (highlighted by an arrow) (ADC value: 1.55) of a #12L lymph node was recognized by DWI, but not by FDG-PET/CT before surgery. A tiny metastatic lesion (a solid line: 2.1 mm) was detected histopathologically in a #12L lymph node (e). Reprinted from [25] Copyright Society of Surgical Oncology.

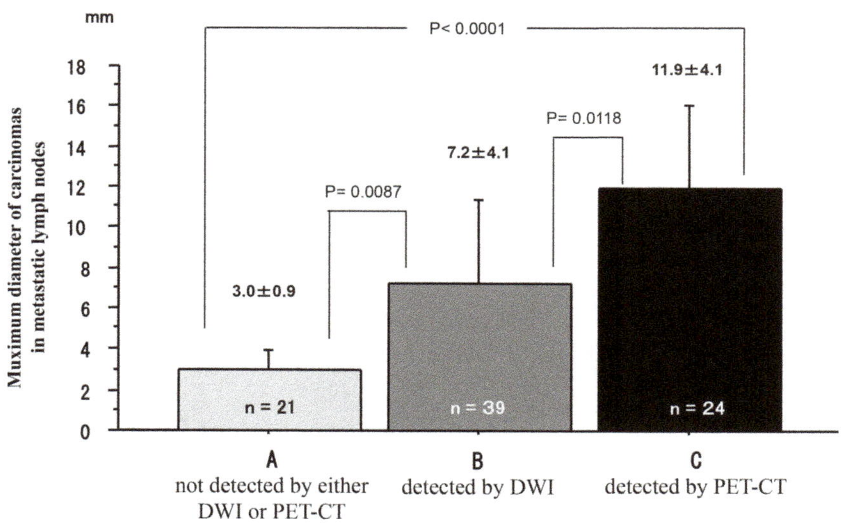

Figure 2.8. The average value of maximum diameter of carcinomas in metastatic lymph node stations not detected by either DWI or PET-CT (A), detected by DWI (B), and detected by PET-CT (C). Maximum diameter of carcinomas in metastatic lymph node stations were 3.0 ±0.9 mm in A, 7.2 ±4.1 mm in B, and 11.9 ±4.1 mm in C. There were significant differences among the groups. Reprinted from [25] Copyright Society of Surgical Oncology.

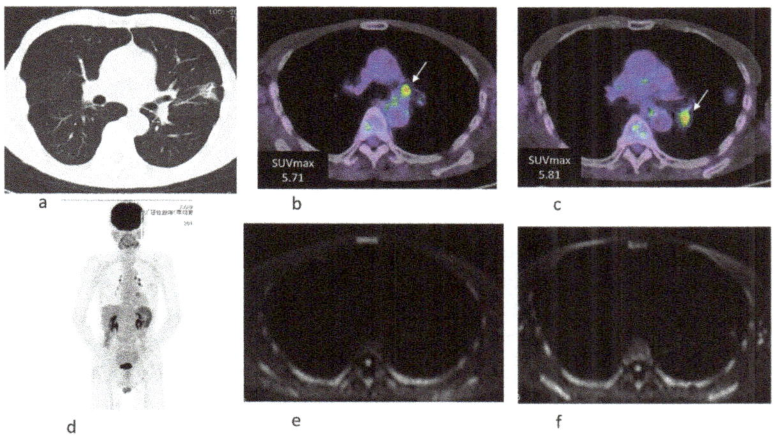

Figure 2.9. Case 7. Pulmonary adenocarcinoma, but no lymph node metastasis. The patient was diagnosed correctly by DWI, not by FDG-PET/CT. The patient was diagnosed with N2 disease by FDG-PET/CT, but N0 disease by DWI. Lymph node station #4L was diagnosed positive by FDG-PET/CT (b), but negative by DWI (e). Lymph node station #11 was diagnosed positive by FDG-PET/CT (c), but negative by DWI (f). The lymph node stations were diagnosed as sarcoidosis pathologically. Reprinted from [28] Copyright Asian Pacific Journal of Cancer Prevention.

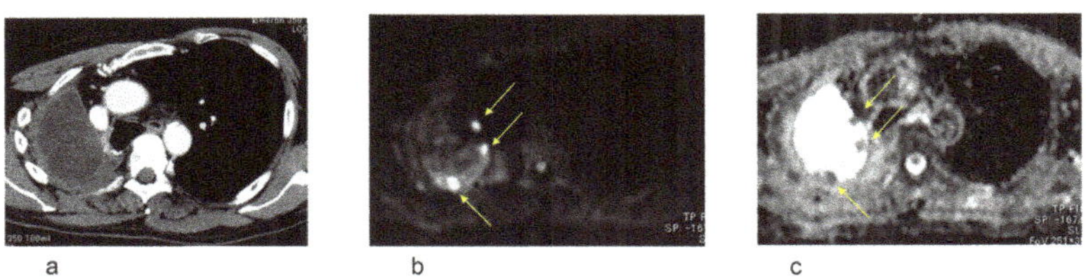

Figure 2.10. Case 8. Pleural dissemination from advanced squamous cell carcinoma. After right pneumonectomy, multiple pleural disseminations had developed. (a) CT, (b) DWI, (c) ADC map, ADC 1.321 $\times 10^{-3}$ $mm^2\ s^{-1}$. Multiple pleural disseminations were shown as high signals on DWI. The metastases to pleura expanded subsequently.

As the diagnostic ability of MRI has consistently improved over time there have been two meta-analyses that have championed the efficacy of DWI for the evaluation of the *N* factor in lung cancer [22]. With the sensitivity being 0.87 and the specificity being 0.88, the meta-analysis of the MRIs by Peerlings *et al* [23] reported a high diagnostic ability for lymph node assessments in non-small cell lung cancer.

When comparing DWI to FDG-PET/CT one of the strengths of the former is in lymph node assessment. When looking at accuracy and sensitivity in terms of evaluating hilar and mediastinal lypmh nodes, DWI scored considerably higher than FDG-PET/CT [24, 25].

With the staging accuracy of DWI at 89% compared to the 78% accuracy of FDG-PET/CT, Nomori *et al* [24] reported that there is less overstaging with DWI. There were some cases of understaging lung cancer in FDG-PET/CT [26]. In 147 lung cancer cases of clinical stage IA by FDG-PET/CT, 21 cases (14.3%) were revealed to be false-negatives, and be pathological N1 to N2 cases [26]. In our report the accuracy (96.2%) of N factor by DWI was remarkably higher than that (94.3%) of FDG-PET/CT in 160 lung cancer cases (figures 2.7 and 2.8) [25]. FDG-PET/CT examinations of tunnellers and miners were described to be inappropriate because of high false-positive rates of lymph nodes by pneumoconiosis [27]. Lymph nodes with silicosis have FDG accumulation in FDG-PET/CT, and they are incorrectly assessed as positive. When there are FDG accumulations of multiple hilar and mediastinal lymph nodes in lung cancer cases it makes it very difficult to get a precise reading with FDG-PET/CT. In lung cancer patients with FDG accumulations of multiple hilar and mediastinal lymph nodes, the specificity and the accuracy of DWI were remarkably higher than those of FDG-PET/CT (figure 2.9) [28]. The etiology of 100 patients who had an FDG accumulation in hilar and mediastinal lymph nodes in FDG-PET/CT consisted of 11 patients with metastases of cancer, 40 with anthracosis, 39 with reactive lymphadenitis, 4 with granulomas and 3 with silicosis [29]. These reports indicate that the diagnostic ability of DWI is equal to or better than that of FDG-PET/CT. That being said, with lymph nodes that had silicosis and granulation in the tissue there were likely to be false positives with DWI [24]. Due to the architectural change, granulation causes the diffusion of the water molecules to decrease when viewed with DWI, showing false positives.

2.4 Recurrence or metastasis from lung cancer (figure 2.11)

CT or FDG-PET/CT have a proven track record of detecting pulmonary metastasis from lung cancer but they have some difficulty when differentiating between pulmonary metastasis and benign lesions. Liver metastasis may be sometimes difficult to detect by plain CT and PET-CT. On the other hand, DWI can diagnose these metastasis of lymph nodes, bone and liver metastasis based on their ADC

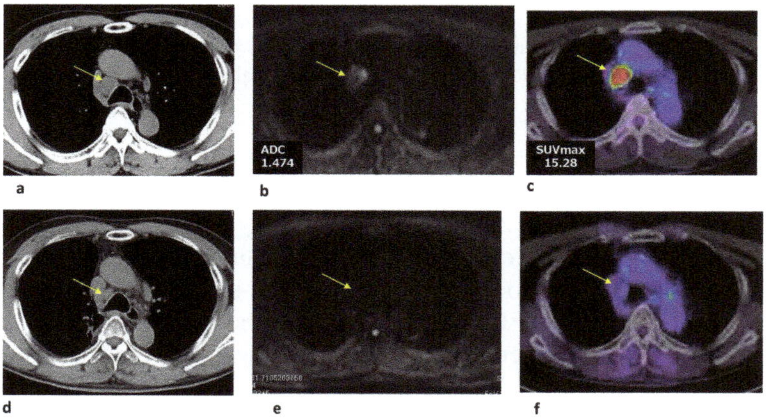

Figure 2.11. Case 9. The patient underwent right upper lobectomy and dissection of lymph nodes for pulmonary adenocarcinoma. Growth of lymph node station #4R was detected by CT (a), DWI (b) and FDG-PET/CT(c). It was diagnosed as the recurrence by EBUS-TBNA. Chemoradiation (RT 50Gy+CBDCA+PTX) was performed. For response evaluation, CT (d) showed PR, but DWI (e) showed CR with no diffusion of the #4R lymph node. FDG-PET/CT(f) also showed CR with little FDG accumulation of the lymph node. Follow-up study showed CR. Reprinted from [37], copyright (2019), with permission from Elsevier.

values [30]. MRI was reported to have a remarkably high degree of sensitivity in the detection of colorectal liver metastasis [31]. Whole-body MRI with DWI can be performed for assessment of bone metastasis of non-small cell lung cancer patients; which is a bit more accurate than bone scintinography and/or FDG-PET/CT [32]. We reported that rates of detection for metastatic lesions from lung cancer were 82% (27/33) in CT, 89% (17/19) in FDG-PET/CT and 100% (36/36) in DWI (figure 2.10) [30]. The detection rate of metastatic lesions of DWI was remarkably higher than that of CT (p=0.0244), but not remarkably higher than that of FDG-PET/CT (p=0.22) [30].

2.5 Diagnosis of lung cancer by whole-body DWI

The diagnostic capability of whole-body DWI (WB-DWI) was reported to be similar to that of FDG-PET/CT [33, 34], and others described that the diagnostic capability of WB-DWI was better than that of FDG-PET/CT [35]. Nowadays clinical staging of lung cancer is usually examined by FDG-PET/CT and cranial MRI. FDG-PET/CT cannot evaluate cranial metastasis because of high metabolism of glucose in the brain, and cranial MRIs make up for the weakpoint of FDG-PET/CT. Diagnostic efficacy of WB-DWI for operable lung cancer was reported to be equivalent to that by FDG-PET/CT + cranial MRI [36]. In the future WB-DWI will be more widely available for the clinical staging of lung cancer.

2.6 Response evaluation to chemotherapy and/or radiotherapy (figure 2.11, table 2.2)

It is a global standard that the response evaluation of chemotherapy and/or radiotherapy is performed with CT. Functional assessment of DWI had better quality than that of CT for the response evaluation of chemotherapy and/or radiotherapy to metastatic tumors of lung cancer (figure 2.11, table 2.2) [37]. DWI was described to be more useful than FDG-PET/CT for the estimation of a tumor's response to therapy in non-small cell lung cancer (NSCLC) patients before chemoradiotherapy [38]. The results of DWI in combination with WB-MRI were equivalent to those of integrated FDG-PET/CT [39]. ADC in DWI can be used as promising data for detecting the early response to or predicting prognosis after chemotherapy of NSCLC [40, 41]. DWI is becoming a more recognized examination for response evaluation of chemotherapy and/or radiotherapy.

2.7 ADC and pathology

ADC value presents diffusion of the tissue, and usually ADCs of lung cancers are lower than that of benign lesions. ADC of lung cancer decreases according to cell differentiation decreasing. Lung cancer can be assessed in terms of quality using DWI.

The ADC ($1.11 \pm 0.26 \times 10^{-3}$ mm^2 s^{-1}) of lung cancer with necrosis was remarkably lower than that ($1.32 \pm 0.33 \times 10^{-3}$ mm^2 s^{-1}) of lung cancer without necrosis [42]. Abscesses and thrombi disturb the diffusivity of water molecules

Table 2.2. Response evaluation to the therapy for recurrence or metastasis of lung cancer. Reprinted from [37], copyright (2019), with permission from Elsevier.

		by DWI				Total cases
		CR	PR	SD	PD	
by CT	CR					
	PR	3	2			5
	SD	1		1		2
	PD				17	17
Total cases		4	2	1	17	24

The response evaluation by CT using RECIST (Response Evaluation Criteria in Solid Tumors) were PR in five patients, SD in two, and PD in the remaining 17 patients. For the response evaluation by DWI, metastatic lesions with no diffusion in DWI or ADC value of more than 1.70×10^{-3} mm^2 s^{-1} after chemotherapy/radiotherapy were judged as CR. The response evaluation by DWI were CR in four patients, PR in two, SD in one, sand PD in the remaining 17 patients. All 4 patients had CR classification by response evaluation of DWI after chemotherapy/radiotherapy was determined, PR in 3 patients and SD in a patient in CT. A follow-up study two years after chemotherapy/radiotherapy revealed response evaluation by DWI were correct.

because they are hyperviscous [43, 44]. Median ADC value (0.877×10^{-3} mm^2 s^{-1}) of abscess was significantly lower than that of (2.118×10^{-3} mm^2 s^{-1}) phlegmon ($p<0.001$), furthermore lower than (3.008×10^{-3} mm^2 s^{-1}) edema ($p<0.01$) [45]. In DWI, 22% of benign lesions exhibited restricted diffusion in images [46]. The article presents that some benign PNMs with abscesses give false-positive results in DWI due to the presence of abscesses and thrombi [46].

The ADC value ($1.91 \pm 0.36 \times 10^{-3}$ mm^2 s^{-1}) of mucinous adenocarcinoma was significantly higher than that ($1.25 \pm 0.25 \times 10^{-3}$ mm^2 s^{-1}) of adenocarcinoma with mucin, furthermore higher than that ($1.24 \pm 0.30 \times 10^{-3}$ mm^2 s^{-1}) of other cell types [42]. Mucinous carcinomas were reported to be hypointense and as a result showed higher ADC values, which could be misjudged as benign lesions in DWI [20]. Mucinous carcinomas showed higher ADC values and lower DWI signal intensity than tubular adenocarcinomas in the anorectal region, because mucinous carcinomas possess lower cellularity than tubular adenocarcinomas [47].

2.8 Medical cost of examinations

The recent rise in medical costs have increasingly become more of an issue for hospitals trying to keep costs down. It is caused by the increasing costs of examinations and therapies as well as by increasing lifespans. For the medical cost, CT costs 10 000 yen (around $ 88) MRI of 1.5T costs 13 300 yen (around $ 116), and MRI of 3T costs 16 000 yen (around $ 140). An extra cost of 5000 yen (around $ 43) is required when using a contrast agent for CT or MRI. In general, examinations using radioisotopes are usually expensive. Bone scintigraphy costs 22 000 yen (around $ 192) and gallium scintigraphy costs 18 000 yen (around $ 157). Furthermore, FDG-PET/CT costs 86 250 yen (around $ 756), which is very expensive. In fact, the cost of an MRI is 81%–84% cheaper than that of

FDG-PET/CT. MRIs are more economical compared to FDG-PET/CT while offering the same or better results and thus provide a superior cost benefit analysis.

2.9 Advantage and disadvantage of MRI

MRI has several advantages against FDG-PET/CT. MRI needs no contrast agents and requires less time for the examination. Furthermore, MRI does not have radiation exposure for patients and is ideal for the examination of children [17]. MRI need a lower cost compared to FDG-PET/CT.

MRI has some disadvantages against FDG-PET/CT. A MRI examination is prohibited for people who have metal implants such as a pacemakers, tattoos or claustrophobia An MRI causes a loud sound which is unpleasant for some patients.

2.10 Future plans

There was no prospective randomized controlled trial between DWI and FDG-PET/CT for PNMs. The result is that the diagnostic capability of DWI is not concluded to be higher, but the diagnostic capability of DWI is compatible with that of FDG-PET/CT for PNMs. Further studies are necessary for to establish the true usefulness of DWI.

2.11 Conclusion

This chapter deals with the latest research of DWI, especially diagnostic advantages of DWI for lung cancer. DWI is useful for differential diagnosis of malignancy or benignity for neoplasm in various organs. Diagnostic abilities of DWI for PNMs, *N* factors and *M* factors of lung cancer are equivalent to or more than that of FDG-PET/CT. DWI has several economic and diagnostic advantages.

References

[1] Le Bihan D, Breton E, Lallemand D, Aubin M L and Vignaud J *et al* 1988 Separation of diffusion and perfusion in intravoxel incoherent motion MR imaging *Radiology* **168** 497–505

[2] Tien R D, Felsberg G J, Friedman H, Brown M and MacFall J 1994 MR imaging of high-grade cerebral gliomas. Value of diffusion-weighted echoplanar plus sequences *AJR* **162** 671–7

[3] Webb W R, Gatsonis C, Zerhouni E A, Heelan R T and Glazer G M *et al* 1991 CT and MR imaging in staging non-small cell bronchogenic carcinoma; Report of the Radiologic Diagnostic Oncology Group *Radiology* **178** 705–13

[4] *Qualitative Imaging, Lung Cancer Practice Guidelines by the EBM Technique on 2018 Version* 2018 Tokyo, Japan: Japanese Lung Cancer Society; Kanehara Publication pp 29–32 (in Japanese)

[5] Padhani A R, Liu G, Koh D M, Chenevert T L, Thoeny H C, Takahara T, Dzik-Jurasz A, Ross B D, Van Sauterne M and Cllins D *et al* 2009 Diffusion-weighted magnetic resonance imaging as a cancer biomarker: consensus and recommendations *Neoplasia* **11** 102–25

[6] Wu L M, Xu J R, Hua J, Gu H Y, Chen J, Haacke E M and Hu J 2013 Can diffusion-weighted imaging be used as a reliable sequence in the detection of malignant pulmonary nodules and masses? *Magn. Reson. Imaging* **31** 235–46

[7] Li B, Li Q, Chen C, Guan Y and Liu S 2014 A systematic review and meta-analysis of the accuracy of diffusion-weighted MRI in the detection of malignant pulmonary nodules and masses *Acad. Radiol.* **21** 21–9
[8] Shen G, Jia Z and Deng H 2016 Apparent diffusion coefficient values of diffusion-weighted imaging for distinguishing focal pulmonary lesions and characterizing the subtype of lung cancer: a meta-analysis *Eur. Radiol.* **26** 556–66
[9] Mori T, Nomori H, Ikeda K, Kawanaka K and Shiraishi S *et al* 2008 Diffusion-weighted magnetic resonance imaging for diagnosing malignant pulmonary nodules/masses. Comparison with positron emission tomography *J. Thoracic Oncol.* **3** 358–64
[10] Ohba Y, Nomori H, Mori T, Ikeda K and Shibata H *et al* 2009 Is diffusion-weighted magnetic resonance imaging superior to positron emission tomography with fludeoxyglucose F 18 in imaging non-small cell lung cancer? *J. Thorac. Cardiovasc. Surg.* **138** 439–45
[11] Usuda K, Zhao X T, Sagawa M, Matoba M and Kuginuki Y *et al* 2011 Diffusion-weighted imaging is superior to PET in the detection and nodal assessment of lung cancers *Ann. Thorac. Surg.* **91** 1689–95
[12] Usuda K, Maeda S, Motono N, Ueno M and Tanaka M *et al* 2015 Diffusion weighted imaging can distinguish benign from malignant mediastinal tumors and mass lesions. comparison with positron emission tomography *Asian Pac. J. Cancer Prev.* **16** 6469–75
[13] Tondo F, Saponaro A, Stecco A, Lombardi M and Casadio C *et al* 2011 Role of diffusion-weighted imaging in the differential diagnosis of benign and malignant lesions of the chest-mediastinum *Radiol. Med.* **116** 720–33
[14] Yamamura J, Salomon G, Buchert R, Hohenstein A and Graessner J *et al* 2011 Magnetic resonance imaging of prostate cancer. Diffusion-weighted imaging in comparison with sextant biopsy *J. Comput. Assist. Tomogr.* **35** 223–8
[15] Fornasa F, Pinali L, Gasparini A, Toniolli E and Montemezzi S 2011 Diffusion-weighted magnetic resonance imaging in focal breast lesions. Analysis of 78 cases with pathological correlation *Radiol. Med.* **116** 264–75
[16] Koike N, Cho A, Nasu K, Seto K and Nagaya S *et al* 2009 Role of diffusion-weighted magnetic resonance imaging in the differential diagnosis of focal hepatic lesions *World J. Gastroenterol.* **15** 5805–12
[17] Darge K, Jaramillo D and Siegel M J 2008 Whole-body MRI in children: current status and future applications *Eur. J. Radiol.* **68** 289–98
[18] Wu L M, Xu J R, Gu H Y, Hua J and Chen J *et al* 2012 Preoperative mediastinal and hilar nodal staging with diffusion-weighted magnetic resonance imaging and fluorodeoxyglucose positron emission tomography/computed tomography in patients with non-small-cell lung cancer: which is better? *J. Surg. Res.* **178** 304–14
[19] Nomori H, Cong Y, Abe M, Sugimura H and Kato Y 2015 Diffusion-weighted magnetic resonance imaging in preoperative assessment of non-small cell lung cancer *J. Thorac. Cardiovasc. Surg.* **149** 991–6
[20] Usuda K, Sagawa M, Motono N, Ueno M and Tanaka M *et al* 2014 Diagnostic performance of diffusion weighted imaging of malignant and benign pulmonary nodules and masses: comparison with positron emission tomography *Asian Pac. J. Cancer Prev.* **15** 4629–35
[21] Roberts P F, Follette D M, von Haag D, Park J A and Valk P E *et al* 2000 Factors associated with false-positive staging of lung cancer by positron emission tomography *Ann. Thoracic Surg.* **70** 1154–9

[22] Shen G, Hu S, Deng H and Kuang A 2016 Performance of DWI in the nodal characterization and assessment of lung cancer: a meta-analysis *Am. J. Roentgenol.* **206** 283–90
[23] Peerlings J, Troost E G, Nelemans P J, Cobben D C and de Boer J C *et al* 2016 The diagnostic value of MR Imaging in determining the lymph node status of patients with non-small cell lung cancer: a meta-analysis *Radiology* **281** 86–98
[24] Nomori H, Mori T, Ikeda K, Kawanaka K and Shiraishi S *et al* 2008 Diffusion-weighted magnetic resonance imaging can be used in place of positron emission tomography for N staging of non-small cell lung cancer with fewer false-positive results *J. Thoracic Cardiovasc. Surg.* **135** 816–22
[25] Usuda K, Sagawa M, Motono N, Ueno M and Tanaka M *et al* 2013 Advantages of diffusion-weighted imaging over positron emission tomography-computed tomography in assessment of hilar and mediastinal lymph node in lung cancer *Ann. Surg. Oncol.* **20** 1676–83
[26] Park H K, Jeon K, Koh W J, Suh G Y and Kim H *et al* 2010 Occult nodal metastasis in patients with non-small cell lung cancer at clinical stage IA by PET/CT *Respirology* **15** 1179–84
[27] Saydam O, Gokce M, Kilicgun A and Tanriverdi O 2012 Accuracy of positron emission tomography in mediastinal node assessment in coal workers with lung cancer *Med. Oncol.* **29** 589–94
[28] Usuda K, Maeda S, Motono N, Ueno M and Tanaka M *et al* 2015 Diagnostic performance of diffusion weighted imaging for multiple hilar and mediastinal lymph nodes with FDG accumulation *Asian Pac. J. Cancer Prev* **16** 6401–6
[29] Koksal D, Demirag F, Bayiz H, Ozmen O and Tatci E *et al* 2013 Apr 4 The correlation of SUVmax with pathological characteristics of primary tumor and the value of tumor/lymph node SUVmax ratio for predicting metastasis to lymph nodes in resected NSCLC patients *J. Cardiothorac. Surg.* **8** 63
[30] Usuda K, Sagawa M, Motono N, Ueno M, Tanaka M and Machida Y *et al* 2014 Recurrence and metastasis of lung cancer demonstrate decreased diffusion on diffusion-weighted magnetic resonance imaging *Asian Pac. J. Cancer Prev.* **15** 6843–8
[31] Blyth S, Blakeborough A, Peterson M, Cameron I C and Majeed A W 2008 Sensitivity of magnetic resonance imaging in the detection of colorectal liver metastases *Ann. R. Coll. Surg. Engl.* **90** 25–8
[32] Takenaka D, Ohno Y, Matsumoto K, Aoyama N, Onishi Y, Koyama H, Nogami M, Yoshikawa T, Matsumoto S and Sugimura K 2009 Detection of bone metastases in non-small cell lung cancer patients: comparison of whole-body diffusion-weighted imaging (DWI), whole-body MR imaging without and with DWI, whole-body FDG-PET/CT, and bone scintigraphy *J. Magn. Reson. Imaging* **30** 298–308
[33] Ohno Y, Koyama H, Onishi Y, Takenaka D and Nogami M *et al* 2008 Non-small cell lung cancer: whole-body MR examination for M-stage assessment – utility for whole-body diffusion-weighted imaging compared with integrated FDG PET/CT *Radiology* **248** 643–54
[34] Sommer G, Wiese M, Winter L, Lenz C and Klarhöfer M *et al* 2012 Preoperative staging of non-small-cell lung cancer: comparison of whole-body diffusion-weighted magnetic resonance imaging and 18F-fluorodeoxyglucose-positron emission tomography/computed tomography *Eur. Radiol.* **22** 2859–67
[35] Laurent V, Trausch G, Bruot O, Olivier P and Felblinger J *et al* 2010 Comparative study of two whole-body imaging techniques in the case of melanoma metastases: advantages of multi-contrast MRI examination including a diffusion-weighted sequence in comparison with PET-CT *Eur. J. Radiol.* **75** 376–83

[36] Usuda K, Sagawa M, Maeda S, Motono N and Tanaka M *et al* 2016 Diagnostic performance of whole-body diffusion-weighted imaging compared to PET-CT plus brain MRI in staging clinically resectable lung cancer *Asian Pac. J. Cancer Prev.* **17** 2393–8

[37] Usuda K, Iwai S, Funasaki A, Sekimura A, Motono N, Matoba M, Doai M, Yamada S, Ueda Y and Uramoto H 2019 Diffusion-weighted magnetic resonance imaging is useful for the response evaluation of chemotherapy and/or radiotherapy to recurrent lesions of lung cancer *Transl. Oncol.* **12** 699–704

[38] Ohno Y, Koyama H, Yoshikawa T, Matsumoto K, Aoyama N, Onishi Y and Sugimura K 2012 Diffusion-weighted MRI versus 18F-FDG PET/CT: performance as predictors of tumor treatment response and patient survival in patients with non-small cell lung cancer receiving chemoradiotherapy *AJR Am. J. Roentgenol.* **198** 75–82

[39] Wu X, Kellokumpu-Lehtinen P L, Pertovaara H, Korkola P, Soimakallio S, Eskola H and Dastidar P 2011 Diffusion-weighted MRI in early chemotherapy response evaluation of patients with diffuse large B-cell lymphoma – a pilot study: comparison with 2-deoxy-2-fluoro-D-glucose-positron emission tomography/computed tomography *NMR Biomed.* **24** 1181–90

[40] Yabuuchi H, Hatakenaka M, Takayama K, Matsuo Y, Sunami S, Kamitani T, Jinnouchi M, Sakai S, Nakanishi Y and Honda H 2011 Non-small cell lung cancer: detection of early response to chemotherapy by using contrast-enhanced dynamic and diffusion-weighted MR imaging *Radiology* **261** 598–604

[41] Nunes T F, Szejnfeld D, Szejnfeld J, Kater C E, Faintuch S, Castro C H and Goldman S M 2016 Assessment of early treatment response with DWI after CT-guided radiofrequency ablation of functioning adrenal adenomas *AJR Am. J. Roentgenol.* **207** 804–10

[42] Usuda K, Iwai S, Yamagata A, Sekimura A, Motono N and Matoba M *et al* 2020 Relationships and qualitative evaluation between diffusion-weighted imaging and pathologic findings of resected lung cancers *Cancers (Basel).* **12** 1194

[43] Kwee T C, Takahara T, Ochiai R, Koh D M, Ohno Y, Nakanishi K, Niwa T, Chenevert T L, Luijten P R and Alavi A 2010 Complementary roles of whole-body diffusion-weighted MRI and ^{18}F-FDG PET. The state of the art and potential application *J. Nucl. Med.* **51** 1549–58

[44] Desprechins B, Stadnik T, Koerts G, Shabana W, Breucq C and Osteaux M 1999 Use of diffusion-weighted MR imaging in differential diagnosis between intracerebral necrotic tumors and cerebral abscesses *Am. J. Neuroradiol.* **20** 1252–7

[45] Chun C W, Jung J Y, Baik J S, Jee W H, Kim S K and Shin S H 2018 Detection of soft-tissue abscess: comparison of diffusion-weighted imaging to contrast-enhanced MRI *J. Magn. Reson. Imaging* **47** 60–8

[46] Feuerlein S, Pauls S, Juchems M S, Stuber T, Hoffmann M H, Brambs H J and Ernst A S 2009 Pitfalls in abdominal diffusion-weighted imaging. How predictive is restricted water diffusion for malignancy *AJR* **193** 1070–6

[47] Nasu K, Kuroki Y and Minami M 2012 Diffusion-weighted imaging findings of mucinous carcinoma arising in the ano-rectal region. Comparison of apparent diffusion coefficient with that of tubular adenocarcinoma *Jpn. J. Radiol.* **30** 120–7

IOP Publishing

Detection Systems in Lung Cancer and Imaging, Volume 1

Ayman El-Baz and Jasjit S Suri

Chapter 3

Computer assisted detection of low/high grade nodule from lung CT scan slices using handcrafted features

Seifedine Kadry and Venkatesan Rajinikanth

3.1 Introduction

The rapid development in science and technology aims to provide better living conditions for the human community irrespective of their age, gender and race. This technological advancement also helped hospitals to improve their environment with recent equipment for the diagnosis, monitoring and the treatment implementation operations. In the current era, for a variety of reasons, disease in humans is gradually improving, most of the undiagnosed disease may cause temporary or permanent disability and some unrecognized disease may lead to death. The report of the World Health Organization (WHO) confirms that cancer in humans is more acute and causes a higher mortality rate compared to other diseases and in particular cancer in the lungs is one of the most acute disease and a major cause of death globally [1, 2].

The lungs are a vital internal organ responsible for circulating air between the other body organs and the atmosphere and problems in the lungs will severely disrupt this process and oxygen shortage will lead to various illnesses. An abnormality in the lungs, such as pneumonia, TB, and nodules arises for various reasons and early detection and treatment will reduce the impact of the disease. The lungs are commonly routinely screened using a prescribed imaging modality and chest radiographs (x-ray) and chest computed tomography (CT) scans are the commonly suggested imaging techniques to record and evaluate abnormalities in lungs [3, 4].

Lung abnormality is one of the medical emergencies in humans and the unrecognized and untreated lung disease can lead to death. Due to its importance, a number of computer assisted detection (CAD) systems are proposed and implemented by researchers to diagnose lung disease with better accuracy [5–7].

doi:10.1088/978-0-7503-3355-9ch3

A summary of the lung abnormality detection procedure discussed in the literature is presented in table 3.1

From table 3.1, it can be observed that a number of techniques are available to detect lung nodules using a suitable technique. Further the reviews also confirm the limitations in the existing methodology and the need for the new disease detection procedure for lung abnormality assessment [27, 28].

In the literature, a number of medical imaging procedures are proposed and implemented by researchers to detect abnormalities using a class of medical imaging modalities [29–37]. The existing methods may work efficiently on a chosen image modality and may provide poor results on other modalities. Further, the choice of a particular image examination methodology depends on the image modality [38–42] and the expertise of the operator who implements the essential procedure to examine the images using the appropriate technique [43–47].

The improved computing facility and the availability of varied hardware and software has helped to develop a range of computing facilities to diagnose the medical images with better detection accuracy. In most modern hospitals image capturing, diagnosis, disease reporting and the treatment suggestions are immediately delivered with the help of the existing computing system and these reports are then once again verified and confirmed by the doctor. The existing methodologies considerably reduce the diagnostic burden on the doctor and in some hospitals, remote diagnosis and treatment planning is also implemented to reduce the existing delay in the traditional disease detection system.

This chapter aims to develop a CAD system to detect the lung nodule using the CT scan slices (CTS). This CAD system will assist the doctor during the disease detection using the existing lung CTS. This work aims to implement a simple and computationally efficient lung nodule detection system without compromising the detection accuracy. The proposed CAD is developed with the following operations; (i) image collection and initial handling, (ii) image pre-processing, (iii) image post-processing, (iv) feature extraction, (v) dominant feature selection, and (vi) classification and validation [48–50].

The major problem in CAD system validation is the unavoidability of the clinical grade images. Since, due to a variety of personal and ethical reasons; the medical images existing in the hospitals are protected with strict copyright and ethical acts. In some cases, the images collected from the volunteers as per the approved ethical norms are summarized in a dedicated location and are permitted to be utilized by the researchers to test and validate their CAD system. The proposed work considered such a dataset available in [51–55]. The RIDER Lung CT dataset consist the CTS of volunteers collected under; (i) normal, (ii) low grade nodule, and (iii) high grade nodule

The existing CT scan images in the RIDER dataset is in three-dimensional (3D) form and the 3D image assessment is computationally complex and time consuming. Hence, in the proposed work, 3D to 2D conversion is achieved using the ITK-Snap software [56, 57]. The ITK-Snap is commonly used by researchers to examine varied modality medical images and the earlier works which considered the ITK-Snap for 3D to 2D conversion can be found in [58, 59]. This is free software and the current version of the ITK-Snap (version 3.8.0) can be downloaded from [54]. ITK-snap helps to convert the 3D lung CT image into various 2D slices, such as axial-view,

Table 3.1. Summary of the lung abnormality assessment using computerized approaches.

References	Methodology implemented
Soliman *et al* [5]	Automated diagnosis of lung injury using 4D-CT chest images.
El-Baz *et al* [6]	Development of a CAD system to detect the malignant lung nodules by integrating the shape feature assessment.
Hammer *et al* [8]	This work discusses a clinical trial to suggest the cancer risk assessment technique based on the assessment of subsolid nodules.
Ardila *et al* [9]	Assessment of lung abnormality based on a 3D deep learning system executed on the low-dose lung CT scan images.
Seijo *et al* [10]	This work presents the role of biomarkers in lung cancer screening methodologies and the challenges to employ the chosen biomarkers.
Ciompi *et al* [11]	Automated technique with deep learning based pulmonary nodule detection is presented with appropriate examples.
Gurcan *et al* [12]	This work implements a computer-aided diagnosis system for lung nodule detection using lung CTS.
Lo *et al* [13]	Assessment of lung nodule using convolution-neural-network (CNN) is presented.
Penedo *et al* [14]	CNN based automated lung nodule detection is discussed using clinical level lung CTS.
Brown *et al* [15]	This work discusses a model assisted detection of the lung nodule using CTS.
Tan *et al* [16]	This work proposes a machine-learning based automated detection of lung nodules from CTS.
Huang *et al* [17]	Presents a detailed assessment of lung nodule recognition in CTS with 3D CNN.
Armato *et al* [18]	Implements an automated lung nodule classification system using machine-learning techniques.
Teramoto and Fujita [19]	Developed and implemented cylindrical nodule-enhancement filter to support fast nodule detection in CTS.
Retico *et al* [20]	This work implements a sequence of techniques for lung nodule detection in low-dose and thin-slice CTS.
Lin *et al* [21]	This work discusses the implementation of two-level neural classification procedure to detect lung nodules with reduced false positives.
Wiemker *et al* [22]	Presents a detailed assessment on computer-aided lung nodule detection using high-resolution CTS.
Tajbakhsh and Suzuki [23]	This work presents a detailed analysis on the CNN based lung nodule detection from the CTS.
Anirudh *et al* [24]	This work implements 3D CNN architecture to detect the lung nodule.
Ko *et al* [25]	This work presents the wavelet assisted nodule detection using lung CTS.
Ali *et al* [26]	Presents a detailed assessment on lung nodule detection using deep reinforcement learning.
Zhang *et al* [27] and Lee *et al* [28]	These works presents detailed reviews on various lung nodule detection techniques available in the literature.

coronal-view and sagittal-view. In most of the earlier lung CTS evaluation procedures, only the axial-view is evaluated and hence, in this research also, the axial-view is considered for the assessment. The complexity of the image increases with its dimension (number of pixels) and hence, in this work, the entire test images of the 2D lung CTS is resized into a standard dimension of 256×256×1 pixels. Normally, the CT scan images are considered to record the lung activity using a radiological technique and this procedure will capture the lungs along with other body parts, such as the heart and bones. In the lung CTS, the infected section (lung nodule) will have better pixel intensity compared to the normal lung section and in order to maintain a better detection of the abnormal section, it is necessary to remove the unwanted sections (artifact) using a chosen technique. In this work, a bi-level threshold filter is initially implemented to divide the test image into the lung nodule and the artifact. The threshold filter helps to divide the image into region of interest (ROI) and artifact based on a chosen threshold and the execution of the threshold filter can be found in earlier works [60–62]. The extracted ROI (nodule division) is then considered for the assessment of the abnormality using the proposed CAD system. The enhanced ROI pixel group is then mined using the commonly adopted level-set procedure called the distance-regularized-level-set (DRLS) technique; which works on an adoptable bounding-box (BB) technique. When the BB is initiated around the lung nodule, it is allowed to shrink towards the edges of the ROI when the iteration in DRLS increases. This process continues until it identifies all the linked pixels and finally, the convergence stops and a binary image is given as the outcome. The essential features, such as the gray-level co-occurrence matrix (GLCM) and the Hu moments are then extracted from this binary image. Further, the essential local-binary-pattern (LBP) features are also extracted from the original test image with the help of the assigned LBP weights of 1,2,3 and 4 respectively. This work also extracts the entropy features from the test image with chosen entropies. The handcrafted features, such as GLCM, Hu, LBP and entropy are combined together to form a single feature vector of a specific length. When a feature size is more, there may be a possibility of the over-fitting problem during the classification and to avoid this problem, a feature selection based on the social-group-optimization (SGO) is executed. This algorithm will compute the hamming distance between two different features sets (normal and abnormal class features) and based on the difference, the principal features are chosen. The selected feature sub-set is then considered to train, test and classify the binary classifiers implemented in this work to separate the lung CTS into three different classes, such as: (i) low grade nodule versus high grade nodule, (ii) normal versus low grade nodule and (iii) normal versus high grade nodule. The proposed experimental investigation is implemented using the MATLAB software and the attained result confirms that, proposed technique works well on the considered test images.

3.2 Computer assisted detection system

This section presents information regarding the proposed CAD system for the lung CTS examination. Figure 3.1 depicts the proposed CAD system to evaluate lung

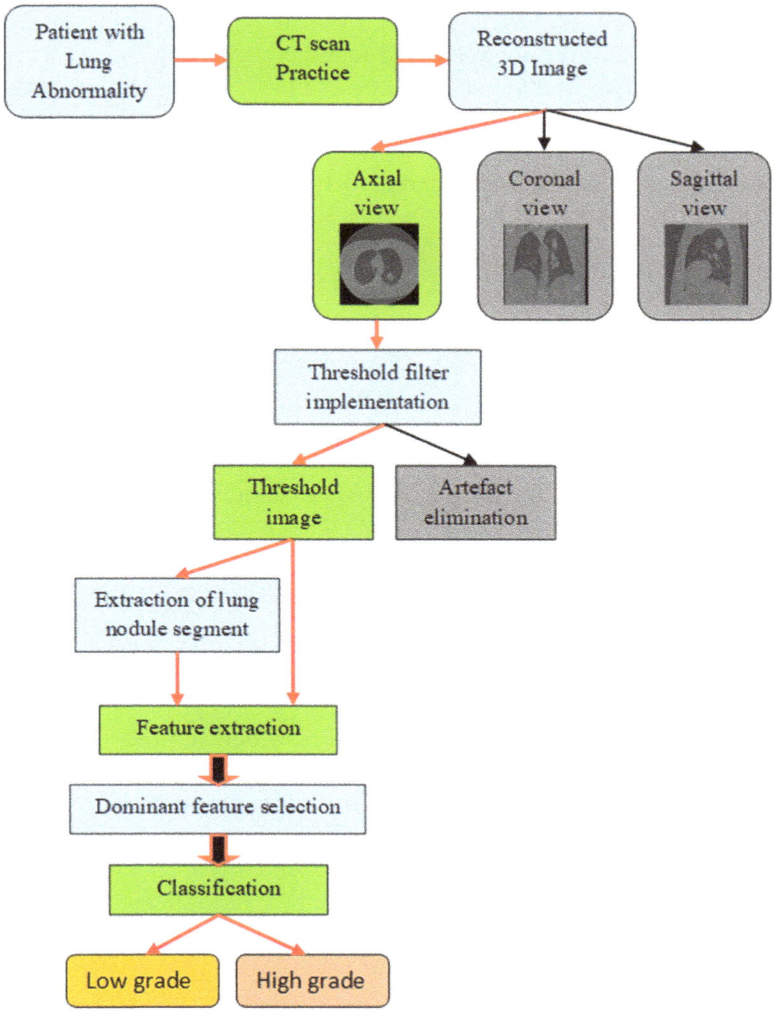

Figure 3.1. Various phases involved in the proposed CAD stream.

abnormality using the CTS. Initially the essential disease screening is performed using CT scan slice and the reconstructed 3D CT is then considered for the experimental evaluation.

Assessment of the 3D CT scan image is quite complex and hence the 3D to 2D conversion is implemented and the converted image is resized into 256×256×1 pixel image for the disease assessment. In the proposed work, the axial-view is considered and the extracted section is then evaluated using a sequence of techniques. Initially, a threshold filter is employed to separate the artifact from the image and the ROI is then considered for the assessment. The DRLS segmentation is then implemented to extract the nodule from the ROI. Later, the essential texture features from the extracted nodule is then mined using the GLCM and Hu techniques. The other related image features (LBP and entropy) are also extracted from the original 2D test image and these features are combined together serially to form a feature vector of finite dimension. The number of features available in the feature vector is very high and hence, a heuristic algorithm based feature selection approach is executed to reduce the feature vector dimension, to avoid the problem of over-fitting. The reduced feature vector is then considered to train, test and validate the classifier implemented to classify the CTS into various sections.

3.2.1 Image collection

Essential images for the experimental investigation are collected from the RIDER Lung CT dataset available at [51–54]. This database consists of low-dose lung CT scan images collected using the prescribed medical protocol and the images are free to use for research purposes. In this work, various class axial lung CT scan slices, such as normal, log grade and high grade nodule are collected and considered to evaluate the performance of the proposed CAD system. The available test images of the RIDER dataset are in the form of 3D and it is very hard to evaluate the conventional image evaluation procedures and needs very high computation cost. Hence, 3D to 2D conversion is implemented in the proposed technique to simplify the disease evaluation process.

3.2.2 3D to 2D conversion

In the literature, the 3D to 2D conversion is widely employed to reduce the computation effort during brain MRI evaluation and lung CTS evaluation tasks [49, 50]. In this work, the ITK-Snap software is considered to convert the existing image into 2D slices and the converted image is then considered for the disease assessment operation. The sample test image considered in this work is depicted in figure 3.2 in which (a) depicts the disease class and (b) to (d) depict the various image orientations, such as axial, coronal and sagittal. In this work, the axial orientation is considered for the assessment and the number of images (axial-view) considered in each case is depicted in table 3.2.

3.2.3 Threshold filter implementation

The major aim in medical image assessment is to achieve better disease detection using the chosen technique. If we consider lung CTS, the detection accuracy is degraded due to the artifact available in the image and hence the lung section to be examined is to be extracted with the help of an appropriate image mask. The mask assisted lung section extraction is also one of the commonly considered approaches to enhance the result and the development of a mask to extract the lung section with better accuracy is time consuming. Hence, this work implemented a threshold filter to enhance the ROI and the implementation of the technique can be found in the earlier works [60–62]. Figure 3.3 depicts the results attained with the proposed technique, in which figure 3.3(a) and (b) shows the image class and sample test images; figure 3.3(c) and (d) presents the artifact and the ROI respectively.

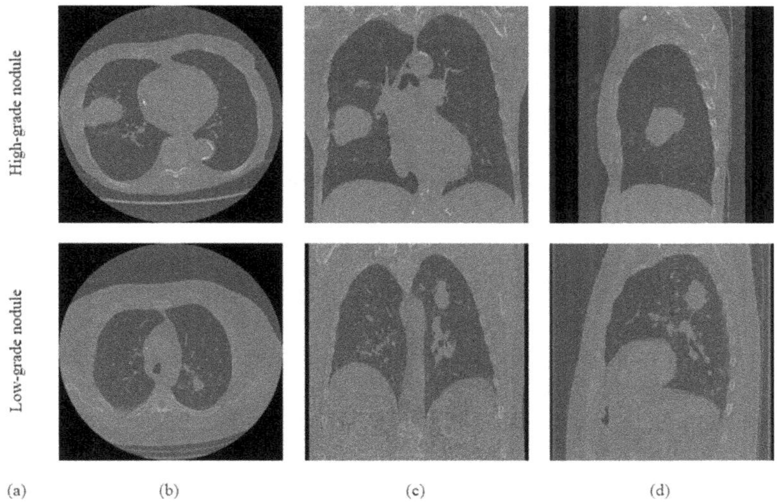

Figure 3.2. Sample test images of RIDER-TCIA database.

Table 3.2. RIDER lung CT scan slices considered to evaluate the proposed system.

Image class	Dimension	Total images	Images for classifier training	Images for classifier testing
Normal	256×256×1	600	420	180
Low grade nodule	256×256×1	600	420	180
High grade nodule	256×256×1	600	420	180

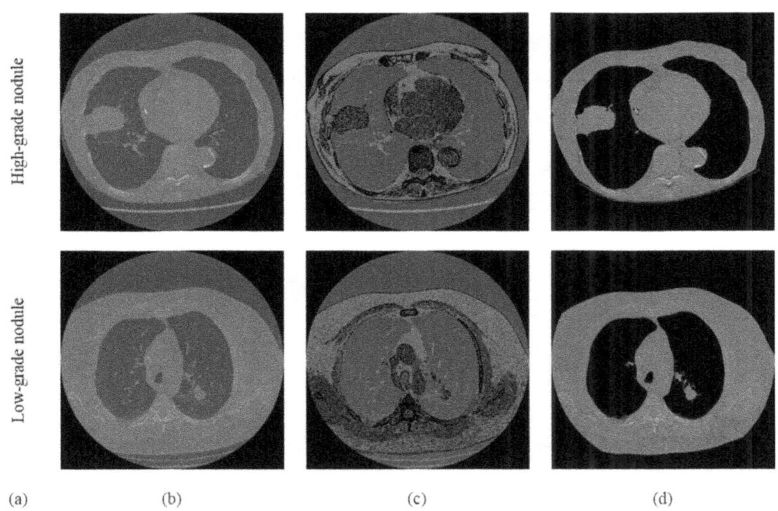

Figure 3.3. Lung CTS tested with the threshold filter.

This work considers the low contrast lung CTS and in this image the visibility of the ROI is very poor and hence, a semi-automated segmentation technique can be considered to extract the abnormal section from the image and then a suitable feature extraction technique can be employed to mine the essential features from the ROI in order to have its scientific/texture/shape information to build the automated disease detection system; which can recognize the lung nodule with better accuracy.

3.2.4 Nodule segmentation

Various image processing phases are employed in the automated disease detection systems and the segmentation is one of the prime phases, which extracts the lung nodule accurately for further assessment. In this work, the extraction of the infected lung section is achieved with a semi-automated segmentation technique known as the distance-regularized level-set (DRLS) proposed in [63–65] (figure 3.4).

The DRLS works with the help of a bounding-box assigned by the user around the abnormal section to be extracted. When the iteration increases, the box will converge toward inside the nodule section and identifies all the possible pixels which are related to the lung nodule. When the identification is achieved, it stops the adjustment and displays the binary image as the output. In the binary image, the background is assigned with a value of 0 (black) and the nodule pixels are assigned with 1 (white). The essential features from this binary image are then extracted using the GLCM and Hu. The working principle of the DRLS can be found in earlier works and in this research, the number of iterations for the DRLS is assigned as 500.

3.2.5 Feature extraction

The overall performance of the automated disease detection using the bio-medical image depends mainly on the features which are considered to train, test and

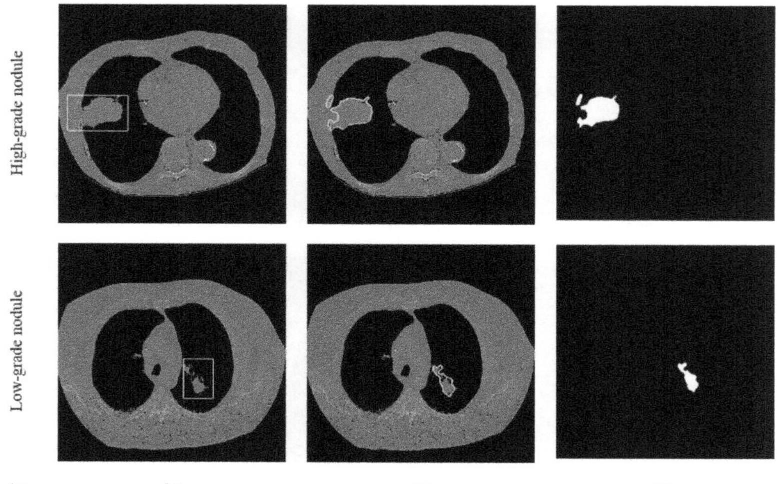

Figure 3.4. Implementation of DRLS segmentation and the corresponding results.

validate the classifiers. In the image processing literature, a considerable number of feature extraction procedures are proposed and implemented to classify a number of medical images and in this work, the feature mining approaches, such as GLCM, Hu, LBP and entropies are considered to extract the vital information from the binary as well as grayscale test images. These features are also termed as the handcrafted features, since each feature extraction approach is to be selected and executed based on the operator's choice.

3.2.5.1 GLCM and Hu moments

In the image processing literature, the GLCM and Hu moments are widely adopted to mine the essential texture information from the test image under examination. The essential information of the GLCM [66, 67] and Hu moments [68, 69] are already discussed in the literature.

The GLCM normally extracts the texture, shape and the scientific information of the image under study and this procedures helps to mine 25 features. Similar to the GLCM, the Hu moments extracts nine pieces of essential information from the image. These two features are extracted from the binary image of the image and the other related information regarding the GLCM and Hu moments can be found in [59].

3.2.5.2 LBP and intropy features

LBP is also a feature extraction procedure, normally considered in the medical image processing task. The complete information regarding the global weighted LBP feature extraction methodology can be found in the recent work of Gudigar *et al* [70] and their work implemented the LBP on the ultrasound-images using the varied weights (R) ranging from 1 to 4. This research work also follows similar methodology to enhance and extract the information from the considered lung CTS using the weighted LBP and the attained results for various image cases are depicted in figure 3.5.

In this work, varied weight levels (R= 1 to 5) are implemented to enhance the texture of the grayscale image to attain the essential information about the abnormalities. Based on the abnormalities, the pixel distribution of the image will vary and this information can be attained from the histogram of the image as depicted in figure 3.6. Figure 3.6(a) depicts the LBP histogram of the normal image case and figure 3.6(b) and (c) shows the LBP histogram of the low and high grade lung nodule cases. After implementing the LBP, from each image, 59 vital LBP features are extracted and the total number of features from a single image case will be around 59×4=236 features.

This procedure is repeated on each image considered for the assessment and the attained features are sequentially arranged to get a one-dimension (1D) feature vector of dimension 1×1×236 and these features are then combined serially with the other handcrafted features, such as the GLCM and the Hu moments.

3.2.6 Feature selection

The total number of raw features available for every image case is large and if these features are used without any additional treatment, the problem of over-fitting will

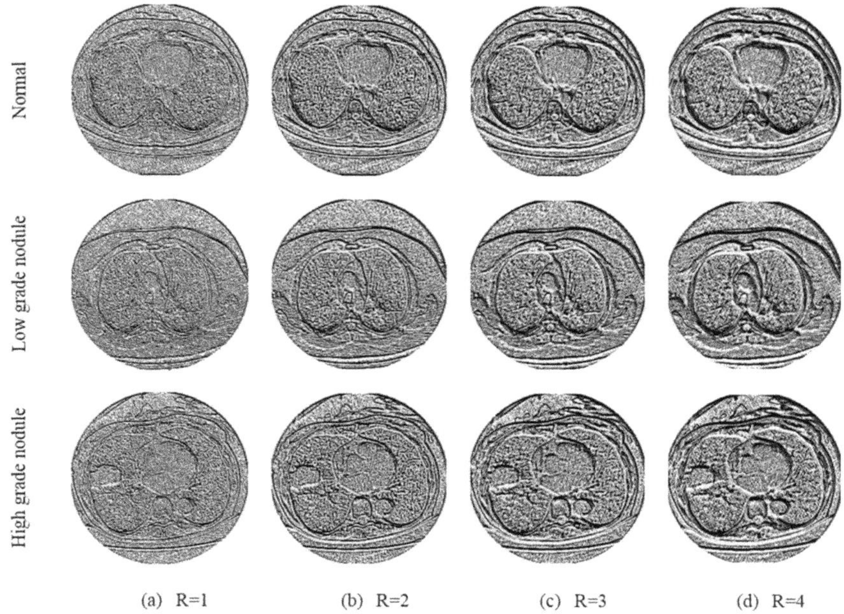

Figure 3.5. LBP results attained for various weights (R = 2 to 4).

happen [71, 72]. To avoid this, a feature reduction or a dominant feature selection technique is implemented and the implemented technique helps to reduce the available raw features to a lower level. In this work, the handcrafted feature vector dimension is larger and it includes the features of the GLCM, Hu and LBP ((1×1×25) + (1×1×9) + (1×1×236) = 1×1×270).

Feature reduction using a traditional statistical technique is time consuming and hence, heuristic algorithm supported techniques are widely adopted by the researchers to identify the dominant features during the automated disease detection process [73–75]. In the proposed work, an SGO algorithm assisted feature selection technique is employed to reduce the number of image features. The working of SGO is based on the mimic of the human decision making concept existing during a group-conversation and the essential information on the SGO can be found in earlier research works [76, 77].

The pseudo-code of the SGO algorithm is depicted below.

Pseudo-code of traditional SGO algorithm
Start
Assume N-agents ($i = 1,2,3,4,N$)
Assign these agents to find the $Gbest_j$ in a D-dimensional search location
Randomly assign the entire agents in the group throughout the examination space during the process
Compute the fitness value
Update the direction of persons for $Gbest_j$= max $\{f(S_i)\}$

Begin the improving stage to change the information of other agents to get the $Gbest_j$
Start the acquiring phase to proceed the information of agents by arbitrarily choosing the agents with finest fitness
Repeat the procedure till entire agents move towards the finest position in the search space
If the agent having roughly similar strength values ($Gbest_j$)
Then
Stop the search and display the final result
Else
Repeat the preceding steps
End
Stop

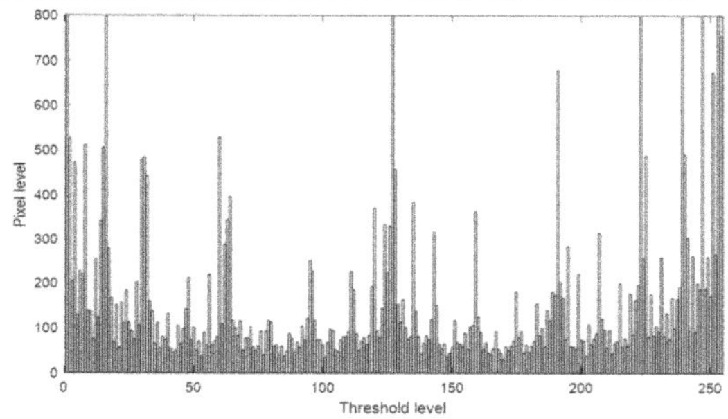

(a) LBP histogram for normal image with R=4

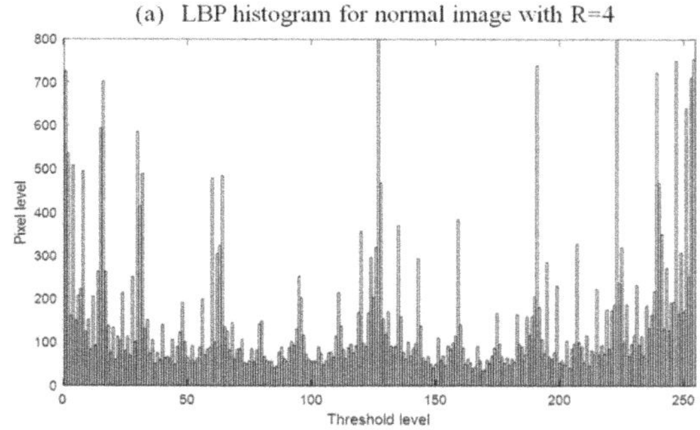

(b) LBP histogram for low grade nodule image with R=4

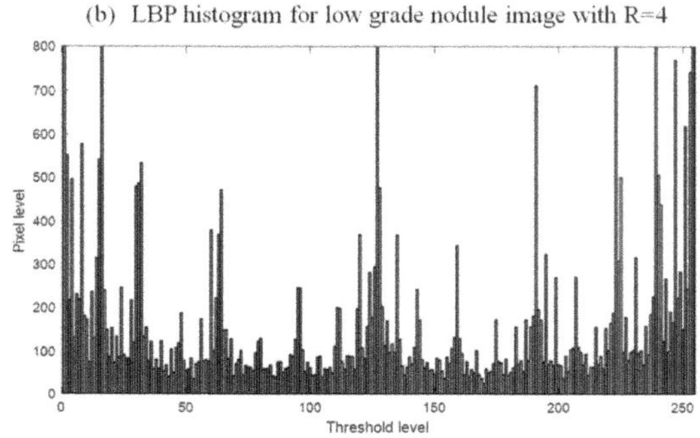

(c) LBP histogram for high grade nodule image with R=4

Figure 3.6. Histogram pattern of LBP images.

The SGO based feature reduction implemented in the proposed work is depicted in figure 3.7 and this process helped to reduce the 1×1×270 number of features into 1×1×24 features and these features are then considered to train, test and validate the classifiers employed in the proposed work.

3.2.7 Classifier implementation

The classifiers play major roles in the automated disease detection using machine-learning and the deep learning systems. In this work, the commonly used traditional classification methods, such as decision-tree (DT), random-forest (RF), *K*-nearest neighbor (KNN) and SVM-RBF are considered to separate the existing image dataset into different classes based on the need.

3.2.7.1 Decision-tree

DT is one if the widely used classifiers applicable for the linear/non-D linear features with a sequence of examination design which progress in the shape of a tree-like flow graph. It employs a unique examination phase as the root and inner nodes, and the class label forms terminal nodes. Once a DT has been created, classification is accomplished by the conclusions reached in every partition of the tree. Other information can be found in [78, 79].

3.2.7.2 Random-forest

RF is an improved procedure and very robust to noise and capable on substantial datasets. It is specified as a set of tree predictors. Each tree relies on a random vector, which is sampled independently and allotted in the same way as tree distribution in the forest. The classical RF technique is widely used in various image classification tasks [80, 81].

3.2.7.3 K-Nearest neighbor

KNN approximates the space from a series of new information to all training data points, and discovers the direct coldness as the best neighbor. The *k* significance is

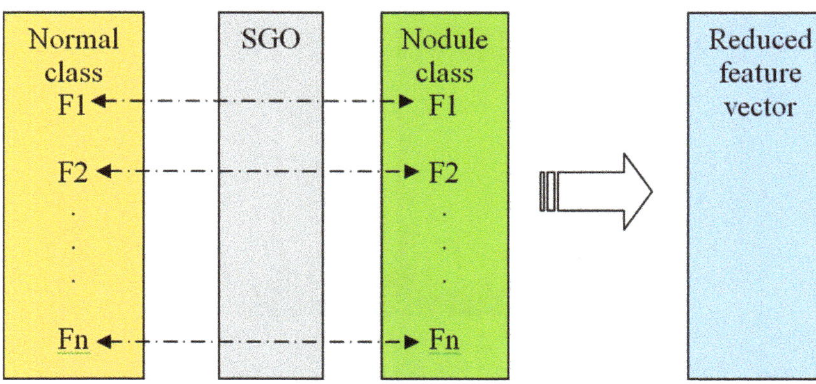

Figure 3.7. SGO assisted feature reduction technique.

empirically computed by means of the training sample's organization error. Further information on KNN can be found in [82, 83].

3.2.7.4 SVM-RBF

SVM is a well-known classifier in the image assessment domain, and in SVM the existing data are separated into various judgment surfaces using a hyperplane. Due to its superiority, the SVM classifiers are widely adopted in a variety of image classification and disease detection tasks [84, 85].

3.2.8 Validation of the CAD system

The performance of the proposed disease detection scheme based on the lung CTS is confirmed by computing the necessary measures presented in equations (3.1)–(3.6) [74, 75]:

$$\text{Accuracy} = \text{ACC} = \frac{T_{+ve} + T_{-ve}}{T_{+ve} + T_{-ve} + F_{+ve} + F_{-ve}} \tag{3.1}$$

$$\text{Precision} = \text{PRE} = \frac{T_{+ve}}{T_{+ve} + F_{+ve}} \tag{3.2}$$

$$\text{Sensitivity} = \text{SEN} = \frac{T_{+ve}}{T_{+ve} + F_{-ve}} \tag{3.3}$$

$$\text{Specitivity} = \text{SPE} = \frac{T_{-ve}}{T_{-ve} + F_{+ve}} \tag{3.4}$$

$$\text{Negative Predictive Value} = \text{NPV} = \frac{T_{-ve}}{T_{-ve} + F_{-ve}} \tag{3.5}$$

$$\text{F1Score} = \text{F1S} = \frac{2T_{+ve}}{2T_{+ve} + \text{F}_{-ve} + \text{F}_{+ve}} \tag{3.6}$$

where F_{+ve}, F_{-ve}, T_{+ve}, and T_{-ve} signify false-positive, false-negative, true-positive, and true-negative respectively.

Table 3.3. Performance measures attained during the classification of normal/low grade nodule class.

Classifier	T+ve	F-ve	T-ve	F+ve	ACC	PRE	SEN	SPE	NPV	F1S
DT	163	17	166	14	91.3889	92.0904	90.5556	92.2222	90.7104	91.3165
RF	168	12	163	17	91.9444	90.8108	93.3333	90.5556	93.1429	92.0548
KNN	167	13	164	16	91.9444	91.2568	92.7778	91.1111	92.6554	92.0110
SVM-RBF	169	11	166	14	93.0556	92.3497	93.8889	92.2222	93.7853	93.1129

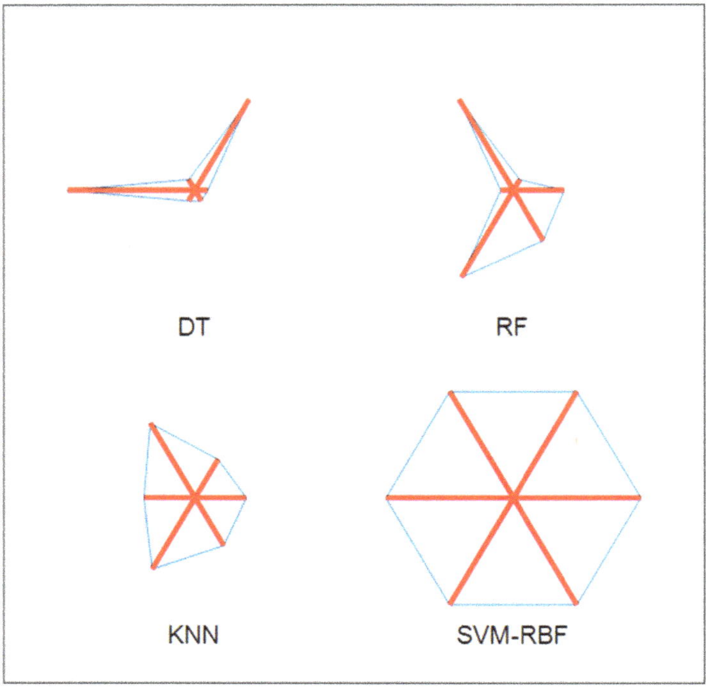

Figure 3.8. Glyph-plot of the normal/low grade class performance measures.

Table 3.4. Performance measures attained during the classification of normal/high grade nodule class.

Classifier	T+ve	F-ve	T-ve	F+ve	ACC	PRE	SEN	SPE	NPV	F1S
DT	163	17	168	12	91.9444	93.1429	90.5556	93.3333	90.8108	91.8310
RF	171	9	168	12	94.1667	93.4426	95.0000	93.3333	94.9153	94.2149
KNN	168	12	164	16	92.2222	91.3043	93.3333	91.1111	93.1818	92.3077
SVM-RBF	166	14	170	10	93.3333	94.3182	92.2222	94.4444	92.3913	93.2584

3.3 Results and discussions

This section of the chapter presents the result attained from this work and its discussion. Experimental investigation of the presented research work is achieved using the MATLAB software.

The proposed research work considered the lung CTS of the normal, low grade and high grade nodule images with dimension 256×256×1 pixels for the investigation. Initially, all the test images were treated using the threshold filter in order to separate the ROI. After separation, the essential low grade and high grade nodule sections (ROI) were then extracted using the DRLS segmentation. The image dimensions were constant; hence the dimension of the bounding-box (BB) was also

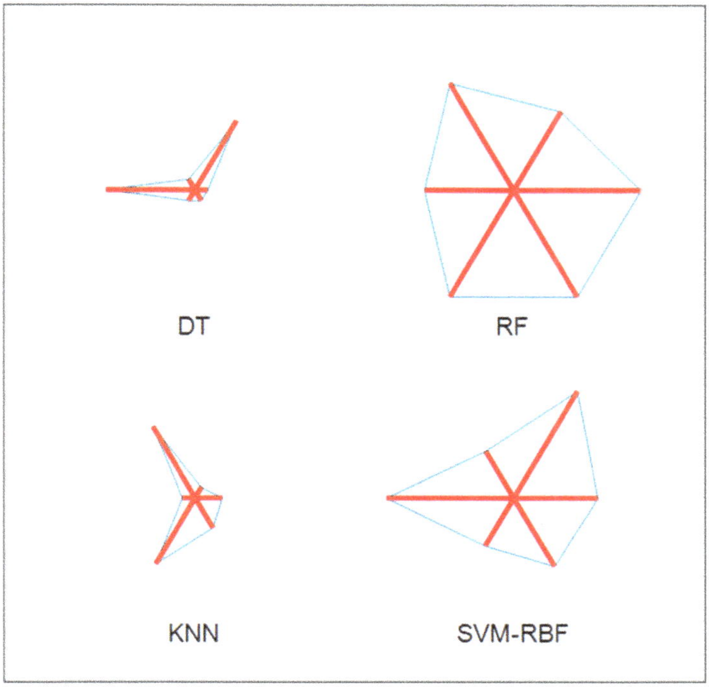

Figure 3.9. Glyph-plot of the normal/high grade class performance measures.

Table 3.5. Performance measures attained during the classification of low grade/high grade nodule class.

Classifier	T+ve	F-ve	T-ve	F+ve	ACC	PRE	SEN	SPE	NPV	F1S
DT	161	19	163	17	90.0000	90.4494	89.4444	90.5556	89.5604	89.9441
RF	158	22	161	19	88.6111	89.2655	87.7778	89.4444	87.9781	88.5154
KNN	163	17	165	15	91.1111	91.5730	90.5556	91.6667	90.6593	91.0615
SVM-RBF	166	14	161	19	90.8333	89.7297	92.2222	89.4444	92.0000	90.9589

fixed during the DRLS implementation. Based on the orientation of the lung nodule, the BB is to be positioned. The converged DRLS extracted the nodule section with better accuracy and the GLCM and Hu moments were then extracted from the binary image of the lung nodule. Further, the essential LBP features were also extracted and then a chosen classifier was implemented to classify the images into normal versus low grade nodule, normal versus high grade nodule and low grade versus high grade nodule. The performance of the implemented classifier was then validated based on the computed classification accuracy in each case.

Table 3.3 presents the performance measure attained during the normal/low grade class detection with the proposed technique with various classifiers. In this work, a 5-fold cross validation is implemented to evaluate the classification

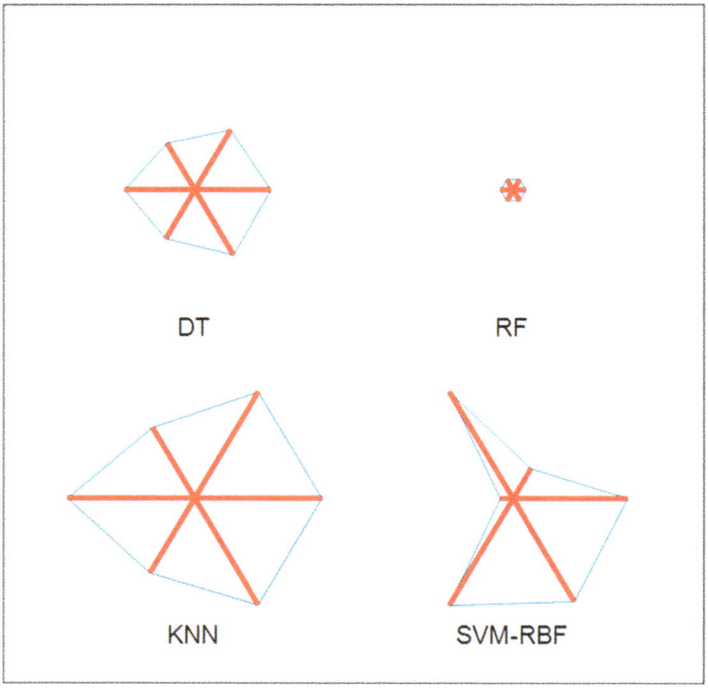

Figure 3.10. Glyph-plot of the low grade/high grade class performance measures.

performance and the best value among the five-trial is chosen as the classification result of the chosen classifier. In this work, the SVM-RBF offered better classification accuracy (93.05%) compared to other methods, such as DT, RF and KNN. In order to identify the overall performance of the proposed technique, a Glyph-plot is then constructed as in figure 3.8 and this figure also confirms the superiority of SVM-RBF compared to other techniques.

A similar procedure is then employed to classify the lung CTS into normal and high grade nodule case using the reduced feature sub-set of dimension 1×1×24 and the obtained result with a 5-fold cross validation is presented in table 3.4 and this confirms that the classification performance of the RF classifier is better when compared to other classifiers considered in this research. The false-negative and false-positive values attained with RF is much less and the overall result of the RF is better as confirmed by a Glyph-plot shown in figure 3.9.

Table 3.5 shows the results obtained with the proposed system with various classifiers and the results of this table depicts that the classification accuracy of KNN is superior when compared to DT, RF and SVM-RBF. The Glyph-plot for this table depicted in figure 3.10 also confirms the overall performance of the proposed system on the considered disease detection task. The results obtained from tables 3.3–3.5 confirm that the classification results during the normal and nodule class are better when compared to the results attained during the low grade/high grade tumor.

This research presents a simple and efficient technique to classify the lung CTS based on the abnormality existing in the test images. This technique offers better classification accuracy (>90%) in all the considered cases. In future, the result by the proposed technique can be improved (i) by employing other image feature extraction techniques, (ii) appropriate feature selection techniques, and (iii) other classifiers existing in the literature.

3.4 Conclusion

The lungs are vital internal organs in human physiology and abnormalities in the lungs are a medical emergencies in humans. Lung nodules is a harsh disease and untreated lung nodules will create severe problems. In the literature, a number of lung nodule detection procedures are already implemented to evaluate the abnormality with better accuracy. This work aims to implement a simple and effective technique to examine the abnormality in lungs using CTS with dimension 256×256×1. This work implemented a separate classification procedure, such as normal/low grade, normal/high grade and low/high grade nodule class and the proposed system helps to attain a better classification accuracy (>90%) in all cases. In future, the performance of the proposed system can be improved by implementing other feature extraction techniques and also other recent classification procedures available in the literature.

References

[1] https://who.int/news-room/fact-sheets/detail/cancer https://wcrf.org/dietandcancer/lung-cancer

[2] Buckler A J, Schwartz L H, Petrick N, McNitt-Gray M, Zhao B, Fenimore C, Reeves A P, Mozley P D and Avila R S 2010 Data sets for the qualification of volumetric CT as a quantitative imaging biomarker in lung cancer *Opt. Express* **18** 15267–82

[3] Bhakta R and Hossain A A 2020 Lung tumor segmentation and staging from CT images using fast and robust fuzzy C-means clustering *Int. J. Image, Graph. Signal Process.* **12** 38

[4] Soliman A, Khalifa F, Shaffie A, Dunlap N, Wang B, Elmaghraby A and El-Baz A 2016 Detection of lung injury using 4D-CT chest images *2016 IEEE 13th Int. Symp. on Biomedical Imaging (ISBI)* (Piscataway, NJ: IEEE) pp 1274–77

[5] El-Baz A S and Nitzken M 2016 Inventors; University of Louisville Research Foundation (ULRF), assignee. Computer aided diagnostic system incorporating shape analysis for diagnosing malignant lung nodules United States Patent US 9,230,320

[6] Soliman A, Elnakib A, Khalifa F, Abou El-Ghar M and El-Baz A 2015 Segmentationof pathological lungs from CT chest images *2015 IEEE Int. Conf. on Image Processing (ICIP)* (Piscataway, NJ: IEEE) pp 3655–9

[7] Hammer M M, Palazzo L L, Kong C Y and Hunsaker A R 2019 Cancer risk in subsolid nodules in the National Lung Screening Trial *Radiology* **293** 441–8

[8] Ardila D *et al* 2019 End-to-end lung cancer screening with three-dimensional deep learning on low-dose chest computed tomography *Nat. Med.* **25** 954–61

[9] Seijo L M *et al* 2019 Biomarkers in lung cancer screening: achievements, promises, and challenges *J. Thorac. Oncol.* **14** 343–57

[10] Ciompi F *et al* 2017 Towards automatic pulmonary nodule management in lung cancer screening with deep learning *Sci. Rep.* **7** 46479

[11] Gurcan M N, Sahiner B, Petrick N, Chan H P, Kazerooni E A, Cascade P N and Hadjiiski L 2002 Lung nodule detection on thoracic computed tomography images: preliminary evaluation of a computer-aided diagnosis system *Med. Phys.* **29** 2552–8
[12] Lo S C, Lou S L, Lin J S, Freedman M T, Chien M V and Mun S K 1995 Artificial convolution neural network techniques and applications for lung nodule detection *IEEE Trans. Med. Imaging* **14** 711–8
[13] Penedo M G, Carreira M J, Mosquera A and Cabello D 1998 Computer-aided diagnosis: a neural-network-based approach to lung nodule detection *IEEE Trans. Med. Imaging* **17** 872–80
[14] Brown M S, McNitt-Gray M F, Goldin J G, Suh R D, Sayre J W and Aberle D 2001 Patient-specific models for lung nodule detection and surveillance in CT images *IEEE Trans. Med. Imaging* **20** 1242–50
[15] Tan M, Deklerck R, Jansen B, Bister M and Cornelis J 2011 A novel computer-aided lung nodule detection system for CT images *Med. Phys.* **38** 5630–45
[16] Huang X, Shan J and Vaidya V 2017 Lung nodule detection in CT using 3D convolutional neural networks *2017 IEEE 14th Int. Symp. on Biomedical Imaging (ISBI 2017)* (Piscataway, NJ: IEEE) pp 379–83
[17] Armato S G III, Altman M B, Wilkie J, Sone S, Li F, Doi K and Roy A S 2003 Automated lung nodule classification following automated nodule detection on CT: a serial approach *Med. Phys.* **30** 1188–97
[18] Teramoto A and Fujita H 2013 Fast lung nodule detection in chest CT images using cylindrical nodule-enhancement filter *Int. J. Comput. Assist. Radiol. Surg.* **8** 193–205
[19] Retico A, Delogu P, Fantacci M E, Gori I and Martinez A P 2008 Lung nodule detection in low-dose and thin-slice computed tomography *Comput. Biol. Med.* **38** 525–34
[20] Lin J S, Lo S C, Hasegawa A, Freedman M T and Mun S K 1996 Reduction of false positives in lung nodule detection using a two-level neural classification *IEEE Trans. Med. Imaging* **15** 206–17
[21] Wiemker R, Rogalla P, Zwartkruis A and Blaffert T 2002 Computer-aided lung nodule detection on high-resolution CT data *Medical Imaging 2002: Image Processing* vol 4684 (Bellingham, WA: Int. Society for Optics and Photonics) pp 677–88
[22] Tajbakhsh N and Suzuki K 2017 Comparing two classes of end-to-end machine-learning models in lung nodule detection and classification: MTANNs vs. CNNs *Pattern Recognit.* **63** 476–86
[23] Anirudh R, Thiagarajan J J, Bremer T and Kim H 2016 Lung nodule detection using 3D convolutional neural networks trained on weakly labeled data *Medical Imaging 2016: Computer-Aided Diagnosis* vol 9785 978532 (Bellingham, WA: Int. Society for Optics and Photonics)
[24] Ko J P, Rusinek H, Naidich D P, McGuinness G, Rubinowitz A N, Leitman B S and Martino J M 2003 Wavelet compression of low-dose chest CT data: effect on lung nodule detection *Radiology* **228** 70–5
[25] Ali I, Hart G R, Gunabushanam G, Liang Y, Muhammad W, Nartowt B, Kane M, Ma X and Deng J 2018 Lung nodule detection via deep reinforcement learning *Front. Oncol.* **8** 108
[26] Zhang G, Jiang S, Yang Z, Gong L, Ma X, Zhou Z, Bao C and Liu Q 2018 Automatic nodule detection for lung cancer in CT images: a review *Comput. Biol. Med.* **103** 287–300
[27] Lee S L, Kouzani A Z and Hu E J 2012 Automated detection of lung nodules in computed tomography images: a review *Mach. Vis. Appl.* **23** 151–63

[28] Abdeltawab H, Khalifa F, Taher F, Alghamdi N S, Ghazal M, Beache G, Mohamed T, Keynton R and El-Baz A 2020 A deep learning-based approach for automatic segmentation and quantification of the left ventricle from cardiac cine MR images *Comput. Med. Imaging Graph.* 101717

[29] Dekhil O, Naglah A, Shaban M, Ghazal M, Taher F and Elbaz A 2019 Deep learning based method for computer aided diagnosis of diabetic retinopathy *2019 IEEE Int. Conf. on Imaging Systems and Techniques (IST)* (Piscataway, NJ: IEEE) pp 1–4

[30] Mesbah S, Shalaby A M, Stills S, Soliman A, Willhite A, Harkema S J, Rejc E and El-Baz A S 2019 Correction: Novel stochastic framework for automatic segmentation of human thigh MRI volumes and its applications in spinal cord injured individuals *PLoS One* **14** e0219810

[31] Shaffie A, Soliman A, Mahmoud A, Ghazal M, Hajjdiab H, Keynton R, Giridharan G, Elmaghraby A, Suri J S and El-Baz A 2019 Lung nodule classification based on the integration of a higher-order Markov-Gibbs random field appearance model and geometric features *Lung Imaging and CADx.* 203

[32] Shaffie A, Soliman A, Khalifeh H A, Taher F, Ghazal M, Dunlap N, Elmaghraby A, Keynton R and El-Baz A 2019 A new system for lung cancer diagnosis based on the integration of global and local CT features *2019 IEEE Int. Conf. on Imaging Systems and Techniques (IST)* (Piscataway, NJ: IEEE) pp 1–6

[33] Shaffie A, Soliman A, Khalifeh H A, Ghazal M, Taher F, Keynton R, Elmaghraby A and El-Baz A 2018 On the integration of CT-derived features for accurate detection of lung cancer *2018 IEEE Int. Symp. on Signal Processing and Information Technology (ISSPIT)* (Piscataway, NJ: IEEE) pp 435–40

[34] Soliman A, Khalifa F, Elnakib A, Abou El-Ghar M, Dunlap N, Wang B, Gimel'farb G, Keynton R and El-Baz A 2016 Accurate lungs segmentation on CT chest images by adaptive appearance-guided shape modeling *IEEE Trans. Med. Imaging* **36** 263–76

[35] Kadry S ed. 2012 Diagnostics and prognostics of engineering systems: methods and techniques: methods and techniques *IGI Global*

[36] Roufayel R and Kadry S 2017 Expression of miR-23a by apoptotic regulators in human cancer: a review *Cancer Biol. Therapy.* **18** 269–76

[37] Ahilan A *et al* 2019 Segmentation by fractional order darwinian particle swarm optimization based multilevel thresholding and improved lossless prediction based compression algorithm for medical images *IEEE Access* **7** 89570–80

[38] Soliman A *et al* 2019 Early assessment of radiation-induced lung injury *Lung Imaging and CADx* 349–70 (Boca Raton, FL: CRC Press)

[39] Ghazal M, Ali S, AlKhodari M and El-Baz A 2019 An unsupervised parametric mixture model for automatic three-dimensional lung segmentation *Lung Imaging and CADx* 307–28 (Boca Raton, FL: CRC Press)

[40] Kadry S and Al-Taie M Z 2014 *Social Network Analysis: An Introduction with an Extensive Implementation to a Large-Scale Online Network Using Pajek* (Bentham Science Publishers)

[41] Bakiya A, Kamalanand K, Rajinikanth V, Nayak R S and Kadry S 2020 Deep neural network assisted diagnosis of time-frequency transformed electromyograms *Multimedia Tools Appl.* **79** 11051–67

[42] Rajinikanth V, Raja N S and Satapathy S C 2016 Robust color image multi-thresholding using between-class variance and cuckoo search algorithm *InInformation Systems Design and Intelligent Applications* (New Delhi: Springer) pp 379–86 https://doi.org/10.1007/978-81-322-2755-7_40

[43] Wang Y, Shi F, Cao L, Dey N, Wu Q, Ashour A S, Sherratt R S, Rajinikanth V and Wu L 2019 Morphological segmentation analysis and texture-based support vector machines classification on mice liver fibrosis microscopic images *Curr. Bioinform.* **14** 282–94

[44] Shree T V, Revanth K, Raja N S and Rajinikanth V 2018 A hybrid image processing approach to examine abnormality in retinal optic disc *Procedia Comput. Sci.* **125** 157–64

[45] Satapathy S C and Rajinikanth V 2018 Jaya algorithm guided procedure to segment tumor from brain MRI *J. Optim.* **2018** 3738049

[46] Rajinikanth V, Satapathy S C, Dey N, Fernandes S L and Manic K S Skin melanoma assessment using Kapur's entropy and level set—a study with bat algorithm *Smart Innov. Syst. Technol.* **104** 193–202

[47] Rajinikanth V, Joseph Raj A N, Thanaraj K P and Naik G R 2020 A customized VGG19 network with concatenation of deep and handcrafted features for brain tumor detection *Appl. Sci.* **10** 3429

[48] Bhandary A, Prabhu G A, Rajinikanth V, Thanaraj K P, Satapathy S C, Robbins D E, Shasky C, Zhang Y D, Tavares J M and Raja N S 2020 Deep-learning framework to detect lung abnormality–A study with chest x-ray and lung CT scan images *Pattern Recognit. Lett.* **129** 271–8

[49] Pugalenthi R, Rajakumar M P, Ramya J and Rajinikanth V 2019 Evaluation and classification of the brain tumor MRI using machine learning technique *J. Control Eng. Appl. Inform.* **21** 12–21 https://wiki.cancerimagingarchive.net/display/Public/RIDER+Lung+CT

[50] Zhao B, Schwartz L H and Kris M G 2015 Data from RIDER_Lung CT *Cancer Imag. Archive.*

[51] Zhao B, James L P, Moskowitz C S, Guo P, Ginsberg M S, Lefkowitz R A, Qin Y, Riely G J, Kris M G and Schwartz L H 2009 Evaluating variability in tumor measurements from same-day repeat CT scans of patients with non–small cell lung cancer 1 *Radiology. Radiological Society of North America (RSNA).*

[52] Clark K *et al* 2013 The Cancer Imaging Archive (TCIA): maintaining and operating a public information repository *J. Digital Imaging* **26** 1045–57

[53] Kalpathy-Cramer J *et al* 2016 Radiomics of lung nodules: a multi-institutional study of robustness and agreement of quantitative imaging features *Tomography* **2** 430–7

[54] http://itksnap.org/pmwiki/pmwiki.php

[55] Yushkevich P A, Piven J, Hazlett H C, Smith R G, Ho S, Gee J C and Gerig G 2006 User-guided 3D active contour segmentation of anatomical structures: Significantly improved efficiency and reliability *Neuroimage* **31** 1116–28

[56] Fernandes S L, Tanik U J, Rajinikanth V and Karthik K A 2020 A reliable framework for accurate brain image examination and treatment planning based on early diagnosis support for clinicians *Neural Comput. Appl.* **32** 15897–908

[57] Dey N, Rajinikanth V, Shi F, Tavares J M, Moraru L, Karthik K A, Lin H, Kamalanand K and Emmanuel C 2019 Social-group-optimization based tumor evaluation tool for clinical brain MRI of Flair/diffusion-weighted modality *Biocybern. Biomed. Eng.* **39** 843–56

[58] Rajinikanth V, Dey N, Raj A N, Hassanien A E, Santosh K C and Raja N 2020 Harmony-search and otsu based system for coronavirus disease (COVID-19) detection using lung CT scan images. arXiv preprint arXiv:2004.03431.

[59] Kadry S, Rajinikanth V, Rho S, Raja N S, Rao V S and Thanaraj K P 2020 Development of a machine-learning system to classify lung CT scan images into normal/COVID-19 class. arXiv preprint arXiv:2004.13122.

[60] Rajinikanth V, Kadry S, Thanaraj K P, Kamalanand K and Seo S 2020 Firefly-algorithm supported scheme to detect COVID-19 lesion in lung CT scan images using Shannon entropy and Markov-random-field. arXiv preprint arXiv:2004.09239.
[61] Li C, Xu C, Gui C and Fox M D 2010 Distance regularized level set evolution and its application to image segmentation *IEEE Trans. Image Process.* **19** 3243–54
[62] Rajinikanth V, Fernandes S L, Bhushan B and Sunder N R 2018 Segmentation and analysis of brain tumor using Tsallis entropy and regularised level set *Proc. of 2nd Int. Conf. on Micro-Electronics, Electromagnetics and Telecommunications* (Singapore: Springer) pp 313–21 https://doi.org/10.1007/978–981–10–4280–5_33
[63] Yang X and Jiang X 2020 A hybrid active contour model based on new edge-stop functions for image segmentation *Int. J. Ambient Comput. Intell. (IJACI).* **11** 87–98
[64] Mohanaiah P, Sathyanarayana P and GuruKumar L 2013 Image texture feature extraction using GLCM approach *Int. J. Sci. Res. Publ.* **3** 1
[65] Xian G M 2010 An identification method of malignant and benign liver tumors from ultrasonography based on GLCM texture features and fuzzy SVM *Expert Syst. Appl.* **37** 6737–41
[66] Otiniano-Rodrıguez K C, Cámara-Chávez G and Menotti D 2012 Hu and Zernike moments for sign language recognition *Proc. of Int. Conf. on Image Processing, Computer Vision, and Pattern Recognition* 1–5
[67] Conseil S, Bourennane S and Martin L 2007 Comparison of Fourier descriptors and Hu moments for hand posture recognition *2007 15th European Signal Processing Conf.* (Piscataway, NJ: IEEE) pp 1960–4
[68] Gudigar A *et al* 2019 Global weighted LBP based entropy features for the assessment of pulmonary hypertension *Pattern Recognit. Lett.* **125** 35–41
[69] Bellamkonda S and Gopalan N P 2020 An enhanced facial expression recognition model using local feature fusion of Gabor wavelets and local directionality patterns *Int. J. Ambient Comput. Intell. (IJACI).* **11** 48–70
[70] Angadi S and Nandyal S 2020 Human identification system based on spatial and temporal features in the video surveillance system *Int. J. Ambient Comput. Intell. (IJACI).* **11** 1–21
[71] Roopini I T, Vasanthi M, Rajinikanth V, Rekha M and Sangeetha M 2018 Segmentation of tumor from brain MRI using fuzzy entropy and distance regularised level set *Computational Signal Processing and Analysis* (Singapore: Springer) pp 297–304 https://doi.org/10.1007/978–981-10–8354-9_27
[72] Jahmunah V, Oh S L, Rajinikanth V, Ciaccio E J, Cheong K H, Arunkumar N and Acharya U R 2019 Automated detection of schizophrenia using nonlinear signal processing methods *Artif. Intell. Med.* **100** 101698
[73] Acharya U R, Fernandes S L, WeiKoh J E, Ciaccio E J, Fabell M K, Tanik U J, Rajinikanth V and Yeong C H 2019 Automated detection of Alzheimer's disease using brain MRI images–a study with various feature extraction techniques *J. Med. Syst.* **43** 302
[74] Satapathy S and Naik A 2016 Social group optimization (SGO): a new population evolutionary optimization technique *Complex Intell. Syst.* **2** 173–203
[75] Dey N, Rajinikanth V, Ashour A S and Tavares J M Social group optimization supported segmentation and evaluation of skin melanoma images *Symmetry* **10** 51
[76] Lu D and Weng Q 2007 A survey of image classification methods and techniques for improving classification performance *Int. J. Remote Sens.* **28** 823–70
[77] Friedl M A and Brodley C E 1997 Decision tree classification of land cover from remotely sensed data *Remote Sens. Environ.* **61** 399–409

[78] Pal M 2005 Random forest classifier for remote sensing classification *Int. J. Remote Sens.* **26** 217–22

[79] Svetnik V, Liaw A, Tong C, Culberson J C, Sheridan R P and Feuston B P 2003 Random forest: a classification and regression tool for compound classification and QSAR modeling *J. Chem. Inf. Comput. Sci.* **43** 1947–58

[80] Peterson L E 2009 K-nearest neighbor *Scholarpedia.* **4** 1883

[81] Denoeux T 2008 A k-nearest neighbor classification rule based on Dempster-Shafer theory *Classic Works of the Dempster-Shafer Theory of Belief Functions* (Berlin: Springer) pp 737–60

[82] Han S, Qubo C and Meng H 2012 Parameter selection in SVM with RBF kernel function *World Automation Congress 2012* (Piscataway, NJ: IEEE) pp 1–4

[83] Kuo B C, Ho H H, Li C H, Hung C C and Taur J S 2013 A kernel-based feature selection method for SVM with RBF kernel for hyperspectral image classification *IEEE J. Sel. Topics Appl. Earth Obs. Remote Sens.* **7** 317–26

IOP Publishing

Detection Systems in Lung Cancer and Imaging, Volume 1

Ayman El-Baz and Jasjit S Suri

Chapter 4

Computer-aided lung cancer screening in computed tomography: state-of the-art and future perspectives

João Pedrosa, Guilherme Aresta and Carlos Ferreira

4.1 Introduction

The diagnosis and follow-up of lung cancer can be performed using several non-invasive imaging procedures, including chest radiography, magnetic resonance imaging (MRI), computed tomography (CT), and positron emission tomography (PET-CT). From these, however, CT is the primary choice due to the simplicity of the procedure and the excellent spatial resolution and contrast of the resulting images [1, 2]. While the use of ionizing radiation is a disadvantage of this technique, it has been determined that low-dose CT for lung cancer screening can be performed with overall average effective doses as low as 2 mSv [3].

In CT, image acquisition is performed using X-photons. The radiation is emitted and measured after travelling through the body and a 3D image is obtained by repeating this measurement along the patient's body. In the end, each voxel of the scan has a corresponding attenuation value (or tissue density value) proportional to the amount of energy that was dispersed during the radiation travel. These values can be standardized via the reference attenuation value of water, resulting in the standard Hounsfield Unit (HU) scale [4] (figure 4.1). This scale enables fast visualization of tissues of different densities during scan assessment. Namely, the majority of the structures of the lung are visible on the HU range [−600, 1000].

Because of the 3D nature of CT, radiologists can never analyze the entire scan at the same time. Commonly, the three major anatomic planes (sagittal, coronal, and transverse) are visualized. Figure 4.2 shows an example of a CT transverse (or axial) slice where the major structures of the lung are visible. For instance, it is noticeable that the lung parenchyma, mainly composed of air, has high contrast with structures of increased density, such as blood vessels and bones. Note that, depending on the acquisition resolution, some structures may be affected by image reconstruction

doi:10.1088/978-0-7503-3355-9ch4

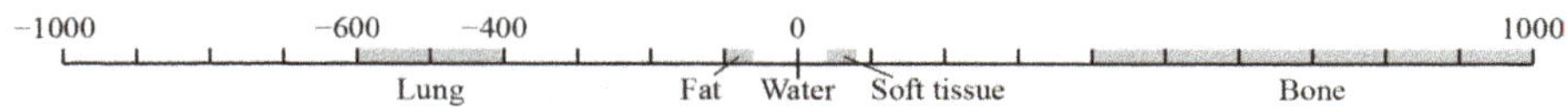

Figure 4.1. Standard Hounsfield Unit scale and intensity ranges of anatomic structures.

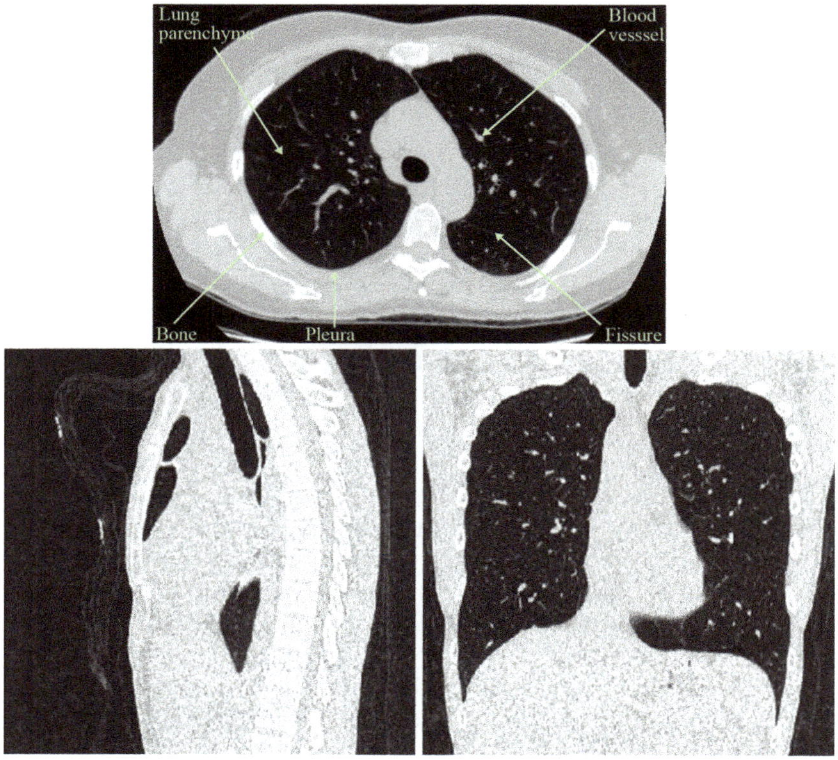

Figure 4.2. Example axial slices of a low dose CT scan and major structures (top row) and coronal (bottom left) and sagital (bottom right) slices.

artifacts. Namely, large values of slice thickness introduce the known partial-volume effect, where the increase in the voxel volume results in higher density averaging and thus blurriness. In order to avoid this hindering effect, most scans have a slice thickness around 1.5 mm or less.

During analysis of a chest CT image, radiologists visually search for relevant indicators of pathology. In the specific case of lung cancer, pulmonary nodules, abnormal sphere-like structures that appear in the lung parenchyma, are the main indicators of the pathology. Usually, this search is done by following either a scanning or drilling search strategy. In scanning, a radiologist searches for nodules on an entire slice before moving to the next, thus having to recur to techniques such as maximum intensity projection (MIP) to assess depth information. Alternatively, in drilling the radiologist focusses on a single quadrant of the volume at a time, scrolling through all slices of the scan to account for 3D information [5, 6].

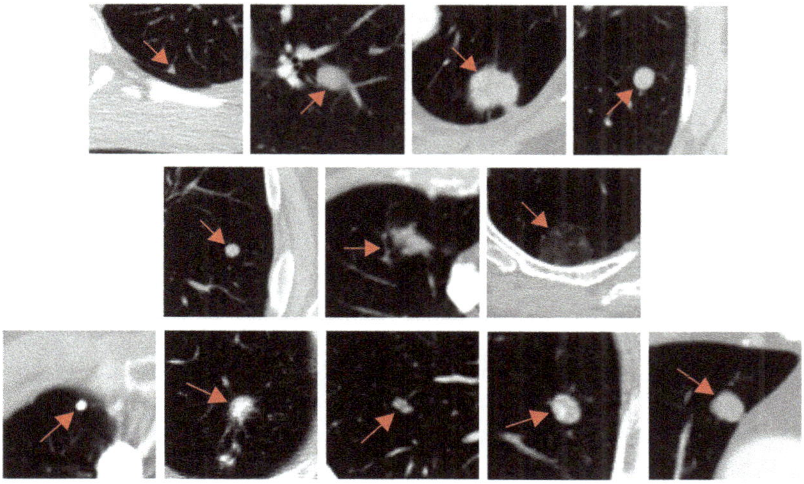

Figure 4.3. Nodule examples in terms of location (first row), texture (second row) and calcification (third row). Central axial slice of each nodule is shown, where red arrows indicates the nodule. First row (from left to right): peri-fissural, juxta-vascular, juxta-pleural and isolated nodule. Second row (from left to right): solid, sub-solid and non-solid nodules. Third row (from left to right): complete, central, popcorn, non-central and absent calcification.

Nevertheless, it is known that radiologists fail at nodule detection and this can happen due to either fixation or recognition errors [7]. Fixation errors, mostly related to stress and fatigue, occur when the expert does not focus on a given region for a long enough period of time to identify potential nodule candidates. On the other hand, recognition errors result from failing to correctly identify a found abnormality as a nodule and depends mostly on the experience of the radiologist [8].

Lung nodules present a wide range of shapes, locations, sizes and appearance. In terms of location, nodules can be classified as peri-fissural, juxta-vascular, juxta-pleural (when attached to a fissure, a blood vessel or the pleura, respectively) or isolated [9]. In terms of texture, nodules are commonly classified as solid, sub-solid or non-solid [10]. Solid nodules have well-defined borders and high contrast with the lung parenchyma, thus usually being the easiest to identify. Non-solid nodules, also known as ground-glass opacities (GGO), have a diffused distribution over the parenchyma, commonly appearing as cloudy structures. Because of this, they present low contrast with the lung parenchyma and their shape is difficult to define properly. Finally, sub-solid nodules combine characteristics of both solid and non-solid abnormalities, with a solid nucleus and diffused boundaries. The presence of calcification is also commonly described as it is a reliable indicator of a benign nodule [11]. Further classification into specific calcification patterns (complete, central, popcorn, non-central or other) is also fairly common. Examples of the discussed nodule types are shown in figure 4.3. Additionally, other features have been used for nodule description and/or classification, namely nodule sphericity, nodule margin (how well-circumscribed is the nodule), the presence of lobulations and spiculations, the internal structure of the nodule—whether it is composed of soft tissue or contains fluid, fat, or air components—and the subtlety of the nodule in the CT image. Nodule size (and growth) is also an important characteristic and an indicator of malignancy and, thus, determinant in patient follow-up. Finally, malignancy of a nodule can also be considered a descriptive feature. Nevertheless, such a description is often subjective and relates to a combination of multiple more low-level features such as the presence of calcifications, nodule texture, spiculations, etc which give an indication of the level of malignancy of a nodule.

As such, the analysis of a chest CT scan for the purposes of lung cancer screening/management is a three-step process: first, radiologists must search the 3D image for the presence of pulmonary nodules; second, each nodule must be characterized in terms of dimension, texture or other features; and third, a patient diagnosis or follow-up is determined based on all findings. This third and final step usually follows well-defined criteria such as the Lung-RADS [12] criterion, which was specifically designed for a screening scenario, the Fleischner guidelines [13] which are designed for incidental nodule findings and the British Thoracic Society (BTS) guidelines [14] which can be used for either screening or incidental findings. Lung-RADS takes the degree of calcification, texture, nodule diameter, and solid diameter size of sub-solid nodules into account for follow-up recommendation. Each nodule is assessed, and patient follow-up is determined according to the 'highest ranking' nodule. Fleischner guidelines, on the other hand are computed at a patient level and depend on the number of nodules found, their sizes (diameter or volume) and texture, as well as patient risk determined by older age, heavy smoking, irregular or spiculated nodule margins and upper lobe location. In both Lung-RADS and Fleischner guidelines, four follow-up recommendations are possible: (1) no follow-up/CT at 12 months; (2) CT at 6 months; (3) CT at 3 months; (4) PET-CT, CT with contrast or biopsy. The BTS guidelines have the particularity of considering a longitudinal assessment for patient management. Based on the largest nodule in a given patient, the BTS guidelines take into account nodule size, growth (namely volume doubling time), texture, spiculation, and nodule location, as well as patient demographics and history. Besides follow-up recommendations similar to Lung-RADS and Fleischner guidelines (discharge, CT at 3 months, 1 year or 2 years), BTS includes specific outputs for imaging and therapeutic interventions. For more detailed information on the specific criteria of Lung-RADS, Fleischner and BTS guidelines, the reader is referred to the original guidelines [12–14].

Despite the established criteria, lung cancer screening in CT is a non-trivial task. The sheer size and dimensionality of the CT image, together with the wide range of nodule locations, textures and shapes makes both lung nodule detection and characterization an experience-dependent and subjective task [13]. CT scans are inherently complex to analyze due to their three-dimensionality and large range of intensities to explore, making the process tiresome and consequently prone to error. The associated fatigue, limitations of the human visual system and stress often coupled with lack of experience severely affect nodule detection performance [15]. Furthermore, small nodules can easily be confused with other lesions such as scars, which rarely have diagnosis relevance. Also, when attached to other structures, such as vessels or the pleura, nodules can be hidden and/or have altered shapes. Even after a correct nodule identification, their characterization is also highly subjective and prone to error. Ideally, to measure a nodule's volume, radiologists would identify all voxels that belong to the nodule and then compute the corresponding volume. However, due to the large amount of work this approach requires, nodular volume is usually approximated by measuring the major axes of the abnormality. These approximations introduce errors on the characterization of the nodules, which can later affect patient follow-up. Furthermore, the characterization of other nodule features such as texture is highly dependent on reader experience and can vary widely between centers.

Given the above reasons and in order to improve radiologist's lung cancer detection performance, reading of each CT by two radiologists has been proposed. Double reading has been shown to increase the average sensitivity of readers to nodule detection [16]—64% versus 79% when comparing single to double reading—and to lead to 19% more reported nodules (though with no improvement to overall lung cancer detection performance) [17]. Nevertheless, such a double reading comes at a significant cost, both in economic terms and in human resources, placing a significant burden on radiologists. As such, automatic second-opinion systems, which would perform automatic nodule detection and characterization and propose these findings to a radiologist, have been proposed as a viable alternative to double reading. These systems, also known as computer-aided diagnosis (CAD) systems, could thus promote a more dedicated analysis of the most important aspects/locations of the 3D CT image, reduce the workload of radiologists and, ultimately, increase lung cancer detection performance.

4.1.1 Computer-aided lung cancer screening

The impact of lung cancer in modern society has motivated the scientific community to develop automatic lung cancer screening algorithms on CT. Given the role of CT in lung cancer screening and the information required for patient diagnosis and follow-up, three main tasks have been addressed in the state-of-the-art: lung nodule detection, lung nodule segmentation and lung nodule feature characterization. Figure 4.4 shows the number of published papers on each of these tasks over the last 15 years, according to PubMeD [18]. First, the abstracts and titles of all papers that matched the search terms lung nodule detection, pulmonary nodule detection, lung nodule segmentation, pulmonary nodule segmentation, lung nodule characterization and pulmonary nodule characterization were retrieved. All duplicates were removed and only the hits that contained the words CT or tomography were kept. This pool was further filtered for the presence of CAD, computer-aided and automatic (writing variations were considered). Detection, segmentation and characterization papers were then classified according to the presence of the words detection, segmentation and characterization, respectively. Deep learning papers were counted by assessing the presence of the expressions artificial intelligence, deep learning, convolutional neural network and CNN (writing variations were considered).

Lung nodule detection has been the most explored task, accumulating the highest number of published works, and this trend continues to this day. This is likely due to

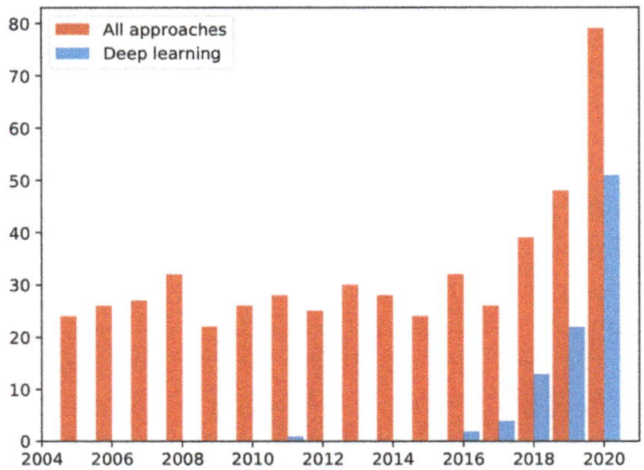

(a) Lung nodule detection.

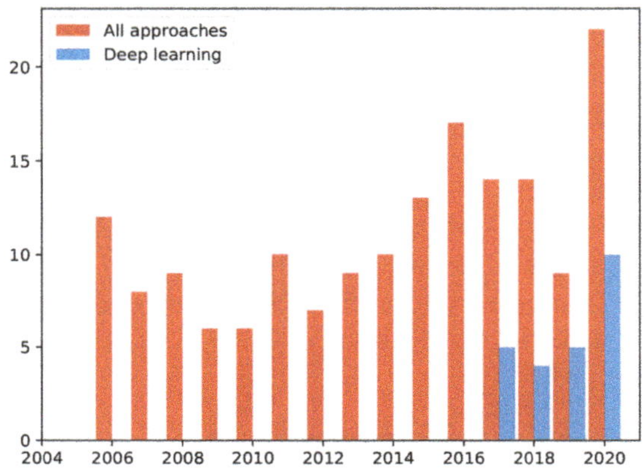

(b) Lung nodule segmentation.

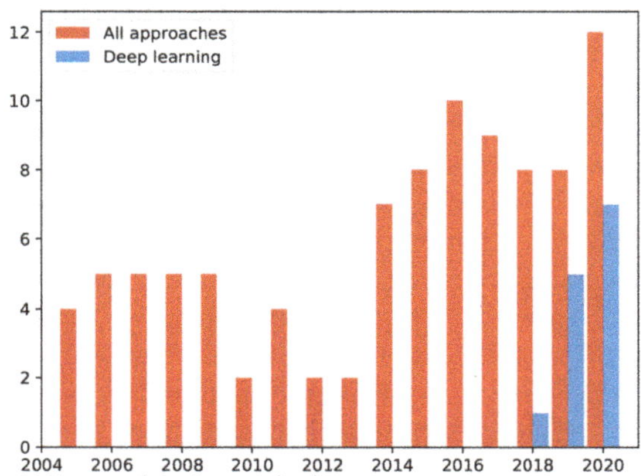

(c) Lung nodule characterization.

Figure 4.4. Number of published scientific papers on lung nodule detection and segmentation since 2005 up to November 2020. Information extracted from PubMed. Number of published scientific papers on lung nodule detection, segmentation and characterization since 2005 up to January 2021 (excluding). Information extracted from PubMed [18].

the fact that, historically, nodule detection has been perceived as the task where an automatic system could have the most impact due to high burden on radiologists and perception error rates. The presence of deep learning approaches on the topic of automatic lung cancer screening has been increasing over the past five years. In fact, in 2020, deep learning has been used on over 50% of the lung cancer detection, segmentation and characterization CAD literature. This increase is most likely related to a combination of deep learning being a trending topic in the computer vision field, the increase of computation power/cost ratio of systems, and the appearance of public datasets and challenges related to the topic (cf section 4.6). Namely, events such as the LUNA16 [19], DSB17 [20] and LNDb [21] challenges, have promoted the progression of novel techniques on the automatic lung cancer screening field.

4.2 Computer-aided lung nodule detection

Automatic lung nodule detection corresponds to the identification of locations on the CT scan where a nodule likely exists. These findings can then be either directly used for diagnosis or first validated by a medical expert. The standard CAD pipeline for nodule detection in CT images is typically composed of two main blocks: (1) initial candidate detection and (2) false positive (FP) reduction, as shown in figure 4.5.

The objective of the initial candidate step is to maximize the number of detected true positive (TP) nodules. However, because lung nodules present a high variety of shapes, sizes and locations, as well as different textures and contrast with the lung parenchyma, this detection step is highly complex. In order to maximize the detection sensitivity, a high number of FPs is detected. These false detections generate the necessity of a second step referred as the FP reduction step. On this stage, features are collected from the candidates and then used for reducing the number of FPs via classification. Ideally, this reduction step would not affect the

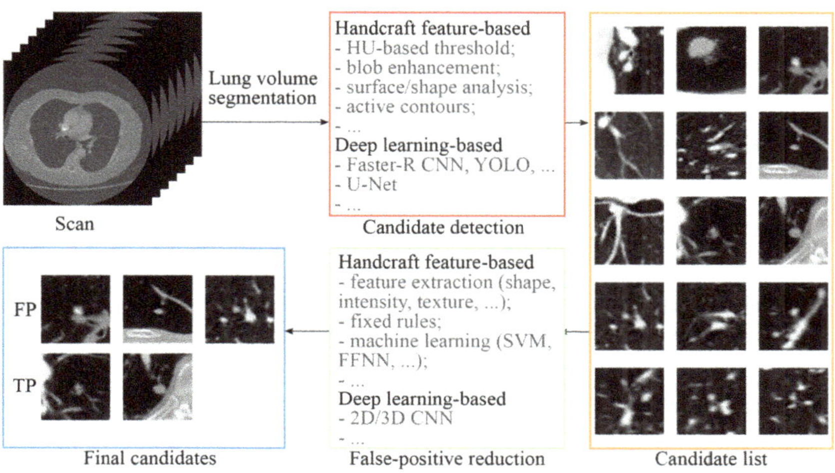

Figure 4.5. Standard lung nodule detection pipeline.

initial candidate sensitivity. In practice, however, CAD detection systems trade-off detection sensitivity and the number of FPs.

A summary of the performance of the methods detailed in this section is available in table 4.1. Most studies report performance in terms of sensitivity (ratio between TPs and total number of nodules) at a given (or several) number of FPs per CT scan. Note that different authors report sensitivity at different FP/scan levels and at different agreement levels (AL) (the number of radiologists that reported a given nodule upon reading the CT), which hinders direct comparisons between methods. Nevertheless, an increasing trend in the reported detection performance (both in terms of higher sensitivity and lower number of FPs per scan) can be seen in table 4.1, specifically when comparing non-deep learning and deep learning approaches, as a result of the increase of interest on the field and the advances in computational power.

Non-deep learning approaches for lung nodule detection are mostly based on field knowledge and involve using and designing features that discriminate lung nodules from other structures present on CT scans. Developing these kinds of approaches require handling samples with large amounts of data due to the volumetric nature of CT scans. Consequently, methods usually consider simpler operations, such as thresholding, while making use of medical and imaging knowledge to detect candidates. For instance, taking advantage of the standard HU and tissue density difference of the parenchyma and other structures, a fixed threshold (e.g., −700 HU) provides a proper detection baseline [23, 37, 39, 50]. Alternatively, this threshold value can be determined based on the histogram of the lung volume using, for instance, a mixture of Gaussians, quality threshold or vector quantization [30, 35, 38, 51]. To solve the issue of multiple nodule textures, detection via threshold can be extended to several HU values [36, 40], resulting in higher sensitivity at the cost of an increased number of FP detections.

Other methods explore the natural sphericity of lung nodules during candidate search. Unlike intensity-based methods, these approaches can allow a better integration of 3D information. For instance, some works detect nodules by searching for regions with high density of overlapping surface normals [26, 28]. These approaches, however, are highly sensitive to image and motion noise and so less strict shape-based search procedures are more common. Namely, Hessian-based approaches allow sphere-like structures to be enhanced in detriment of vessel-like structures without relying too heavily on border definition [22, 25, 27, 52]. The shape-index and curvedness metrics have been commonly applied for this purpose.

The discussed candidate detection systems produce either a centroid or a rough segmentation of the structure. However, under/poor segmentation can often hinder the FP reduction step. As a consequence, it is common to include candidate segmentation improvement as a step within nodule detection. To do so, some authors use morphological operations to detach nodules from high intensity structures such as vessels and the pleura [23, 37, 40, 50]. Other methodologies consider intensity region growing for candidate refinement [25, 34, 35, 39, 40]. Alternatively, active contours can also be used for candidate boundary refinement [32, 42, 53].

Table 4.1. Performance of selected automatic lung nodule detection algorithms. Method: whether the nodule candidate detection method is 2D, 2.5D or 3D as well as DL when deep learning techniques are used. Performance: sensitivity/[FP/scan] (number of scans used for evaluation).

Author	Method	Dataset	Performance	Comments
Dehmeshki *et al* 2007 [22]	3D	Private	0.9/15 (70)	
Enquobahrie *et al* 2007 [23]	3D	Private	0.94/7.1 (250)0.91/6.9 (250)	Isolated nodules;$r>2$ mm
Hirose *et al* 2008 [24]	3D	Private	0.71/1.0 (21)	
Li *et al* 2008 [25]	3D	Private	0.75/1.6 (117)	
Golosio *et al* 2009 [26]	3D	LIDC	0.79/4 (83)	AL 4
Murphy *et al* 2009 [27]	3D	NELSON	0.8/4.2 (813)	
Retico 2009 *et al* [28]	3D	Private	0.44/1 (42)	Juxta-pleural
Súarez-Cuenca *et al* 2009 [29]	3D	Private	0.8/7.7 (22)	
da Silva Sousa *et al* 2010 [30]	3D	Private	0.85/0.4 (33)	
Tan *et al* 2011 [31]	3D	LIDC-IDRI	0.88/4 (125)	
Cascio *et al* 2012 [32]	3D	LIDC	0.88/2.5 (84)	
Teramoto *et al* 2013 [33]	3D	LIDC	0.8/4.2 (84)	$r>2.5$ mm
Brown *et al* 2014 [34]	3D	LIDC-IDRI	0.79/1 (108)	AL $\geqslant 3$
de Carvalho Filho *et al* 2014 [35]	2D	LIDC-IDRI	0.86/1.8 (28)	Isolated nodules
Choi *et al* 2014 [36]	3D	LIDC-IDRI	0.98/6.8 (84)	
Jacobs *et al* 2014 [37]	3D	NELSON	0.8/1 (109)	Sub-solid
Santos *et al* 2014 [38]	3D	LIDC-IDRI	0.91/1.2 (28)	
Lopez Torres *et al* 2015 [39]	3D	LIDC-IDRI	0.7/8 (899)0.8/8 (899)	
Setio *et al* 2015 [40]	3D	LIDC-IDRI	0.94/1 (888)	Solid $r>5$ mm
Van Ginneken *et al* 2015 [41]	2.5D-DL[a]	LUNA16	0.73/1 (865)	
Wang *ct al* 2015 [42]	3D	LIDC-IDRI	0.88/4 (108)	
Setio *et al* 2016 [43]	2.5D-DL[a]	LUNA16	0.85/1 (888)	
Ding *et al* 2017 [44]	2.5D-DL	LUNA16	0.92/1 (888)	
Dou *et al* 2016 [45]	3D-DL[a]	LUNA16	0.85/1 (888)	
Aresta *et al* 2018 [46]	2.5D-DL	LUNA16	0.93/0.25 (88)	$r \geqslant 2$ mm
Zheng *et al* 2020 [47]	2.5D-DL	LUNA16	0.93/1 (888)	
Kaluva *et al* 2020 [48]	3D-DL	LNDb	0.71 (58)	AL $\geqslant 2$
Katz *et al* 2020 [49]	3D-DL	LNDb	0.58/1 (58)	AL $\geqslant 2$

[a] FP reduction only

The complexity of the chest CT scans leads to a high number of FP detections during the initial candidate detection. These correspond mainly to blood vessels (which in the axial plane may appear as circular structures) as well as other abnormalities, such as scars. In fact, it is common to achieve a 1:10 or higher ratio between TP and FP detections. As a result, a proper FP reduction step is critical for CAD performance.

Historically, FP reduction has shifted from simple fixed rule-based candidate filtering to handcraft feature engineering. More recently, the increase on computational (namely graphical) power has enabled the use of deep learning methods to do this task, significantly reducing the need for manual feature design. Specifically, fixed rules are usually shape-related, thus complementing the intensity-based detection schemes. Since the main objective is to distinguish vessels from nodules, it is common to filter candidates using metrics such as elongation, volume and sphericity [22, 23]. Nevertheless, other works also consider intensity, gradient, Hessian features and even location for FP reduction [24, 25, 29].

Using fixed rules is only useful for coarse candidate reduction, as it is difficult to represent nodules with such few metrics. Furthermore, there is a high risk of overfit, especially with a small number of nodules. Because of this, the majority of the approaches use instead a two-step FP reduction. First, fixed rules are used for removing obvious FPs, which usually correspond to large vessels or poorly segmented portions of the lung volume. The remaining candidates are then used for training single or multiple classifiers. Here, most of the approaches opt for either support-vector machine or feed-forward neural network for the refined candidate reduction. Consequently, proper feature design is a key element of the system's performance. With that in mind, the majority of the studies aim at replicating visual features that physicians observe during the screening process. For instance, features related with shape, intensity, texture and gradient (namely border information) are commonly used [31, 33, 37, 40, 54]. Besides these, location and Hessian features are also considered, since they provide further insight on the context and shape of the nodules. Likewise, Hessian features can be used for deriving surface normal descriptors, which help to better characterize and distinguish between spheres, cylinders and planes [36]. The number and type of features have a high influence on the performance of the system, and most of the published research aims at creating, selecting and refining these feature sets. Consequently, some works focus at automatizing the optimization process. For that purpose, multi-kernel learning can be used [55]. In this kind of scheme, the objective is to weight the contribution of different classification kernels (e.g., linear and quadratic in support-vector machines) and thus improve the overall classification result.

Despite the relative success of field knowledge-based methods for the complex task of lung nodule detection in CT images, the performance of CAD systems using non-deep learning schemes is often too low for proper clinical application. Recently, the advances on computational power have enabled the application of deep learning approaches for computer vision and medical imaging problems. This kind of approach significantly reduces the need for field knowledge by learning a multi-step mapping from the raw input to an easy to solve feature space. CNNs have, in fact, been used successfully for both lung nodule initial candidate detection and FP reduction and feature prominently on the leaderboards of recent challenges such as LUNA16 and LNDb. Indeed, the lack of field knowledge of CNNs eases the application of more generic schemes for initial candidate detection. On the other hand, these types of approach require large amounts of data to train and avoid overfit and their training is computationally heavy. Computational requirements are especially high when dealing with 3D data, such as CT scans, and thus methods often tend to use 2D representations of the scans for nodule detection. For instance, the U-Net [56] has been used with some degree of success for initial candidate detection [19]. Specifically, one of the participants of the LUNA16 challenge, ZNET, trained a U-net on axial slices containing nodules. Nodule candidates were then predicted scan-wise by inferring on all slices in a sliding fashion, resulting in a 3D probability map. After thresholding and morphological erosion, each connected component was considered as a possible nodule. As previously mentioned, this results in a high number of candidates, requiring *a posterior* FP reduction step. However, the complexity of chest CT images and the lack of proper 3D context due to limitations in computational power hindered the performance of the model, which resulted in little increase in performance when compared to handcrafted feature-based methods.

Because of this, other authors have applied dedicated object detection networks, such as the Faster R-CNN [57], achieving high performance on candidate detection [44] by assessing axial slices in a depth-wise sliding fashion. The outline of the detection model is depicted in figure 4.6. First, a neural network performs near pixel-wise feature extraction. The extracted feature maps serve as input of a sub-model responsible for proposing regions of interest (ROIs) likely to contain objects of interest. A second fully convolutional network is used for analyzing small regions of this feature map. For each of these small patches, different rectangular regions in the corresponding input space are compared in order to account for different object sizes and scales. The regions with higher classification score and similarity with the ground truth are kept as ROIs for the final object detection process. At the region proposal step, ROI proposal is achieved by using two fully-connected networks of shared weights responsible for evaluating and refining the quality of the bounding box and the prediction (i.e., if it matches the ground truth in both location and content). Each of the candidate ROIs is then sampled to a standard size and once again evaluated by a pair of fully-connected networks in terms of bounding and

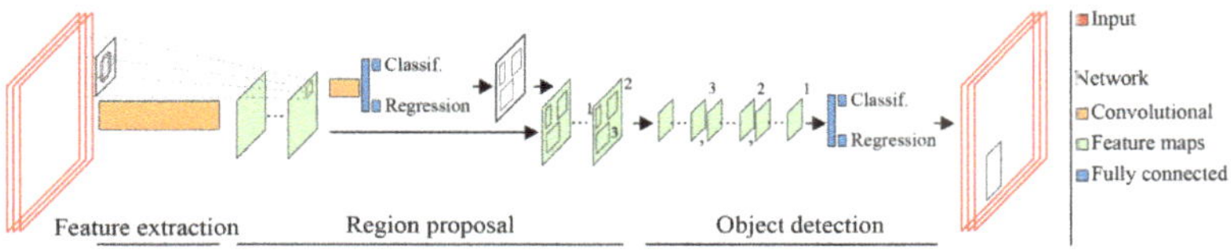

Figure 4.6. Schematic representation of the Faster R-CNN network for object detection.

content quality. This method is capable of, via an end-to-end training, proposing and filtering a set of ROIs to properly distinguish between background and relevant occurrences. To adapt the Faster R-CNN for lung nodule detections, the authors added an upsample layer that changes the output of the feature map to be more suitable to the small size of the nodules relative to the scan. Also, to provide 3D context to the network, the authors use as input an image composed of three adjacent axial slices. The resulting candidate list must then be reduced via a FP reduction step, following the standard detection pipeline. More recently, it has been suggested that the YOLO object detection framework [58] can also be used for nodule detection without the need for FP reduction [46]. Similarly to Ding *et al* [44], stacks of axial images for 3D context are used. However, slices at higher distances were used instead of adjacent ones to help to distinguish nodules from blood vessels. The network is then trained with a hard sample mining scheme, predicting both nodules and nodule confounders. Other authors suggest using MIP instead of axial slices stacks for 3D context [47].

CNNs have also shown promising results in the FP reduction task, while significantly reducing the need for field knowledge. In fact, features of models trained with natural images can be used as is for FP reduction [41]. However, this approach seems not to be as good as training a network from scratch since the achieved FP reduction performance is the same as that of handcrafted feature-based methods. In fact, Arindra *et al* showed that carefully designing and training a CNN from scratch can easily achieve state-of-the-art results [43]. For that, the network was designed to account for 3D context by analyzing multiple 2D slices of a cubic patch centered on the candidate centroid. A patch size of 50×50×50mm ensures that all nodules are completely visible and each slice is analyzed by a dedicated CNN block composed of convolutional-pooling layers pairs followed by a fully-connected layer. The number of layers, maps and other hyperparameters are manually tuned using a smaller dataset and overfit is avoided by using dropout and artificial data augmentation. Following a similar strategy, [45] considered a multi-scale approach for the same FP reduction task. The model analyses 3D patches at different scales by altering the size and stride of the pooling layers. The outputs of each network are then combined with the learned weights to produce a final candidate classification.

Recently, there have been efforts to improve the integration of CAD systems on the clinical practice by combining the assessment of the radiologist with the output of the system. For instance, it was shown that the gaze of the radiologists during the nodule search task can be used for establishing a set of nodule candidates, which can then be classified by a deep learning system as nodule/non-nodule with state-of-the-art performance [59]. Even though this approach allows the workload of specialists to be reduced during screening, it may not contribute to increase the quality of early diagnosis. Indeed, since using the radiologists gaze as an initial candidate detection only allows recognition errors to be mitigated, other studies aimed at assessing the value of the *a posteriori* combination of the radiologists gaze with the CAD outputs. Namely, offline experiments suggest that providing CAD outputs only for regions with low attention times allows improvement of the overall nodule detection performance to the same performance level of two radiologists [60].

4.3 Computer-aided lung nodule segmentation

Lung nodule segmentation corresponds to the identification of the voxels of a given ROI (resulting, for instance, from automatic detection) that belong to a nodule (figure 4.7). As discussed in section 4.1, full 3D nodule segmentation is rarely performed in a clinical setting and radiologists typically assess nodule size by measuring the largest axial diameter of the nodule as full 3D manual segmentation is extremely time consuming. Patient follow-up criteria such as Lung-RADS and Fleischner have also been designed with this limitation in mind and report both 3D volume thresholds as well as axial diameters. Nevertheless, the geometrical assumptions of a single axial diameter measurement can introduce errors and a full 3D segmentation can significantly improve the description of a nodule's size and shape. If performed automatically, 3D nodule segmentation could then improve the extracted information without introducing a significant time overhead, which has motivated the development of the methods described in this section.

Table 4.2 presents a summary of the performance of the methods discussed in this section. Performance is most often reported in terms of the intersection over union (IoU) (also known as Jaccard index) or Dice coefficient (DC) [61]. Other reported metrics are mean absolute distance or Hausdorff distance [62] between predicted and ground truth nodule surfaces. Note that the definition of the segmentation ground truth tends to vary between authors, and it is sometimes not clear whether performance metrics were computed in 2D or 3D. Because of this, a direct comparison between methods is not always possible.

Although manual segmentation is typically done on the axial planes, 3D segmentation has been the most adopted by the scientific community as it allows the perception of the entire nodule geometry. Nevertheless, 2D or 2.5D based methods (where multiple CT slices are used for 3D context) have also been proposed given the additional complexity and computational burden of 3D segmentation.

Similarly to lung nodule detection using non-deep learning methods, segmentation methods usually take advantage of the natural characteristics of solid nodules, which commonly have high contrast with the lung parenchyma and a spherical

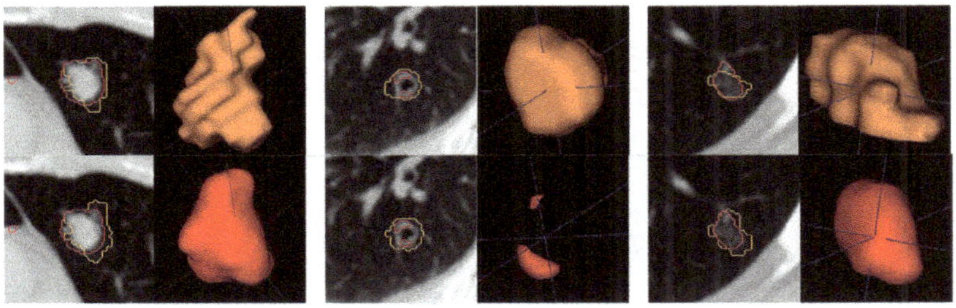

Figure 4.7. Manual and automatic nodule segmentation examples. For each 2 × 2 block, the figure shows the central axial slice of the nodule with automatic (red) and manual (orange) segmentations by two different experts on the top and bottom left quadrants as well as the 3D representations of the manual and automatic segmentations on the top right and bottom right quadrants respectively. Adapted from [63].

Table 4.2. Performance of selected automatic lung nodule segmentation algorithms. NA: not available. Method: whether the method is 2D, 2.5D or 3D as well as DL when deep learning techniques are used. Performance: IoU/DC (number of nodules used for evaluation).

Author	Method	Dataset	Performance	Comments
Ye *et al* 2010 [64]	3D	Private	NA/0.85 (181)	
Tan *et al* 2013 [65]	3D	Private; LIDC-IDRI	0.65/NA (23)	
Messay *et al* 2015 [66]	3D	LIDC-IDRI	0.74/NA (66)	AL⩾3
Zhao *et al* 2015[67]	2D	Private	0.89/NA (281)	
Gonçalves *et al* 2016 [68]	3D	LIDC-IDRI	0.65/NA (569)	
Feng *et al* 2017 [69]	2D-DL	LIDC-IDRI	NA/0.76 (1390)	
Wang *et al* 2017 [70]	2.5D-DL	LIDC-IDRI	0.71/0.82 (493)	
Aresta *et al* 2018 [46]	2D-DL	LIDC-IDRI	0.63/0.79 (NA)	
Jung *et al* 2018 [71]	3D	SNUH;LIDC-IDRI	0.68/0.85 (58); 0.64/0.78 (18)	Sub-solid
Tong *et al* 2018 [72]	2D-DL	LIDC-IDRI	NA/0.74 (1245)	
Wang *et al* 2018 [73]	3D-DL	LIDC-IDRI	NA/0.95 (NA)	
Wu *et al* 2018 [74]	3D-DL	LIDC-IDRI	NA/0.74 (1404)	
Aresta *et al* 2019 [63]	3D-DL	LIDC-IDRI	0.48/NA (2284)	
Huang *et al* 2019 [75]	2D-DL	LIDC-IDRI	NA/0.79 (1186)	
Atwal *et al* 2020 [76]	3D-DL	LNDb	0.40/NA (127)	
Cao *et al* 2020 [77]	2.5D-DL	LIDC-IDRI	NA/0.83 (986)	
Dong *et al* 2020 [78]	2.5D-DL	LIDC-IDRI	NA/0.93 (874)	
Galdran *et al* 2020 [79]	3D-DL	LNDb	0.57/NA (127)	
Rassadin *et al* 2020 [80]	3D-DL	LNDb	0.51/NA (127)	
Rocha *et al* 2020 [81]	2D; 2D-DL; 2D-DL	LIDC-IDRI	NA/0.67 (2653); NA/0.83 (531); NA/0.82 (531)	
Shi *et al* 2020 [82]	3D-DL	LIDC-IDRI	NA/0.85 (1154)	
Tian *et al* 2020 [83]	3D-DL	LNDb	0.57/NA (127)	
Usman *et al* 2020 [84]	2.5D-DL	LIDC-IDRI	NA/0.88 (893)	
Wu *et al* 2020 [85]	2D-DL;3D-DL	LIDC-IDRI	NA/0.80 (200)	

shape. Traditional image processing tools such as thresholding and morphological methods [86] have been employed in the past, as well as region-growing approaches [67, 87–90], deformable and level-set methods [71, 91, 92] and graph-cut algorithms [64]. Alternatively, voxel-wise segmentation has also been proposed by extracting intensity [65] and shape-related features, namely from Hessian matrices [68], and training classifiers such as support-vector machines or neural networks [66] to obtain the final result. However, the handcrafted nature of these approaches makes their extension for non-solid and sub-solid nodules a hard and tedious process [89] due to the cloudy texture, irregular shape and reduced contrast with the parenchyma of non-solid nodules and the diffused boundaries of sub-solid nodules.

Following the tendency of other computer vision and medical image analysis applications, recent approaches for lung nodule segmentation mostly rely on deep learning. For instance, Wang *et al* proposed a multi-scale CNN that performs voxel-wise predictions, inside a cube containing a lung nodule [70]. Each predicted voxel corresponds to the center of a fixed size patch to be processed by the network and thus predicting an entire segmentation requires the evaluation of a high number of patches. Furthermore, this model has an inherent lack of global context, since the network only evaluates patches, and thus the 3D reconstruction of the nodule may be affected. Huang *et al* implemented a fully-connected network for segmenting 2D axial slices, which is no longer common, since this architecture can cause loss of information in the convolutional layers [75]. The most common solution is to adapt 2D or 3D U-Net [93] architectures, since they allow to consider both local and global context, and different variations of these architectures have been used by multiple authors [46, 48, 72, 76–79, 81, 84, 85].

Multi-task approaches, combining segmentation with additional tasks, particularly the prediction of other nodule characteristics, have also been designed. Wu *et al* proposed a multi-task scheme for pulmonary nodule segmentation together with the prediction of the nodules' malignancy, achieving state-of-the-art performance in both tasks [74]. This malignancy prediction is performed by concatenating and processing, via a set of fully-connected layers, the features of the segmentation network's bottleneck with a convolved version of the produced segmentation prediction. Other works have followed similar strategies but combining segmentation, based on a U-Net architecture, with texture prediction, which is more closely related to segmentation features [80, 83].

Given the high requirements of the above methods in terms of annotated data for training, weakly or non-supervised methods as well as synthetic data have also been explored. Feng *et al* proposed the use of slice-level labels—indicating the presence (or absence) of a nodule in each slice—instead of the typical voxel-wise ground truth [69]. Active self-paced learning, where the model iteratively labels unannotated data which is used for training in the next iteration, has also been proposed [73]. The generation of synthetic data for training has been proposed by Shi *et al*, where a style-based generative adversarial network is used to generate augmented samples from real semantic labels using random styles, which are then fed to a 3D U-Net architecture for segmentation [82].

Despite the high performance of deep learning methods, their application in the medical field is often criticized due to (1) the inherent lack of explanations behind the decision and, (2) the production of deterministic outputs, ignoring the existing interobserver variability of the annotations and inhibiting the medical specialist to interact and change the decisions of the system. With this in mind, Aresta *et al* proposed an architecture, iW-Net, that allows experts to correct automatic nodule segmentations with minimal interaction [63]. The model is composed of a sequence of two 3D encoder–decoder networks with a structure similar to a U-Net. The first block predicts an initial segmentation proposal, which is shown to the user. This segmentation can then be corrected by marking two points on the expected diameter of the nodule. These points are converted to a weight map which, together with the initial segmentation, are used for the second encoder–decoder block, resulting in a corrected segmentation. Simulated experiments have shown that this kind of interaction allows significant improvment of the segmentation performance on all nodule types, but specially on challenging GGO and small nodules.

4.4 Computer-aided lung nodule characterization

Lung nodule characterization refers to the description or classification of any nodule characteristic beyond those already obtained in the detection and segmentation steps, i.e., location and volume. As described in section 4.1, a wide range of characteristics have been used to describe and classify pulmonary nodules. Early literature on nodule characterization was mostly focused on malignancy classification as this was considered to be the ultimate clinical endpoint. However, the subjective nature of this assessment has motivated the development of approaches for the prediction of other features, in particular for texture characterization since it is strongly related to nodule malignancy. Furthermore, since texture is featured on both Lung-RADS and Fleischner guidelines, a texture characterization model could be used to aid clinicians in obtaining patient follow-up. The prediction of other features has also been proposed, mostly in multi-task scenarios where several nodule features (including malignancy) are predicted. Besides nodule malignancy and patient follow-up, the prediction of features to guide specific segmentation or detection architectures has also been an additional motivation which has fueled the development of nodule characterization methods.

4.4.1 Malignancy characterization

Table 4.3 presents a summary of the performance of the methods for malignancy characterization discussed in this subsection. Performance is reported in terms of accuracy and area under the curve (AUC) on the receiver operating characteristic curve since these are the most widely used metrics in literature. Note that due to the different number of classes and data selection criteria used, direct comparisons between authors cannot be performed.

Malignancy classification has mostly been approached as a binary classification problem (i.e., benign versus malignant), although occasionally classification with more classes or regression has been reported. Importantly, most studies rely on

Table 4.3. Performance of selected automatic malignancy classification algorithms. NA indicates data not available. Method: whether the method is 2D, 2.5D or 3D as well as DL when deep learning techniques are used. Source: R when the ground truth is based on visual assessment of the CT by radiologists and D when the ground truth was obtained by an external diagnostics method such as biopsy. Output: Number of classes considered followed by C or R depending on if classification or regression was used. Performance: accuracy/AUC (number of nodules used for evaluation).

Author	Method	Source	Output	Dataset	Performance
Zinovev *et al* 2011 [94]	2D	R	2C	LIDC-IDRI	0.495/0.642 (914)
Chen *et al* 2011 [95]	2D	R	3C	LIDC-IDRI	0.787/NA (47)
Han *et al* 2015 [96]	3D	R	2C	LIDC-IDRI	NA/0.927 (906)
Buty *et al* 2016 [97]	2.5D-DL	R	5C	LIDC-IDRI	0.750/NA (2054)
Chen *et al* 2016 [98]	2D-DL	R	5R	LIDC-IDRI	NA/NA (2400)
Shen *et al* 2017 [99]	2D-DL	R	2C	LIDC-IDRI	0.871/0.930 (1375)
Sun *et al* 2017 [100]	2D-DL	R	2C	LIDC-IDRI	0.818/0.899 (NA)
Song *et al* 2017 [101]	2D-DL	R	2C	LIDC-IDRI	0.842/NA (NA)
Hussein *et al* 2017 [102]	3D-DL	R	2C	LIDC-IDRI	0.913/NA (1144)
Liu *et al* 2017 [103]	2D-DL	D	2C; 3C	LIDC-IDRI	0.946/0.981 (776); 0.861/NA (776)
Kang *et al* 2017 [104]	3D-DL	D	2C; 3C	LIDC-IDRI	0.953/0.990 (776); 0.922/NA (776)
Xie *et al* 2017 [105]	2D-DL	R	2C	LIDC-IDRI	0.934/0.978 (1357)
Gonçalves *et al* 2018 [106]	2D	R; D	2C; 2C	LIDC-IDRI	NA/0.962 (300); 0.684/0.905 (157)
Wei *et al* 2018 [107]	2D	R	2C	LIDC-IDRI	0.858/NA (746)
Dey *et al* 2018 [108]	3D-DL	R	2C	LIDC-IDRI	0.868/0.901 (686)
da Nóbrega *et al* 2018 [109]	2.5D-DL	R	2C	LIDC-IDRI	0.884/0.932 (1536)
Dai *et al* 2018 [110]	3D-DL	R	2C	LIDC-IDRI	0.915/0.969 (1011)
Wu *et al* 2018 [74]	3D-DL	R	4C	LIDC-IDRI	0.976/NA (1404)
Shen *et al* 2019 [111]	3D-DL	R	2C	LIDC-IDRI	0.842/0.856 (NA)
Wang *et al* 2019 [112]	2D-DL	R	5R	LIDC-IDRI	NA/NA (2632)
Liu *et al* 2019 [113]	2D-DL	R	2C	LIDC-IDRI	0.935/0.979 (1000)
Xiao *et al* 2020 [114]	2D-DL	R	2C	LIDC-IDRI	0.931/0.820 (NA)
Veasey *et al* 2020 [115]	3D-DL	R; D	2C; 2C	LIDC-IDRI; NLST	NA/0.939 (647); NA/0.806 (857)
Wang *et al* 2020 [116]	3D-DL	R	5C	LIDC-IDRI	0.685/NA (1882)

radiologist annotations based on visual assessment of CT images for ground truth malignancy references, whereas only a minority of studies report malignancy classification performance in comparison to additional diagnostic methods such as biopsy, surgical resection, and progression or reviewal of previous radiological images to assess nodule evolution in time. In spite of the fact that visual assessment in a single time point is known to be a highly subjective task and other diagnostic methods give a significantly higher degree of certainty, this type of data is notoriously difficult to obtain, which has hindered the use of this reference method. In order to avoid the uncertainty is visually assessed labels, the exclusion of uncertain cases, when radiologist labels vary widely or are given uncertain labels are often excluded from training and/or validation [111].

Most approaches rely on the extraction of an ROI around the nodule, and 2D, 2.5D and 3D approaches have been proposed, though this does not appear to have a significant impact to performance (table 4.3). This may be related to the fact that radiologists mainly base their classification on the axial slice and resort only occasionally to other planes.

In non-deep learning methods, handcrafted features based on the intensity, texture, size, and shape of the nodules extracted from the nodule segmentation have been proposed. Nodule classification was then performed using methods such as decision trees [94], linear regression [107], neural networks [95], and SVMs [96, 107].

Regarding deep learning architectures, those widely used in literature for different types of classification/regression tasks have been adopted for the prediction of malignancy, such as VGGNet [97, 100, 101, 103], InceptionNet [104], DenseNet [110, 116] and ResNet [113]. Methodologies based on custom CNNs [99, 108] and ensemble classification models [105, 114, 115] have also been proposed.

Hybrid methods have also been proposed, combining the advantages of deep learning and handcrafted features. These often combine handcrafted ones related to shape [97] and intensity [98] to deep learning features for classification. da Nóbrega *et al* used a CNN for feature extraction followed by standard classification methodologies such as naive Bayes, multilayer perceptron, SVMs, KNN, and random forest.

The characterization of nodule malignancy in multi-task scenarios has also been proposed, namely as an additional task to nodule segmentation and/or in multi-feature classification. Joint segmentation and malignancy classification has been proposed using a 3D U-Net architecture [74], where a malignancy classification branch is added from the encoded U-Net features. In terms of multi-feature classification approaches, these can be roughly divided into two groups: either the features extracted from the image are used to predict both malignancy and other nodule characteristics in parallel [98, 110, 113], or the predicted nodule characteristics are used themselves as the features for malignancy prediction [74, 102, 113], though sometimes combined with features directly derived from the image [111, 113]. While the second approach guarantees that the network has access to information that is clinically relevant for malignancy characterization (e.g., texture and calcification), a direct cause-and-effect relationship cannot be established if additional features from the image are added. Nevertheless, such approaches undeniably provide a degree of supervision, though perhaps not explainability per se, on the interpretation of the image by the network.

Given the limited data available, artificial generation of nodule samples based on a generative adversarial network has been proposed by Wang *et al* [112] where oversampling of minority classes based on additional nodules features (such as texture, calcification, spiculation, etc) was performed to balance the data during training.

4.4.2 Other nodule features

Table 4.4 presents a summary of the nodule characterization methods discussed in this subsection, describing the features and discretization used in each strategy. Given that LIDC-IDRI has the most extensive nodule features characterization, most works are based on this dataset.

Fully dedicated methods for nodule characterization are scarce and most approaches are designed in multi-task scenarios with the purpose of malignancy characterization, as described in section 4.1. Specific methods for nodule characterization have been limited to the characterization of either texture [48, 79, 83, 117, 119–121] or spiculation [118, 122]. While most of the nodule features described in LIDC-IDRI are annotated in a 1–5 scale (calcification and internal structure are annotated in a 1–6 and 1–4 scales respectively), classification in a binary scale has also been employed [94, 99, 102, 111, 118]. When the full scale is used, both classification and regression methods have been employed. However, internal structure and calcification are, by nature, not in an ordinal scale and their prediction through regression [98, 113] must be interpreted carefully.

As seen for malignancy characterization, while radiologists tend to visualize nodules on the axial slices only, the use of the full 3D ROI surrounding the nodule [48, 74, 83, 94, 102, 110, 111, 117] or multiple 2D slices—axial, coronal and sagittal [79, 119, 120] or also diagonal slices [121]—for a more complete description of nodule features is common in literature.

In terms of non-deep learning approaches, dependent on handcrafted features, the differences in HU intensity across different nodule classes have motivated the use of nodule intensity features [94, 117] as well as textural features [94] and shape features [118] in traditional classifiers as decision trees [94] and k-nearest-neighbor [117] for texture characterization tasks. Nevertheless, and as in the previous sections, recent approaches tend to favor deep learning architectures. In terms of the architectures used, most works propose custom CNN architectures, though widely used classification networks such as such as DenseNet [110, 116] or ResNet [48, 79, 113] are also used, which have the advantage that pretrained weights are easily available when compared to custom CNNs. Tian *et al* avoided this issue by applying Models Genesis, a learning method which can be used for pretraining through self-supervised reconstruction of random CT cubes with added augmentations [83].

Table 4.4. Description of selected automatic nodule feature classification algorithms. Method: whether the method is 2D or 3D as well as DL when deep learning techniques are used. Nodule Features: the nodule features characterized in each approach where the number of classes considered followed by C or R depending on if classification or regression was used is given.

			Nodule features								
Author	Method	Dataset	Cal	ISt	Mar	Lob	Sph	Spi	Sub	Tex	Others
Zinovev *et al* 2011 [94]	2D	LIDC-IDRI (914)	2C		2C	2C	2C	2C	2C	2C	Mal
Jacobs *et al* 2015 [117]	3D	NELSON (150)								3C	
Niehaus *et al* 2015 [118]	2D	LIDC-IDRI (2660)						2C			
Chen *et al* 2016 [98]	2D-DL	LIDC-IDRI (2400)	6R	4R	5R	5R	5R	5R	5R	5R	Mal
Ciompi *et al* 2017 [119]	2.5D-DL	MILD;DLCST (639)								6C	
Hussein *et al* 2017 [102]	3D-DL	LIDC-IDRI (1144)	2C		2C	2C	2C	2C		2C	Mal
Shen *et al* 2017 [99]	2D-DL	LIDC-IDRI (756)			2C				2C		Mal
Tu *et al* 2017 [120]	2D-DL;2.5D-DL	LIDC-IDRI (570)								3C	
Dai *et al* 2018 [110]	3D-DL	LIDC-IDRI (1011)	6C	4C	5C	5C	5C	5C	5C	5C	Mal
Ferreira *et al* 2018 [121]	2.5D-DL	LIDC-IDRI (907)								3C	
Wu *et al* 2018 [74]	3D-DL	LIDC-IDRI (1404)	6C	4C	5C	5C	5C	5C	5C	5C	Mal;Seg
Shen *et al* 2019 [111]	3D-DL	LIDC-IDRI (NA)	2C		2C		2C		2C	2C	Mal
Wang *et al* 2019 [112]	2D-DL	LIDC-IDRI (2632)			5C	4C	4C	4C	5C	5C	Mal
Galdran *et al* 2020 [79]	2.5D-DL	LNDb (178)								3C	
Kaluva *et al* 2020 [48]	3D-DL	LNDb (178)								3C	
Liu *et al* 2020 [113]	2D-DL	LIDC-IDRI (1000)	6R	4R	5R	5R	5R	5R	5R	5R	Mal
Tian *et al* 2020 [83]	3D-DL	LNDb (178)								3C	Seg
Qiu *et al* 2020 [122]	2D-DL	LIDC-IDRI (2084)						2C			

Cal: calcification; ISt: internal structure; Mal: malignancy; Mar: margin; Lob: lobulation; Seg: segmentation; Sph: sphericity; Spi: spiculation; Sub: subtlety; Tex: texture.

As described in subsection 4.1, the characterization of nodule features in multi-task scenarios has also been proposed, particularly combined with nodule segmentation [74, 83] and malignancy characterization (cf section 4.1).

Given the relationship between these features and nodule malignancy, it is not surprising that most authors have combined nodule feature characterization with malignancy prediction, seeking to introduce a degree of explainability/interpretability to their models. However, even stand-alone feature characterization can be a suitable tool for clinical use, particularly for nodule features that are used in clinical guidelines such as nodule texture, spiculation and calcification. While the first two have received some attention in literature, calcification is notoriously absent. This might be due to the fact that a binary classification of calcification can be easily obtained through thresholding (typically using a threshold of 200 HU). While there could be clinical value in different calcification patterns—such as those are described in LIDC-IDRI—these do not feature very prominently in clinical guidelines.

4.5 Computer-aided lung cancer patient diagnosis/management

While most works in the literature on CAD methods for lung cancer in CT have addressed the three aspects described in sections 4.2, 4.3 and 4.4 and relatively promising results have been obtained, the final goal of any lung cancer CAD system will be to improve patient-level diagnosis and management. However, the detached nature of independent solutions for nodule detection, segmentation and characterization/classification has hindered the adoption of these methods in clinical practice, thus limiting their impact to the scientific community. In order to solve this issue, several authors have proposed methods for patient-level diagnosis or management, either based on novel tools specifically designed for this purpose or by concatenating CAD nodule detection, segmentation and/or characterization modules to obtain a patient-level recommendation. These approaches can be divided into two main groups depending on the clinical goal in mind: the first, aims to determine whether a certain patient/CT has or will have lung cancer within a certain period of time, whereas the second uses validated clinical criteria (such as Lung-RADS or Fleischner guidelines) to predict a patient-level recommendation of follow-up. While the first group is particularly attractive and could be extremely interesting if correctly validated, a yes/no decision on the presence of cancer is far removed from the current reality of clinical practice where patients are routinely followed at different intervals depending on their risk factors. Following such recommendations allows radiologists to make knowledge-based decisions regarding nodule findings for better patient management while reducing the number of unnecessary follow-up examinations.

4.5.1 Lung cancer patient diagnosis

Table 4.5 presents a summary of the performance of the methods for lung cancer patient diagnosis discussed in this subsection. Performance has mostly been reported in terms of AUC on the receiver operating characteristic curve. The DSB17

Table 4.5. Performance of selected automatic lung cancer diagnosis algorithms. Method: the different components of the solution proposed by the authors (D for detection, S for segmentation, C for classification and E for end-to-end solution) as well as DL when deep learning techniques are used. Performance: AUC for patient-level classification (number of scans used for evaluation).

Author	Method	Dataset	Performance
Alakwaa *et al* 2017 [123]	S+C DL	LUNA16; DSB17	0.83 (506)
Chon *et al* 2017 [124]	S+C DL	LUNA16; DSB17	0.757 (420)
Tafti *et al* 2018 [125]	E DL	Private; DSB17	0.926 (3397)
Ardila *et al* 2019 [126]	E DL	NLST	0.944 (6716)
Liao *et al* 2019 [127]	D+C DL	LUNA16; DSB17	0.875 (505)
Ozdemir *et al* 2019 [128]	S+C DL	LIDC-IDRI; DSB17	0.87 (506)
Trajanovski *et al* 2021 [129]	D+C DL	Private; NLST; DSB17	0.886 (505)

challenge has been the main reference in this topic and most works have been based in the data associated to this challenge. Unfortunately, this data is no longer publicly available, which may restrict future research in this topic.

Most solutions published in the literature or proposed in the DSB17 challenge rely on solutions similar to those explored in sections 4.2–4.4 employing state-of-the-art deep learning architectures such as ResNet, DenseNet, VGG and U-Net, among others [130]. Most methods proposed are composed of two parts, the first of which aims at localizing ROIs through a detection or segmentation module, followed by a malignancy classification module based on the ROIs detected by the previous module.

Both Alakwaa *et al* and Chon *et al* proposed U-Nets for nodule segmentation, followed by custom 3D CNN networks for malignancy classification and ultimately classifying the CT scan as positive or negative for lung cancer [123, 124]. Ozdemir *et al* proposed a cascade of 3D CNNs which perform nodule segmentation at CT level followed by nodule ranking and malignancy prediction of each nodule candidate providing as output a per-patient malignancy classification probability, per-nodule malignancy scores, and segmented lung nodule candidates [128].

A similar approach, based on two subsequent 3D patch-based U-Net-like architectures was proposed by Liao *et al* and this solution obtained the first place on the DSB17 challenge [127]. This approach was extended by Trajanovski *et al* with additional training data and by sorting the top-ten nodules in any given scan in terms of nodule size (as predicted by the nodule detector), improving patient-level classification performance [129].

End-to-end patient-level classification has also been proposed and might have additional advantages by allowing a full exploration of CT image features to deep learning methodologies, and both end-to-end solutions published in the literature present the best results in terms of AUC. However, the quantity of available data is a significant constraint to these kinds of approaches, and both works had to employ additional largescale datasets. Tafti *et al* proposed a multi-scale 3D CNN for end-to-end diagnostic classification of lung CT images [125]. Ardila *et al* proposed an end-to-end solution which receives as input a primary CT scan and, if available, a prior CT scan of the same patient and produces as output a probability of malignancy, as well as cancer localization bounding boxes and lung cancer malignancy scores. The solution relies on three CNN components: (i) a 3D CNN for feature extraction of a single CT scan; (ii) a 3D CNN for detection of ROIs; (iii) a CNN that receives the output from the two first components and performs patient-level diagnosis.

4.5.2 Patient follow-up recommendation

Table 4.6 presents a summary of the performance of the methods for patient follow-up recommendation discussed in this subsection. Performance is reported in terms of accuracy or kappa [131] as these two measures have been the most widely used in the literature. Note that due to the different number of classes and data selection criteria used, direct comparisons between authors cannot be performed.

In terms of the prediction of patient follow-up, approaches for follow-up predictions according to both Lung-RADS and Fleischner guidelines have been proposed but, to the authors' best knowledge, automatic follow-up prediction algorithms according to the BTS guidelines have not yet been proposed. One method for patient referral according to NLST criteria has also been proposed.

Regarding Lung-RADS, the fact that it can be applied nodule-wise means that nodule-wise training and validation has been performed in literature and a full patient-level approach and validation has not been reported in the literature. Nevertheless, such approaches could easily be coupled to existing nodule detection models for a fully automatic patient-level referral. Given the recent nature of these solutions, deep learning classification architectures have been employed by all authors. State-of-the-art CNNs have been used, namely VGG-16 [132], ResNet [133] and DenseNet [134] architectures. Modifications of the exact Lung-RADS classification have been used, with the more complex guidelines being reduced to either two [133] or three [132] classes, though a more recent work by Ferreira *et al* considers the full range of Lung-RADS outcomes. One of the main challenges with

Table 4.6. Performance of selected automatic lung cancer patient follow-up recommendation algorithms. NA indicates data not available. Method: the different components of the solution proposed by the authors (D for detection, S for segmentation and C for classification) as well as DL when deep learning techniques are used. Output: Guidelines considered (number of classes). Performance: accuracy/kappa (number of scans/nodules used for evaluation).

Author	Method	Output	Dataset	Performance
Aresta *et al* 2018 [46]	D+S DL	NLST (3)	NLST; DSB17	NA/NA (500 scans)
Nishio *et al* 2018 [132]	C DL	Lung-RADS (3)	Private	0.680/NA (123 nodules)
Ferreira *et al* 2019 [133]	C DL	Lung-RADS (2)	LIDC-IDRI	0.870/NA (950 nodules)
Ferreira *et al* 2020 [134]	C DL	Lung-RADS (5)	LIDC-IDRI	0.724/NA (2666 nodules)
Kaluva *et al* 2020 [48]	D+S+C DL	Fleischner(4)	LNDb	NA/0.464 (58 scans)
Kim 2021 [21]	S DL	Fleischner (4)	LNDb	NA/0.580 (58 scans)

Lung-RADS is that it relies on data that is not currently available in public datasets, specifically the measurement of the solid diameter of part-solid nodules, which has likely hindered the development of further work on this topic.

Regarding classification according to Fleischner guidelines, the LNDb challenge was set up to include nodule detection, segmentation and texture characterization with the goal of performing patient-level follow-up recommendation according to Fleischner guidelines [21]. Nevertheless, the recent nature of this challenge means that few works on this topic have been published so far. Kaluva *et al* proposed a method based on the fact that the follow-up prediction can be defined from an accurate description of all nodules in a CT [48]. In this way, the authors used nodule detection, segmentation and characterization strategies, followed by a rule-based approach to predict follow-up. An SVM-based approach was also proposed by Kaluva *et al* but could not outperform the rule-based approach. Kim proposed the use of a 3D U-Net variant, nnU-Net, for simultaneous nodule segmentation and texture characterization in the full 3D scan, followed again by a rule-based module for follow-up prediction [21].

Finally, Aresta *et al* proposed a single-step nodule detection system based on YOLOv2, followed by a U-Net for nodule segmentation [46]. A referral decision was then obtained according to NLST criteria which rely on the presence of nodules, their diameters and the calcified area (obtained through thresholding at 70 HU).

4.6 Available datasets

The evaluation and validation of CAD systems require a large amount of annotated data. Methods can be developed and tested using private datasets, but the usage of publicly available datasets eases algorithm benchmarking. This section describes publicly available chest CT datasets commonly used for the development of lung cancer CAD systems, and a summary is available on table 4.7.

4.6.1 ANODE09 dataset

The ANODE09 dataset [9] is composed of 55 nearly isotropic CT scans randomly selected from the NELSON study [138]. The dataset was annotated by two observers, and findings were either considered relevant, i.e., nodules with diameter

Table 4.7. Datasets commonly used for lung cancer screening algorithm development. NS: number of CT scans; NAn: number of annotators per scan; NN: number of nodules ($r > 1.5$ mm); S: voxel-wise segmentation available; C: nodule-wise characterization available; PM: patient medical history available. NA indicates data not available.

Dataset	Year	NS	NAn	NN	S	C	PM
ANODE09 [9]	2010	55	2	246			
LIDC-IDRI [135]	2011	1018	4	2699	✓	✓	
NLST [136]	2011	5994[a]	1	9028			✓
LUNA16 [19]	2016	888	4	1186			
DSB17 [20]	2017	1903	NA	NA			
LNDb [137]	2019	294	2	946	✓	✓	

[a] Number does not include CT scans with no findings.

$\geqslant$ 4 mm and irrelevant findings, corresponding to findings that have nodule-like characteristics but that experts believe not be a nodule, as well as small and benign nodules. In the end, a total of 246 nodules and 464 irrelevant findings.

4.6.2 Lung image database consortium image collection dataset

The LIDC-IDRI [135] is one of the most used datasets for the development of chest CT lung cancer CAD algorithms due to the quality of the annotations, large variety of acquisition conditions and high number of scans.

The LIDC-IDRI is composed of 1018 annotated scans. The standard size of the CT volumes is 512×512 voxels with 150–300 axial slices or more, corresponding to a slice thickness range of approximately 1.5–3.5 mm. Each scan is annotated by 4 out of 12 experienced thoracic radiologists. Each specialist was asked to annotate abnormal structures of interest on a chest CT scan as (1) nodule with diameter $<$ 3 mm, (2) nodule with diameter $\geqslant$ 3 mm, and (3) non-nodule with diameter $\geqslant$ 3 mm. Furthermore, radiologists were asked to ignore lesions considered as obviously benign. Non-nodules are lesions, such as scars, that even though have no direct cancerous manifestation, may be of interest for the diagnosis of lung cancer or other pathologies.

The dataset provides manual/semi-automatic volumetric segmentations for nodules with diameter $\geqslant$ 3 mm and only centroids for the other structures. Furthermore, the number of annotations per physician for nodules with diameter $\geqslant$ 3 mm was limited to 6 and a scan may not contain any nodules. During the annotation process, each radiologist was also asked to subjectively evaluate each delineated nodule on several characteristics: (1) subtlety, (2) internal structure (3) calcification, (4) sphericity, (5) margin (6) spiculation, (7) texture, and (8) malignancy assuming a 60-year-old male smoker. No location-based classification (juxta-pleural, juxta-vascular, peri-fissural or isolated) is provided.

The annotations were performed in two steps. First, each specialist performed a blind reading where no access to the work of the other radiologists was provided. During the annotation procedure, segmentations were done manually or with the help of a semi-automatic software. Then, on a second, open, phase, specialists voluntarily refined their annotations based on the work of the others. In the end, each nodule was assigned an AL according to the number of specialists that delimited it. With this, the dataset is composed of 2669 nodules with diameter $\geqslant$ 3 mm and 4702 $<$ 3 mm nodules, on a total of 7371 nodules.

4.6.3 Luna16 dataset

The LUNA16 dataset [19] is a curated version of the LIDC-IDRI dataset. This dataset is composed of 888 scans with slice thickness $\leqslant$ 3 mm, following 2014 ACR-STR screening recommendations [139]. The LIDC-IDRI annotations are simplified to the nodule centroid and its respective equivalent radius to ease data handling. Furthermore, only nodules with AL of 3 or higher are considered. Non-nodules, nodules with diameter $<$ 3 mm and detections with lower AL are all regarded as irrelevant findings i.e., CAD detections on these structures should neither be considered FP nor TP. To ease comparisons between studies, the dataset is divided in 10 folds with a similar number of scans in each. The dataset contains 1186 nodules and 31 617 irrelevant findings.

4.6.4 National lung screening trial dataset

The National Lung Screen Trial dataset [136] results from a randomized controlled trial to assess the potential of chest CT for reducing lung cancer mortality in comparison to chest radiography. The study had 53 454 participants and 26 722 were enrolled on the CT arm and were followed over 3 years. The prevalence of lung cancer is approximately 3%. During the trial, a CT scan was considered screening positive if at least one non-calcified nodule with major axis dimension $\geqslant 4$ mm on the axial view was found. Consequently, there can be multiple scans for the same patient on different time points, allowing to study the evolution of the patient with time. No follow-up scans were performed if a malignant abnormality was found or upon death of the participant. Information regarding the patients' medical history is also available. From all participants, there are 2284 patients with findings related to lung cancer, but only the slice-wise location of the nodule/finding is available. Note that this dataset is available for use for scientific research after formal request.

4.6.5 Kaggle data Science Bowl 2017 dataset

The Kaggle Data Science Bowl 2017 dataset [20] (DSB17) was temporarily made available during the Kaggle Data Science Bowl 2017 competition. The dataset is composed of 1397 training and 506 test chest CT scans and only binary cancer/non-cancer scan-wise labels are available. All data is provided by the National Cancer Institute (USA). Approximately 25% of the cases are lung cancer positive. Note that it is not mandatory that these scans contain lung nodules. Also, the lack of nodule-wise annotations makes impossible for direct CAD system assessment, but good performance on this dataset may still prove that a given system is usable for screening purposes.

4.6.6 LNDB dataset

The LNDb dataset [137] is composed of 294 CT images by several Siemens models at Centro Hospitalar de São João, Porto, Portugal. The median number of slices and slice thickness is 318.5 and 1.0 mm, respectively. The CT scan selection criteria and annotation procedure are similar to the LIDC-IDRI dataset, with the exception that only a single blind annotation round was performed. With this in mind, all scans have voxel-wise annotations (single blind) of nodules and most of the volumes were assessed by at least two radiologists. Furthermore, each abnormality is also subjectively characterized following the same criteria of the LIDC-IDRI.

4.7 Conclusion and future perspectives

As shown throughout this chapter, a significant amount of research has been developed in the field of computer-aided lung cancer screening in CT. Given that lung cancer currently remains the most lethal cancer, largely due to late detection of nodules, the development of effective screening strategies remains of the utmost importance and CAD could play a significant clinical role in the near future. Nevertheless, the main body of work has targeted the individual tasks that compose patient screening—lung nodule detection, segmentation and characterization—while the final goal of patient diagnosis/follow-up has received relatively little attention. This trend may however soon be inverted due to the saturation of nodule detection, segmentation and characterization performances, increasing computational power and the release of relevant datasets and challenges directed at patient-level tasks such as DSB17 and LNDb. Such a shift would allow CAD systems to play a role which is significantly closer to clinical reality, approach the problem in a more holistic way and ultimately simplify the adoption of CAD systems in lung cancer screening.

Unquestionably, one of the biggest challenges that lies ahead is the collection and public release of large international multi-center datasets that properly represent the variety and complexity of the problem, allowing for the creation of more robust algorithms and, at the same time, improving validation efforts. Specifically, future datasets should aim at collecting CT scans of different sources and equipment annotated by medical experts from different clinical backgrounds to better encode the diversity both of the manifestations of the pathology as well as the corresponding medical opinions. Interestingly, current CAD systems for nodule detection, segmentation and characterization may already provide an important baseline for the creation of these datasets, reducing the time needed for annotation. The relatively high perceptual error of radiologists in nodule detection is well known and the use of current CAD systems could decrease the number of radiologists needed to obtain a solid reference standard, leveraging the ability of automatic systems to quickly assess a full CT scan with high sensitivity and delegating the task of recognition (i.e., distinguishing nodules from FPs) to radiologists. Also in segmentation, current CAD systems could play a role by proposing an initial segmentation to be refined by radiologists. A semi-automatic approach has in fact already been used in LIDC-IDRI [135] but current interactive 3D segmentation tools such as proposed by Aresta *et al* [63] could go one step further in improving workflow, while simultaneously decreasing radiologist variability. Nodule characterization could also be initially performed by a CAD system and subsequently reviewed by a radiologist, particularly in distinguishing the relatively more common nodule types—solid isolated and spherical nodules—from other nodule types which require additional radiologist interpretation. In any of these cases however, clinical oversight is imperative to guarantee that existing biases and errors made by current CAD systems are not propagated to the final annotations and the dataset adequately represents the radiologists' interpretation of the image.

The framing of future datasets within public challenges could also play a significant role by allowing direct benchmarking of algorithms in a hidden representative test set, focusing the community in solving specific problems and attracting additional researchers. Nevertheless, any such challenge must be carefully designed to ensure that the results are relevant to the community both in terms of the challenge motivation and goals as well as the evaluation metrics and ranking strategy [140].

As described in the beginning of this section, most research has targeted the individual tasks of lung nodule detection, segmentation and characterization, while the final goal of patient diagnosis/follow-up has received relatively little attention. More recent literature has already indicated a shift towards patient-level CAD strategies and future datasets and methodologies should follow this approach, bringing CAD systems closer to clinical reality. As seen in section 4.5, two different approaches are possible: either following existing clinical guidelines to predict patient follow-up or management, or performing direct patient diagnosis. Closely following existing clinical guidelines has several advantages, namely making the adoption of CAD systems in clinical practice much more straightforward (both at a pragmatic level as in terms of radiologists' acceptance) and would ensure that the decisions made by CAD systems are based on validated clinical evidence. Nevertheless, direct patient diagnosis is particularly attractive and could be extremely interesting if correctly validated. While patient-level presence/absence of lung cancer has been previously targeted, such as in the DSB17 challenge, long-term risk stratification—such as determining if a given patient will develop cancer after a certain amount of time or predicting patient survival is particularly interesting from a clinical point of view, requiring however long-term follow-up of patients, and the collection of these datasets may involve significant costs and resources. Akin to malignancy prediction, as described in section 4.1, the use of diagnostic information for training and validation—instead of radiologist image interpretation—would also increase trust in the resulting algorithms. Development of these systems for patient-level long-term prediction could not only prove useful but even give further insights into how lung cancer patient screening and follow-up should be managed at a population level. Importantly, both approaches are non-exclusive and a dataset directed towards one could feasibly be converted to the other, if sufficient annotated data is available. Independently of the approach favored, there is one important aspect that must be present in any future lung cancer screening dataset effort, and that is the ensured active participation in radiologists in the framing of the problem, interpretation of the data and the solutions developed. As the community moves away from direct tasks and into more complex goals, which are ever closer to clinical reality, the ability to distinguish what is most important and what is most clinically relevant becomes crucial.

Besides the aforementioned paradigm shift in terms of the patient-level goal definition, the development of these end-to-end approaches would allow for additional aspects to be explored. While current algorithms focus on the direct manifestations of lung cancer, i.e. pulmonary nodules, through detection, segmentation and characterization, other radiological features can also be related to patient outcome. The use of the complete CT scan as input to a decision network, rather than structuring the decision around nodule findings, would allow for other features to be explored by the network, potentially with improved performance at patient level. Such radiomics approaches have been used in CT lung cancer characterization, for example in the prediction of mutation status to determine therapy [141], but have not been explored in lung cancer screening to the authors' knowledge.

Another additional and important aspect that would derive from patient-level approaches and that warrants further research is the longitudinal analysis of CT scans from the same patient. Nodule size is naturally a relevant indicator of malignancy, but is inherently limited as it represents a single point of data in time. Nodule growth, however, would give a more complete description of the malignancy of a nodule. Guidelines such as BTS already highlight the importance of nodule growth through nodule volume doubling time, which gives an easily understandable measure of how quickly a nodule is growing. Besides nodule size/growth, other features that change in time could also be important in indicating malignancy and patient cancer risk. To the authors' knowledge, automatic CT longitudinal analysis has been limited, mostly due to a lack of sufficient quality data, though the work of Ardila *et al* is a notable exception [126].

To further improve the applicability of CAD in lung cancer screening, the incorporation of patient data such as age, smoking history and patient history, would also be a significant step forward in bringing CAD systems closer to clinical practice. To the best of the authors' knowledge, there is still very limited research on combining both patient data and radiological manifestations to provide a robust prediction of lung cancer risk.

In addition to the above challenges related to patient-level analysis, the human aspect of the screening process must be better taken into account through the development of algorithms that keep radiologists in the loop and work in symbiosis with their abilities and limitations. Again, the active participation of radiologists in this effort is essential in a two-way learning process: first, so that the development of algorithms is tailored to radiologists' needs and second, so that radiologists are 'trained' in what these solutions could be able to provide. Indeed, a basic knowledge of the functioning of machine/deep learning systems could be important for a successful adoption of automatic systems by radiologists. The integration of these tools in the workflow of radiologists is also an important research line where, for instance, the combination of eyetracking tools and deep learning-based lung nodule detection approaches could be used for a greater symbiosis between automatic methods and radiologists as already shown in literature [59, 60], but also as a learning tool for medical students and radiology interns. Furthermore, and particularly for end-to-end patient-level decision systems, CADs should be able to transmit to the user the reasoning behind the decision. Without this ability, radiologists' trust in these algorithms can quickly degrade, and examples where the algorithm inexplicably fails in a single seemingly simple case (such as missing a particularly large nodule) can effectively prevent a CAD system from being adopted independently of its performance at a population level. Researchers should thus place an additional importance in adding explainability and/or uncertainty mechanisms to their algorithms, as that may prove essential for a successful incorporation of CAD systems in clinical practice.

Finally, extensive validation of these algorithms must be conducted to ensure that they serve the purpose for which they were designed and catastrophic failure upon deployment is avoided. As mentioned earlier in this section, data from multiple centers, equipments, annotators and populations should be used, particularly for deep learning solutions that are prone to dataset bias. Furthermore, future approaches should consider more detailed validation to ensure that performance is stable throughout different data and nodule types. For instance, the reporting of nodule detection or segmentation mechanisms should go beyond a unique value and ensure that performance is robust to size, nodule texture (solid versus sub-solid), location (isolated vrsus juxta-pleural) and other factors.

It is the authors' belief that, if properly designed and planned, future solutions will pave the way for adoption of CAD in lung cancer screening and the promising results obtained in literature thus far are encouraging. Nevertheless, there is still significant work ahead in improving and collecting datasets and challenges, developing algorithms that work together with radiologists and that perform full-volume analysis for patient-level long-term decisions which are explainable to human readers. In this way, future approaches designed with and for radiologists will be closer to the clinical reality from their very origin, ensuring their adoption and hopefully improving the quality of healthcare by reducing the burden on radiologists and associated costs, improving detection rates and, first and foremost, improve lung cancer patient outcomes.

References

[1] Swensen S J, Jett J R, Hartman T E, Midthun D E, Sloan J A, Sykes A-M, Aughenbaugh G L and Clemens M A 2003 Lung cancer screening with CT: Mayo Clinic experience *Radiology* **226** 756–61

[2] Bach P B *et al* 2012 Benefits and harms of CT screening for lung cancer *JAMA* **307** 2418–29

[3] Larke F J, Kruger R L, Cagnon C H, Flynn M J, McNitt-Gray M M, Wu X, Judy P F and Cody D D 2011 Estimated radiation dose associated with low-dose chest CT of average-size participants in the National Lung Screening Trial *Am. J. Roentgenol.* **197** 1165–9

[4] Holmes E J, Forrest-Hay A C and Misra R R 2008 *Interpretation of Emergency Head CT.* (Cambridge: Cambridge University Press)

[5] Drew T, Vo M L-H, Olwal A, Jacobson F, Seltzer S E and Wolfe J M 2013 Scanners and drillers: characterizing expert visual search through volumetric images *J. Vision* **13** 3

[6] Diaz I, Schmidt S, Verdun F R and Bochud F O 2015 Eye-tracking of nodule detection in lung CT volumetric data *Med. Phys.* **42** 2925–32

[7] Krupinski E A 2010 Current perspectives in medical image perception *Attent. Percept. Psychophys.* **72** 1205–17

[8] Brunyé T T, Nallamothu B K and Elmore J G 2019 Eye-tracking for assessing medical image interpretation: a pilot feasibility study comparing novice vs expert cardiologists *Perspect. Med. Educ.* **8** 65–73

[9] van Ginneken B *et al* 2010 Comparing and combining algorithms for computer-aided detection of pulmonary nodules in computed tomography scans: the ANODE09 study *Med. Image Anal.* **14** 707–22

[10] McNitt-Gray M F *et al* 2007 The Lung Image Database Consortium (LIDC) data collection process for nodule detection and annotation *Acad. Radiol.* **14** 1464–74

[11] Erasmus J J, Connolly J E, McAdams H P and Roggli V L 2000 Solitary pulmonary nodules: Part I. Morphologic evaluation for differentiation of benign and malignant lesions *Radiographics* **20** 43–58

[12] American College of Radiology 2019 *Lung-RADS Assessment Criteria* https://acr.org/Clinical-Resources/Reporting-and-Data-Systems/Lung-Rads
[13] MacMahon H *et al* 2017 Guidelines for management of incidental pulmonary nodules detected on CT images: from the Fleischner Society 2017 *Radiology* **284** 228–43
[14] Callister M, Baldwin D, Akram A, Barnard S, Cane P, Draffan J, Franks K, Gleeson F, Graham R and Malhotra P *et al* 2015 British Thoracic Society guidelines for the investigation and management of pulmonary nodules: accredited by NICE *Thorax* **70** ii1–54
[15] Matsumoto S, Ohno Y, Aoki T, Yamagata H, Nogami M, Matsumoto K, Yamashita Y and Sugimura K 2013 Computer-aided detection of lung nodules on multi-detector CT in concurrent-reader and second-reader modes: a comparative study *Eur. J. Radiol.* **82** 1332–7
[16] Wormanns D, Ludwig K, Beyer F, Heindel W and Diederich S 2005 Detection of pulmonary nodules at multirow-detector CT: effectiveness of double reading to improve sensitivity at standard-dose and low-dose chest CT *Eur. Radiol.* **15** 14–22
[17] Wang Y *et al* 2012 No benefit for consensus double reading at baseline screening for lung cancer with the use of semi-automated volumetry software *Radiology* **262** 320–6
[18] National Center for Biotechnology Information 2020 PubMed https://pubmed.ncbi.nlm.nih.gov/
[19] Setio A A A *et al* 2017 Validation, comparison, and combination of algorithms for automatic detection of pulmonary nodules in computed tomography images: the LUNA16 challenge *Med. Image Anal.* **42** 1–13
[20] Hamilton B 2017 Data Science Bowl 2017 https://kaggle.com/c/data-science-bowl-2017
[21] Pedrosa J, Aresta G, Ferreira C, Atwal G, Phoulady H A, Chen X, Chen R, Li J, Wang L and Galdran A *et al* 2021 LNDb challenge on automatic lung cancer patient management *Med. Image Anal.* **70** 102027
[22] Dehmeshki J, Ye X, Lin X, Valdivieso M and Amin H 2007 Automated detection of lung nodules in CT images using shape-based genetic algorithm *Comput. Med. Imaging Graph.* **31** 408–17
[23] Enquobahrie A A, Reeves A P, Yankelevitz D F and Henschke C I 2007 Automated detection of small pulmonary nodules in whole lung CT scans *Acad. Radiol.* **14** 579–93
[24] Hirose T, Nitta N, Shiraishi J, Nagatani Y, Takahashi M and Murata K 2008 Evaluation of Computer-aided Diagnosis (CAD) software for the detection of lung nodules on Multidetector Row Computed Tomography (MDCT). JAFROC study for the improvement in radiologists' diagnostic accuracy *Acad. Radiol.* **15** 1505–12
[25] Li Q, Li F and Doi K 2008 Computerized detection of lung nodules in thin-section CT images by use of selective enhancement filters and an automated rule-based classifier *Acad. Radiol.* **15** 165–75
[26] Golosio B *et al* 2009 A novel multithreshold method for nodule detection in lung CT *Med. Phys.* **36** 3607
[27] Murphy K, van Ginneken B, Schilham A, de Hoop B, Gietema H and Prokop M 2009 A largescale evaluation of automatic pulmonary nodule detection in chest CT using local image features and k-nearest-neighbour classification *Med. Image Anal.* **13** 757–70
[28] Retico A, Fantacci M E, Gori I, Kasae P, Golosio B, Piccioli A, Cerello P, Nunzio G D and Tangaro S 2009 Pleural nodule identification in low-dose and thin-slice lung computed tomography *Comput. Biol. Med.* **39** 1137–44

[29] Súarez-Cuenca J J, Tahoces P G, Souto M, Lado M J, Remy-Jardin M, Remy J and Vidal J J 2009 Application of the iris filter for automatic detection of pulmonary nodules on computed tomography images *Comput. Biol. Med.* **39** 921–33

[30] da Silva Sousa J R F, Silva A C, de Paiva A C and Nunes R A 2010 Methodology for automatic detection of lung nodules in computerized tomography images *Comput. Methods Programs Biomed.* **98** 1–14

[31] Tan M, Deklerck R, Jansen B, Bister M and Cornelis J 2011 A novel computer-aided lung nodule detection system for CT images *Med. Phys.* **38** 5630

[32] Cascio D, Magro R, Fauci F, Iacomi M and Raso G 2012 Automatic detection of lung nodules in CT datasets based on stable 3D mass–spring models *Comput. Biol. Med.* **42** 1098–109

[33] Teramoto A and Fujita H 2013 Fast lung nodule detection in chest CT images using cylindrical nodule-enhancement filter *Int. J. Comput. Assist. Radiol. Surg* **8** 193–205

[34] Brown M S, Lo P, Goldin J G, Barnoy E, Kim G H J, McNitt-Gray M F and Aberle D R 2014 Toward clinically usable CAD for lung cancer screening with computed tomography *Eur. Radiol.* **24** 2719–28

[35] de Carvalho Filho A O, de Sampaio W B, Silva A C, de Paiva A C, Nunes R A and Gattass M 2014 Automatic detection of solitary lung nodules using quality threshold clustering, genetic algorithm and diversity index *Artif. Intell. Med.* **60** 165–77

[36] Choi W-J and Choi T-S 2014 Automated pulmonary nodule detection based on three-dimensional shape-based feature descriptor *Comput. Methods Programs Biomed.* **113** 37–54

[37] Jacobs C *et al* 2014 Automatic detection of sub-solid pulmonary nodules in thoracic computed tomography images *Med. Image Anal.* **18** 374–84

[38] Santos A M, De Carvalho Filho A O, Silva A C, De Paiva A C, Nunes R A and Gattass M 2014 Automatic detection of small lung nodules in 3D CT data using Gaussian mixture models, Tsallis entropy and SVM *Eng. Appl. Artif. Intell.* **36** 27–39

[39] Lopez Torres E, Fiorina E, Pennazio F, Peroni C, Saletta M, Camarlinghi N, Fantacci M E and Cerello P 2015 Large scale validation of the M5L lung CAD on heterogeneous CT datasets *Med. Phys.* **42** 1477–89

[40] Setio A A A, Jacobs C, Gelderblom J and Van Ginneken B 2015 Automatic detection of large pulmonary solid nodules in thoracic CT images *Med. Phys.* **42** 5642–53

[41] van Ginneken B, Setio A A A, Jacobs C and Ciompi F 2015 Off-the-shelf convolutional neural network features for pulmonary nodule detection in computed tomography scans *2015 IEEE 12th Int. Symp. on Biomedical Imaging (ISBI)* (Piscataway, NJ: IEEE) **4** pp 286–9

[42] Wang B, Tian X, Wang Q, Yang Y, Xie H, Zhang S and Gu L 2015 Pulmonary nodule detection in CT images based on shape constraint CV model *Med. Phys.* **42** 1241–54

[43] Setio A A A, Ciompi F, Litjens G, Gerke P, Jacobs C, Van Riel S J, Winkler Wille M M, Naqibullah M, Sánchez C I and Van Ginneken B 2016 Pulmonary nodule detection in CT images: false positive reduction using multi-view convolutional networks *IEEE Trans. Med. Imaging* **35** 1160–9

[44] Ding J, Li A, Hu Z and Wang L 2017 Accurate pulmonary nodule detection in computed tomography images using deep convolutional neural networks *Int. Conf. on Medical Image Computing and Computer-Assisted Intervention* (Berlin: Springer) pp 559–67

[45] Dou Q, Chen H, Yu L, Qin J and Heng P A 2016 Multi-level contextual 3D CNNs for false positive reduction in pulmonary nodule detection *IEEE Trans. Biomed. Eng.* **PP** 1558–67

[46] Aresta G, Araújo T, Jacobs C, van Ginneken B, Cunha A, Ramos I and Campilho A 2018 Towards an automatic lung cancer screening system in low dose computed tomography *Image Analysis for Moving Organ, Breast, and Thoracic Images* (Berlin: Springer) pp 310–18

[47] Zheng S, Guo J, Cui X, Veldhuis R N, Oudkerk M and Van Ooijen P M 2020 Automatic pulmonary nodule detection in CT scans using convolutional neural networks based on maximum intensity projection *IEEE Trans. Med. Imaging* **39** 797–805

[48] Kaluva K C, Vaidhya K, Chunduru A, Tarai S, Nadimpalli S P P and Vaidya S 2020 An automated workflow for lung nodule follow-up recommendation using deep learning *Int. Conf. on Image Analysis and Recognition* (Berlin: Springer) pp 369–77

[49] Katz O, Presil D, Cohen L, Schwartzbard Y, Hoch S and Kashani S 2020 Pulmonary-nodule detection using an ensemble of 3D SE-ResNet18 and DPN68 models *Image Analysis and Recognition* ed A Campilho, F Karray and Z Wang (Cham: Springer Int. Publishing) pp 378–85

[50] Messay T, Hardie R C and Rogers S K 2010 A new computationally efficient CAD system for pulmonary nodule detection in CT imagery *Med. Image Anal.* **14** 390–406

[51] Ciompi F, Jacobs C, Scholten E T, Wille M M W, de Jong P A, Prokop M and van Ginneken B 2015 Bag-of-frequencies: a descriptor of pulmonary nodules in computed tomography images *IEEE Trans. Med. Imaging* **34** 962–73

[52] Li Q, Sone S and Doi K 2003 Selective enhancement filters for nodules, vessels, and airway walls in two- and three-dimensional CT scans *Med. Phys.* **30** 2040

[53] Chan T F and Vese L A 2001 Active contours without edges *IEEE Trans. Image Process.* **10** 266–77

[54] Han H, Li L, Han F, Song B, Moore W and Liang Z 2015 Fast and adaptive detection of pulmonary nodules in thoracic CT images using a hierarchical vector quantization scheme *IEEE J. Biomed. Health Inform.* **19** 648–59

[55] Cao P, Liu X, Zhang J, Zhao D, Huang M and Zaiane O 2017 '2,1 norm regularized multi-kernel based joint nonlinear feature selection and over-sampling for imbalanced data classification *Neurocomputing* **234** 38–57

[56] Ronneberger O, Fischer P and Brox T 2015 U-net: convolutional networks for biomedical image segmentation *Medical Image Computing and Computer-Assisted Intervention - MICCAI 2015* (Lecture Notes in Computer Science (including subseries Lecture Notes in Artificial Intelligence and Lecture Notes in Bioinformatics) vol 9351 (Berlin: Springer) **9351** 234–41

[57] Ren S, He K, Girshick R and Sun J 2017 Faster R-CNN: towards real-time object detection with region proposal networks *IEEE Trans. Pattern Anal. Mach. Intell.* **39** 1137–49

[58] Redmon J and Farhadi A 2017 YOLO9000: better, faster, stronger *Proc. of the IEEE Conf. on Computer Vision and Pattern Recognition* 7263–71

[59] Khosravan N, Celik H, Turkbey B, Jones E C, Wood B and Bagci U 2019 A collaborative computer aided diagnosis (C-CAD) system with eye-tracking, sparse attentional model, and deep learning *Med. Image Anal.* **51** 101–15

[60] Aresta G *et al* 2020 Automatic lung nodule detection combined with gaze information improves radiologists' screening performance *IEEE J. Biomed. Health Inform* **24** 2894–901

[61] Bertels J, Eelbode T, Berman M, Vandermeulen D, Maes F, Bisschops R and Blaschko M B 2019 Optimizing the dice score and jaccard index for medical image segmentation: theory and practice *Int. Conf. on Medical Image Computing and Computer-Assisted Intervention* (Berlin: Springer) pp 92–100

[62] Huttenlocher D P, Klanderman G A and Rucklidge W J 1993 Comparing images using the Hausdorff distance *IEEE Trans. Pattern Anal. Mach. Intell.* **15** 850–63

[63] Aresta G, Jacobs C, Araújo T, Cunha A, Ramos I, van Ginneken B and Campilho A 2019 iW-Net: an automatic and minimalistic interactive lung nodule segmentation deep network *Sci. Rep.* **9** 1–9

[64] Ye X, Beddoe G and Slabaugh G 2010 Automatic graph cut segmentation of lesions in CT using mean shift superpixels *Int. J. Biomed. Imaging* **2010** 983963

[65] Tan Y, Schwartz L H and Zhao B 2013 Segmentation of lung lesions on CT scans using watershed, active contours, and Markov random field *Med. Phys.* **40** 043502

[66] Messay T, Hardie R C and Tuinstra T R 2015 Segmentation of pulmonary nodules in computed tomography using a regression neural network approach and its application to the Lung Image Database Consortium and Image Database Resource Initiative dataset *Med. Image Anal.* **22** 48–62

[67] Zhao J-J, Ji G H, Xia Y and Zhang X L 2015 Cavitary nodule segmentation in computed tomography images based on self–generating neural networks and particle swarm optimisation *Int. J. Bio-Inspir. Com.* **7** 62–7

[68] Gonçalves L, Novo J and Campilho A 2016 Hessian based approaches for 3D lung nodule segmentation *Expert Syst. Appl.* **61** 1–15

[69] Feng X, Yang J, Laine A F and Angelini E D 2017 Discriminative localization in cnns for weakly-supervised segmentation of pulmonary nodules *Int. Conf. on Medical Image Computing and Computer-Assisted Intervention* (Berlin: Springer) pp 568–76

[70] Wang S, Zhou M, Liu Z, Liu Z, Gu D, Zang Y, Dong D, Gevaert O and Tian J 2017 Central focused convolutional neural networks: developing a data-driven model for lung nodule segmentation *Med. Image Anal.* **40** 172–83

[71] Jung J, Hong H and Goo J M 2018 Ground-glass nodule segmentation in chest CT images using asymmetric multi-phase deformable model and pulmonary vessel removal *Comput. Biol. Med.* **92** 128–38

[72] Tong G, Li Y, Chen H, Zhang Q and Jiang H 2018 Improved U-Net network for pulmonary nodules segmentation *Optik* **174** 460–9

[73] Wang W, Lu Y, Wu B, Chen T, Chen D Z and Wu J 2018 Deep active self-paced learning for accurate pulmonary nodule segmentation *Int. Conf. on Medical Image Computing and Computer-Assisted Intervention* (Berlin: Springer) pp 723–31

[74] Wu B, Zhou Z, Wang J and Wang Y 2018 Joint learning for pulmonary nodule segmentation, attributes and malignancy prediction *2018 IEEE 15th Int. Symp. on Biomedical Imaging (ISBI 2018)* (Piscataway, NJ: IEEE) pp 1109–113

[75] Huang X, Sun W, Tseng T-L B, Li C and Qian W 2019 Fast and fully-automated detection and segmentation of pulmonary nodules in thoracic CT scans using deep convolutional neural networks *Comput. Med. Imaging Graph.* **74** 25–36

[76] Atwal G and Phoulady H A 2020 Automatic lung cancer follow-up recommendation with 3D deep learning *Int. Conf. on Image Analysis and Recognition* (Berlin: Springer) pp 406–18

[77] Cao H, Liu H, Song E, Hung C-C, Ma G, Xu X, Jin R and Lu J 2020 Dual-branch residual network for lung nodule segmentation *Appl. Soft Comput.* **86** 105934

[78] Dong X, Xu S, Liu Y, Wang A, Saripan M I, Li L, Zhang X and Lu L 2020 Multi-view secondary input collaborative deep learning for lung nodule 3D segmentation *Cancer Imag.* **20** 1–13

[79] Galdran A and Bouchachia H 2020 Residual networks for pulmonary nodule segmentation and texture characterization *Int. Conf. on Image Analysis and Recognition* (Berlin: Springer) pp 396–405
[80] Rassadin A 2020 Deep residual 3D U-Net for joint segmentation and texture classification of nodules in lung *Int. Conf. on Image Analysis and Recognition* (Berlin: Springer) pp 419–27
[81] Rocha J, Cunha A and Mendonça A M 2020 Conventional filtering versus U-Net based models for pulmonary nodule segmentation in CT images *J. Med. Syst.* **44** 1–8
[82] Shi H, Lu J and Zhou Q 2020 A novel data augmentation method using style-based GAN for robust pulmonary nodule segmentation *2020 Chinese Control And Decision Conf. (CCDC)* (Piscataway, NJ: IEEE) pp 2486–91
[83] Tian Z, Jia Y, Men X and Sun Z 2020 3DCNN for pulmonary nodule segmentation and classification *Int. Conf. on Image Analysis and Recognition* (Berlin: Springer) pp 386–95
[84] Usman M, Lee B-D, Byon S-S, Kim S-H, Lee B I and Shin Y-G 2020 Volumetric lung nodule segmentation using adaptive ROI with multi-view residual learning *Sci. Rep.* **10** 1–15
[85] Wu W, Gao L, Duan H, Huang G, Ye X and Nie S 2020 Segmentation of pulmonary nodules in CT images based on 3D-UNet combined with three-dimensional conditional random field optimization *Med. Phys.* **47** 4054–63
[86] Mukhopadhyay S 2016 A segmentation framework of pulmonary nodules in lung CT images *J. Digital Imaging.* **29** 86–103
[87] Kalpathy-Cramer J, Zhao B, Goldgof D, Gu Y, Wang X, Yang H, Tan Y, Gillies R and Napel S 2016 A comparison of lung nodule segmentation algorithms: methods and results from a multi-institutional study *J. Digital Imaging* **29** 476–87
[88] Kubota T, Jerebko A K, Dewan M, Salganicoff M and Krishnan A 2011 Segmentation of pulmonary nodules of various densities with morphological approaches and convexity models *Med. Image Anal.* **15** 133–54
[89] Lassen B C, Jacobs C, Kuhnigk J M, Van Ginneken B and Van Rikxoort E M 2015 Robust semi-automatic segmentation of pulmonary sub-solid nodules in chest computed tomography scans *Phys. Med. Biol.* **60** 1307–23
[90] Moltz J H, Bornemann L, Kuhnigk J-M, Dicken V, Peitgen E, Meier S, Bolte H, Fabel M, Bauknecht H-C and Hittinger M *et al* 2009 Advanced segmentation techniques for lung nodules, liver metastases, and enlarged lymph nodes in CT scans *IEEE J. Sel. Top. Signal Process.* **3** 122–34
[91] Awad J, Owrangi A, Villemaire L, O'Riordan E, Parraga G and Fenster A 2012 Three-dimensional lung tumor segmentation from x-ray computed tomography using sparse field active models *Med. Phys.* **39** 851–65
[92] Farag A A, Abd El Munim H E, Graham J H and Farag A A 2013 A novel approach for lung nodules segmentation in chest CT using level sets *IEEE Trans. Image Process.* **22** 5202–13
[93] Çiçek O, Abdulkadir A, Lienkamp S S, Brox T and Ronneberger O 2016 3D U-Net: learning dense volumetric segmentation from sparse annotation *Medical Image Computing and Computer-Assisted Intervention—MICCAI 2016* ed S Ourselin, L Joskowicz, M R Sabuncu, G Unal and W Wells (Cham: Springer) pp 424–32
[94] Zinovev D, Feigenbaum J, Furst J and Raicu D 2011 Probabilistic lung nodule classification with belief decision trees *2011 Annual Int. Conf. of the IEEE Engineering in Medicine and Biology Society* (Piscataway, NJ: IEEE) pp 4493–8

[95] Chen H, Wu W, Xia H, Du J, Yang M and Ma B 2011 Classification of pulmonary nodules using neural network ensemble *Int. Symp. on Neural Networks* (Berlin: Springer) pp 460–6

[96] Han F, Wang H, Zhang G, Han H, Song B, Li L, Moore W, Lu H, Zhao H and Liang Z 2015 Texture feature analysis for computer-aided diagnosis on pulmonary nodules *J. Digital Imaging* **28** 99–115

[97] Buty M, Xu Z, Gao M, Bagci U, Wu A and Mollura D J 2016 Characterization of lung nodule malignancy using hybrid shape and appearance features *Int. Conf. on Medical Image Computing and Computer-Assisted Intervention* (Berlin: Springer) pp 662–70

[98] Chen S, Qin J, Ji X, Lei B, Wang T, Ni D and Cheng J-Z 2016 Automatic scoring of multiple semantic attributes with multi-task feature leverage: a study on pulmonary nodules in CT images *IEEE Trans. Med. Imaging* **36** 802–14

[99] Shen W, Zhou M, Yang F, Yu D, Dong D, Yang C, Zang Y and Tian J 2017 Multi-crop convolutional neural networks for lung nodule malignancy suspiciousness classification *Pattern Recognit.* **61** 663–73

[100] Sun W, Zheng B and Qian W 2017 Automatic feature learning using multichannel ROI based on deep structured algorithms for computerized lung cancer diagnosis *Comput. Biol. Med.* **89** 530–39

[101] Song Q, Zhao L, Luo X and Dou X 2017 Using deep learning for classification of lung nodules on computed tomography images *J. Healthcare Eng.* **2017** 8314740

[102] Hussein S, Cao K, Song Q and Bagci U 2017 Risk stratification of lung nodules using 3D CNN-based multi-task learning *Int. conference on information processing in medical imaging* (Berlin: Springer) pp 249–60

[103] Liu K and Kang G 2017 Multi-view convolutional neural networks for lung nodule classification *Int. J. Imaging Syst. Technol.* **27** 12–22

[104] Kang G, Liu K, Hou B and Zhang N 2017 3D multi-view convolutional neural networks for lung nodule classification *PLoS One* **12** e0188290

[105] Xie Y, Xia Y, Zhang J, Feng D D, Fulham M and Cai W 2017 Transferable multi-model ensemble for benign-malignant lung nodule classification on chest CT *Int. Conf. on Medical Image Computing and Computer-Assisted Intervention* (Berlin: Springer) pp 656–64

[106] Gonçalves L, Novo J, Cunha A and Campilho A 2018 Learning lung nodule malignancy likelihood from radiologist annotations or diagnosis data *J. Med. Biol. Eng.* **38** 424–42

[107] Wei G, Ma H, Qian W, Han F, Jiang H, Qi S and Qiu M 2018 Lung nodule classification using local kernel regression models with out-of-sample extension *Biomed. Signal Process. Control* **40** 1–9

[108] Dey R, Lu Z and Hong Y 2018 Diagnostic classification of lung nodules using 3D neural networks *2018 IEEE 15th int. symposium on biomedical imaging (ISBI 2018)* (Piscataway, NJ: IEEE) pp 774–8

[109] da Nóbrega R V M, Rebouças Filho P P, Rodrigues M B, da Silva S P, Junior C M D and de Albuquerque V H C 2018 Lung nodule malignancy classification in chest computed tomography images using transfer learning and convolutional neural networks *Neural Comput. Appl.* **32** 11065–82

[110] Dai Y, Yan S, Zheng B and Song C 2018 Incorporating automatically learned pulmonary nodule attributes into a convolutional neural network to improve accuracy of benign-malignant nodule classification *Phys. Med. Biol.* **63** 245004

[111] Shen S, Han S, Aberle D, Bui A and Hsu W 2019 An interpretable deep hierarchical semantic convolutional neural network for lung nodule malignancy classification *Expert Syst. Appl.* **128** 84–95
[112] Wang Q, Zhou X, Wang C, Liu Z, Huang J, Zhou Y, Li C, Zhuang H and Cheng J-Z 2019 WGAN-based synthetic minority over-sampling technique: improving semantic fine-grained classification for lung nodules in CT images *IEEE Access* **7** 18450–63
[113] Liu L, Dou Q, Chen H, Qin J and Heng P-A 2019 Multi-task deep model with margin ranking loss for lung nodule analysis *IEEE Trans. Med. Imaging* **39** 718–28
[114] Xiao N, Qiang Y, Bilal Zia M, Wang S and Lian J 2020 Ensemble classification for predicting the malignancy level of pulmonary nodules on chest computed tomography images *Oncol. Lett.* **20** 401–8
[115] Veasey B, Farhangi M M, Frigui H, Broadhead J, Dahle M, Pezeshk A, Seow A and Amini A A 2020 Lung nodule malignancy classification based on NLSTx data *2020 IEEE 17th Int. Symp. on Biomedical Imaging (ISBI)* (Piscataway, NJ: IEEE) pp 1870–4
[116] Wang W, Chakraborty G and Chakraborty B 2020 3D multi-scale DenseNet for malignancy grade classification of pulmonary nodules *2020 11th Int. Conf. on Awareness Science and Technology (iCAST)* (Piscataway, NJ: IEEE) pp 1–4
[117] Jacobs C, van Rikxoort E M, Scholten E T, de Jong P A, Prokop M, Schaefer-Prokop C and van Ginneken B 2015 Solid, part-solid, or non-solid?: classification of pulmonary nodules in low-dose chest computed tomography by a computer-aided diagnosis system *Invest. Radiol.* **50** 168–73
[118] Niehaus R, Raicu D S, Furst J and Armato S 2015 Toward understanding the size dependence of shape features for predicting spiculation in lung nodules for computer-aided diagnosis *J. Digital Imag.* **28** 704–17
[119] Ciompi F, Chung K, Van Riel S J, Setio A A A, Gerke P K, Jacobs C, Scholten E T, Schaefer-Prokop C, Wille M M and Marchiano A *et al* 2017 Towards automatic pulmonary nodule management in lung cancer screening with deep learning *Sci. Rep.* **7** 1–11
[120] Tu X, Xie M, Gao J, Ma Z, Chen D, Wang Q, Finlayson S G, Ou Y and Cheng J-Z 2017 Automatic categorization and scoring of solid, part-solid and non-solid pulmonary nodules in CT images with convolutional neural network *Sci. Rep.* **7** 1–10
[121] Ferreira C A, Cunha A, Mendonça A M and Campilho A 2018 Convolutional neural network architectures for texture classification of pulmonary nodules *Iberoamerican Congress on Pattern Recognition.* (Berlin: Springer) pp 783–91
[122] Qiu B, Furst J, Rasin A, Tchoua R and Raicu D 2020 Learning latent spiculated features for lung nodule characterization *2020 42nd Annual Int. Conf. of the IEEE Engineering in Medicine & Biology Society (EMBC)* (Piscataway, NJ: IEEE) pp 1254–7
[123] Alakwaa W, Nassef M and Badr A 2017 Lung cancer detection and classification with 3D convolutional neural network (3D-CNN) *Lung Cancer* **8** 409
[124] Chon A, Balachandar N and Lu P 2017 Deep convolutional neural networks for lung cancer detection Standford University
[125] Tafti A P, Bashiri F S, LaRose E and Peissig P 2018 Diagnostic classification of lung CT images using deep 3D multi-scale convolutional neural network *2018 IEEE Int. Conf. on Healthcare Informatics (ICHI)* (Piscataway, NJ: IEEE) pp 412–14
[126] Ardila D, Kiraly A P, Bharadwaj S, Choi B, Reicher J J, Peng L, Tse D, Etemadi M, Ye W and Corrado G *et al* 2019 End-to-end lung cancer screening with three-dimensional deep learning on low-dose chest computed tomography *Nat. Med.* **25** 954–61

[127] Liao F, Liang M, Li Z, Hu X and Song S 2019 Evaluate the malignancy of pulmonary nodules using the 3-D deep leaky noisy-or network *IEEE Trans Neural Netw. Learn. Syst.* **30** 3484–95
[128] Ozdemir O, Russell R L and Berlin A A 2019 A 3D probabilistic deep learning system for detection and diagnosis of lung cancer using low-dose CT scans *IEEE Trans. Med. Imaging* **39** 1419–29
[129] Trajanovski S, Mavroeidis D, Swisher C L, Gebre B G, Veeling B S, Wiemker R, Klinder T, Tahmasebi A, Regis S M and Wald C *et al* 2021 Towards radiologist-level cancer risk assessment in CT lung screening using deep learning *Comput. Med. Imaging Graph.* **90** 101883
[130] Yu K-H, Lee T-L M, Yen M-H, Kou S, Rosen B, Chiang J-H and Kohane I S 2020 Reproducible machine learning methods for lung cancer detection using computed tomography images: algorithm development and validation *J. Med. Internet Res.* **22** e16709
[131] Fleiss J L, Cohen J and Everitt B S 1969 Large sample standard errors of kappa and weighted kappa. *Psycho. Bull.* **72** 323
[132] Nishio M, Sugiyama O, Yakami M, Ueno S, Kubo T, Kuroda T and Togashi K 2018 Computer-aided diagnosis of lung nodule classification between benign nodule, primary lung cancer, and metastatic lung cancer at different image size using deep convolutional neural network with transfer learning *PLoS One* **13** e0200721
[133] Ferreira C A, Aresta G, Cunha A, Mendonça A M and Campilho A 2019 Wide residual network for Lung-RADS^{TM} screening referral *2019 IEEE 6th Portuguese Meeting on Bioengineering (ENBENG)* (Piscataway, NJ: IEEE) pp 1–4
[134] Ferreira C A, Aresta G, Pedrosa J, Rebelo J, Negrão E, Cunha A, Ramos I and Campilho A 2020 Classification of lung nodules in CT volumes using the Lung-RADSTM guidelines with uncertainty parameterization *2020 IEEE 17th Int. Symp. on Biomedical Imaging (ISBI)* (Piscataway, NJ: IEEE) pp 791–4
[135] Armato S G *et al* 2011 The Lung Image Database Consortium (LIDC) and Image Database Resource Initiative (IDRI): a completed reference database of lung nodules on CT scans *Med. Phys.* **38** 915
[136] The National Lung Screening Trial Research Team 2011 Reduced lung-cancer mortality with low-dose computed tomographic screening *New Engl. J. Med.* **365** 395–409
[137] Pedrosa J *et al* 2019 LNDb: a lung nodule database on computed tomography *arXiv preprint* arXiv:1911.08434
[138] van Klaveren R J *et al* 2009 Management of lung nodules detected by volume CT scanning *New Engl. J. Med.* **361** 2221–9
[139] Kazerooni E A, Austin J H M, Black W C, Dyer D S, Hazelton T R, Leung A N, McNitt-Gray M F, Munden R F and Pipavath S 2014 ACR-STR practice parameter for the performance and reporting of lung cancer screening thoracic computed tomography (CT): 2014 (Resolution 4) *J. Thorac. Imaging* **29** 310–16
[140] Maier-Hein L, Eisenmann M, Reinke A, Onogur S, Stankovic M, Scholz P, Arbel T, Bogunovic H, Bradley A P and Carass A *et al* 2018 Why rankings of biomedical image analysis competitions should be interpreted with care *Nat. Commun.* **9** 1–13
[141] Pinheiro G, Pereira T, Dias C, Freitas C, Hespanhol V, Costa J L, Cunha A and Oliveira H P 2020 Identifying relationships between imaging phenotypes and lung cancer-related mutation status: EGFR and KRAS *Sci. Rep.* **10** 1–9

IOP Publishing

Detection Systems in Lung Cancer and Imaging, Volume 1

Ayman El-Baz and Jasjit S Suri

Chapter 5

Radiation therapy in lung cancer treatment

Mary McGunigal, Jonathan W Lischalk, Pamela Randolph-Jackson and Puja Gaur Khaitan

Radiation therapy is a core pillar of oncologic care in both curative and palliative settings. Radiation has a well-established role in treatment paradigms for lung cancer, ranging from cure of inoperable early-stage non-small cell lung cancer (NSCLC) and locally advanced disease to ameliorating symptomatology in the palliative setting for intracranial metastases and painful bone lesions [1]. The landscape of systemic agents available to patients has shifted considerably with the advent of immunotherapy; in addition there has been great progress in radiation technology that has allowed radiation to be delivered with increasingly greater precision and accuracy than ever before [2]. In both planning and delivering of therapy, radiation oncologists must balance the goals of maximizing dose to the tumor target to achieve the desired effect of cure or palliation while minimizing dose and thereby toxicity to the normal surrounding structures, known as optimization of the therapeutic window.

Despite radiation therapy being a cornerstone of a significant proportion of lung cancer patients' care, the logistics of treatment and reasoning behind radiation modality choice may at times be opaque to those outside the field of radiation oncology. In this chapter, we aim to 'demystify' radiation oncology by providing a broad overview of the fundamentals of radiation therapy for lung cancer. This will include discussion of the most common radiation modalities used to treat lung cancer and their associated acute and chronic toxicities.

Radiation therapy (RT) works by using high energy particles, such as photons (x-rays) or charged particles (for example, protons) to attack cancer cells by exacting DNA damage. Dose is prescribed in units of gray (Gy) and is selected based on several factors, including goal of treatment (i.e., curative or palliative), extent and location of disease, and radiosensitivity of the tumor histology. For instance, small cell lung cancer (SCLC) is more sensitive to radiation than NSCLC. The dose is split up into a pre-set number of daily treatments (usually over a course of weeks), termed

doi:10.1088/978-0-7503-3355-9ch5

'fractions' [3]. Delivering the total dose over the course of a number of fractions, rather than all in one session, is both safe—it allows the tissue of normal surrounding structures (termed organs at risk, or OARs) time to undergo sublethal damage repair in between fractions—and efficacious, as delivering over multiple sessions will allow tumor cells opportunities to 'cycle into' more radiosensitive phases of the cell cycle. The radiobiological trade-off, however, is that increased fractionation means a lower dose per treatment is delivered.

A firm diagnosis established via biopsy with tissue confirmation is typically a prerequisite to consideration of radiation treatment. In select cases, treatment of patients with repeated non-diagnostic biopsies may be recommended after review by a multidisciplinary team if there is consensus of appropriately high suspicion of malignant lesion with additional factors supporting a likely cancer diagnosis (smoking history, lesion size and change over time, spiculated appearance, and PET avidity) to warrant treatment. Conventional fractionation for definitive treatment of locally advanced NSCLC is typically 1.8–2 Gy daily, Monday through Friday, for 5–7 weeks, to a total dose of 60–70 Gy for locally advanced NSCLC or limited stage SCLC (LS-SCLC); 1.5 Gy delivered twice-daily to a total dose of 45 Gy for LS-SCLC may also be used. Treatments are quick (usually 15–30 min in total, including setup time) and painless and only require of the patient to lie flat and motionless; no sedation is needed. A helpful way to describe treatment to patients at initial consultation is that it will be much like undergoing a CT scan, but with a higher dose of radiation.

For locally advanced NSCLC, chemoradiation is the standard of care and the most common pattern of treatment failure is distant [4]. However, local recurrence is still a concern, highlighting the need for close monitoring with follow-up and surveillance scans and fueling investigation into dose escalation as a potential means of improving local control outcomes [5]. RTOG 0617 was a phase III trial that compared standard dose (60 Gy) with high-dose (74 Gy) radiation for stages IIIA-B NSCLC. The dose escalation arm had worse toxicity, inferior overall survival, and poorer local control rates (30.7% versus 38.6% at 2 years) [6]. Efforts are ongoing to elucidate the ideal balance of high-dose with reasonable toxicity profile, including RTOG 1106, a phase II trial which randomized 138 patients with stage III NSCLC between the standard 60 Gy versus the use of 'adaptive' radiation using PET/CT performed midway through treatment (after delivery of the first 40–46 Gy) to dose-escalate up to 80.4 Gy to a smaller, PET-avid volume [3]. Publication of results is pending, however, recent presentation of initial data revealed similar overall 2-year local-regional tumor progression-free time (27.5 months for the standard dose versus 28.4 months for the adaptive arm) albeit with a 17% difference in primary tumor control at 2 years, at the cost of higher rates of grade 2 esophagitis in the adaptive arm [7]. Further data is needed on the benefit of adaptive radiation approaches in locally advanced NSCLC, and per current consensus guidelines, dose escalation beyond the standard should be avoided, especially in patients that are already very frail from a cardiopulmonary standpoint [3].

Radiation therapy is considered a local treatment and in this sense is more akin to surgery, another local therapy, as opposed to chemotherapy. Radiation 'fields' (i.e., the area of the body where the radiation will be delivered) for lung cancer were historically far larger and more generous, encompassing the mediastinum and ipsilateral hilum electively in addition to covering the area involved by the primary tumor. Modern practice guidelines recommend omission of any elective coverage of the mediastinum and do not recommend any elective nodal irradiation (ENI) as there is presently no strong data to support its use [3, 8, 9]. The standard of care is to cover the primary tumor and any nodal areas positive on pre-treatment staging (including PET/CT) [8]. This enables safe dose escalation with improved normal tissue-sparing of smaller fields. Adjuvant, or post-operative radiation therapy (PORT) is generally indicated for positive margins and N2 disease, however, the initial results of the LungART trial have challenged the role of PORT in N2 disease as no disease-free survival benefit was demonstrated in completely resected stage IIIA NSCLC; however, final publication of results of this trial is pending [3, 10].

Development of clinical radiation therapy occurred rather rapidly after the discovery of x-rays in 1895 by German physicist Wilhelm Conrad Roentgen—a revolutionary breakthrough for the fields of both physics and medicine which would earn him the first Nobel Prize for Physics in 1901; just weeks later, they were used therapeutically to treat an ulcerated breast tumor [11]. It was not until the 1950s that radiation was used to cure lung cancer [12]. Modern radiotherapy in concert with imaging techniques have come a long way since the pre-CT era—which consisted of planning based on 2D x-rays using bony landmarks as guideposts and hand-drawn blocking—and has evolved to include not only routine use of CT scanning for treatment planning (often with the additional assistance of PET/CT and MRI scans) but also computerized 3D reconstructions of images and optimization algorithms [13].

External beam radiation therapy (EBRT) is the most common form of radiation delivered to treat lung cancer. It is delivered externally from a machine source termed a linear accelerator (LINAC) or particle accelerator. High energy rays ('beams') are aimed and delivered at various angles to travel to and deposit dose at the tumor target. The beam emerges from a part of the LINAC termed the 'gantry' which can rotate around the patient. EBRT has advanced from simple two-dimensional (2D) radiotherapy—which aimed single beams arranged from one to four different directions (for instance, two opposed lateral beams or four-field 'boxes' comprised of AP/PA and opposed laterals)—to 3D conformal, CT-based planning. In the early days of radiation oncology, beams simply matched the height and width of the tumor, thereby exposing large swaths of adjacent healthy tissue to radiation. Routine use of blocks was later incorporated to improve precision of the field shape; molten metal (Cerrobend) blocks were designed, custom-poured and then mounted on the gantry to sculpt the radiation beam shape to match that of the target [13]. By the 1980s, CT-based treatment planning became standard as did the use of multileaf collimators (MLCs), small metallic leaves built into the collimator of each LINAC that continuously move to alter the field shape during treatment and replaced the far most time-consuming and labor intensive Cerrobend blocks (which had to be custom-made and manually installed for each patient's treatments) [13]. 3D conformal radiation therapy (3D-CRT), which involves drawing out treatment volumes on a computer using a planning CT as a template, became widely accepted by the late 1990s [14].

A critical first step in any EBRT treatment is a CT simulation, which means obtaining a CT scan to be used as a template for treatment planning. Appropriate superior and inferior anatomical borders for scanning are selected and the patient is scanned in a position which they will replicate for daily treatments (for lung cancer patients, this typically means supine with arms up), and depending on the location of the treatment volume, different devices may be used to immobilize the patient. Radiation oncologists will then 'contour' the intended target volumes as well as OARs on the planning CT scan, axial slice by slice. This is performed with planning software and then beams will be designed to conform to the physician's contours. Simulation scans are typically fused with relevant prior scans (for example PET/CT) that may aid in guiding accurate target volume delineation. Once contours are complete, physicians collaborate with physicists and dosimetrists to use computer optimization algorithms in creating beam arrangements and a finalized plan to maximize dose coverage to the target volumes as while keeping dose to the OARs as low as is feasible.

Intensity-modulated radiation therapy (IMRT) is a distinct treatment technique which came about after the genesis of 3D-CRT. As in 3D-CRT, the tumor and OARs are contoured on the planning scan, however, there is an even greater degree of conformality achieved with the added step of 'modulating' the intensity of the beam across the field such that it is non-uniform. While 3D-CRT relies upon forward planning, IMRT uses 'inverse planning' where the desired dose objectives and constraints and their respective priority levels are fed into the computer and then optimization algorithms work to create a plan that will meet all pre-designated objectives. [15]. This garners improved conformality with decreased dose to OARs and translates to clinical benefit of reduced toxicity as a result of the improved dose-sparing. IMRT technique became standard of care for locally advanced NSCLC managed with definitive chemoradiation after a secondary analysis of NRG Oncology/ RTOG 0617 by Chun *et al* demonstrated IMRT is associated with lower rates of Grade 3+ pneumonitis along with decreased heart dose compared to 3D-CRT [16].

With decreased toxicity from more conformal treatment, there is the added potential advantage of widening the therapeutic window of safer dose escalation to improve outcomes of local control. Volumetric modulated arc therapy (VMAT), an IMRT technique first introduced in 2007, is a form of rotational delivery where radiation is given with both MLCs and the gantry, the main body of the LINAC, in motion as the radiation source rotates around the patient during treatment [17]. While VMAT reduces overall treatment time, which theoretically could be beneficial in minimizing the patient's respiratory variation, studies in NSCLC reveal no clear advantage of one IMRT technique over another [17]. Further, the dosimetric advantages of IMRT are especially advantageous in the setting of certain cases, including larger tumors, tumors with bilateral mediastinal involvement, tumors adjacent to an OAR (for example, abutting the spinal cord) or in patients with extensive pre-existing comorbidities, all scenarios where maximizing treatment conformality is crucial [14, 16].

Stereotactic body radiation therapy (SBRT) is a newer form of EBRT used in the treatment of both primary tumor and metastatic lesions in lung, among many other, cancers. SBRT employs larger doses of radiation than conventional long-course EBRT in far fewer fractions (typically 1–5) and is termed 'stereotactic' for its emphasis on image guidance to localize tumors and thereby treat with ultra-precise beams and sharp dose fall-off gradient [18]. Similar to other forms of EBRT, it is delivered with use of both tumor motion management strategies and reliance on daily imaging for setup verification [19]. Image guidance is critical in any radiation modality, as thoracic tumors are particularly susceptible to respiratory motion. There are two categories of motion to contend with: intrafraction motion (changes in the position of the target volume during the actual delivery of the radiation treatment) and interfraction motion (day-to-day differences in the target position between fractions due to differences in patient setup) [20]. After the gross tumor is contoured, a small expansion is placed on to account for such motion uncertainties, although this treatment planning practice of adding margin is not unique to SBRT treatment [21].

One common motion management strategy is obtaining a 4D CT scan (the '4th dimension' is time), in which an infrared camera tracks the movement of a reflective marker to measure phases of the respiratory cycle [21]. Multiple discrete 3D CT scans are then reconstructed to create a 'movie' of the respiratory cycle which will capture the entire path of the tumor throughout such that contours can be created to encompass the tumor regardless of the phase of respiratory cycle it is treated in [22]. Another method, called respiratory 'gating' utilizes a computer software to activate and deactivate treatment based on tumor position. In other words, when the tumor enters a pre-specified region, the 'gate' is opened the beam is turned on, and when the tumor exits that region, the x-rays are turned off [23].

There are also a number of methods used for tumor tracking, including routine use of daily on-board imaging. In lung SBRT, this is often aided by placing intralesional fiducials—gold markers—that are used as guideposts to verify accurate patient setup prior to treatment, to ensure precise delivery of radiation [24]. This can allow for reduced treatment margins and obviate the need for patient immobilization devices as compared to other LINAC-based SBRT approaches [25]. Although patients are often staged with PET/CT and biopsy alone prior to SBRT, at many institutions nodal staging (usually performed via bronchoscopy) is also routinely performed prior to radiation, with fiducial placement done at the same time as mediastinal nodal sampling. Long-term data from our own institutional experience has demonstrated this method of fiducial placement for tumor tracking to have clinically comparable outcomes to other LINAC-based SBRT approaches in terms of local control, locoregional control, and overall survival [25].

Unlike in conventionally fractionated therapy, where radiation is typically delivered in small doses over several weeks, SBRT is comprised of higher doses of radiation delivered over 1–5 fractions which equates to biologically effective doses higher than 100 Gy in conventional 2 Gy fractions [26, 27]. Data from both phase II single institution trials and matched cohort studies support SBRT as a non-surgical option for cure of early-stage inoperable NSCLC and local control rates exceed 90% with minimal pulmonary toxicity [28, 29]. However, distant failure remains a concern. Randomized controlled trials are currently ongoing to investigate the question of whether benefit may be gleaned from the addition of systemic therapy following SBRT in this setting, to mitigate this risk. Given the decrease in metastatic progression seen with the addition of immunotherapy in stage III NSCLC, there is intense interest in whether immunotherapy may hold similar promise in changing patterns of failure for stage I NSCLC [30]. Ongoing trials include PACIFIC-4, which is investigating SBRT +/– durvalumab in early-stage NSCLC and KEYNOTE-867 which is examining the addition of pembrolizumab after SBRT also in early-stage unresected NSCLC. In addition to early-stage disease, numerous trials are underway examining combination of radiation with immunotherapy in locally advanced and metastatic NSCLC.

There is a phenomenon, first described approximately 50 years ago, called the abscopal effect, and an alluring concept to many radiation oncologists in which local radiation therapy may be associated with regression of metastatic cancer distant from the irradiated site—possibly through a mechanism of aiding the immune system in recognizing and then eliminating micrometastatic disease—however, understanding of this idea is still evolving [31]. Pre-clinical studies have shown evidence of interplay between tumors and the immune system augmented by radiation. While it has been posited that the immunostimulatory properties of radiation therapy may in part account for the improved survival with SBRT demonstrated in the much-criticized STARS and ROSEL pooled analysis, this is merely speculative and as of yet, there is no randomized evidence to support practice-changing inclusion of SBRT as an option for early-stage NSCLC.

The possibility of a role for SBRT in the case of operable or borderline operable patients remains controversial. A combined analysis of the STARS and ROSEL trials revealed improved 3-year survival with SBRT over lobectomy (95% versus 79%) without a difference in recurrence free survival [32]. A caveat in interpreting this data is that both studies had very weak accrual (58 patients in total) and the 90-day mortality rate in the surgical arm was higher as compared to other studies in stage I NSCLC [32]. This question is now being further explored in multiple ongoing randomized trials including VALOR (Veterans Affairs Lung cancer surgery or stereotactic radiotherapy trial) in the United States and SABRtooth in the United Kingdom [33]. However, the current standard of care is still surgery for medically operable early-stage NSCLC patients.

Another question that has been raised is appropriate size cutoffs for lung SBRT. By definition, SBRT is only standard of care in early-stage NSCLC and for tumors larger than 5 cm, per consensus guidelines SBRT is conditionally recommended if surgery is not a possibility and an acceptable therapeutic ratio may be achieved [34]. That said, there is a dearth of high-quality randomized data to guide treatment decisions in tumors of this size as the large, multi-institutional RTOG studies only included tumors under 5 cm. There are current clinical trials underway posing the question of SBRT in larger tumors, such as the VOLUMES trial in the Netherlands, that may be able to shed additional light on this question once data has matured [34].

All forms of radiation previously discussed in this chapter are delivered by photons (x-rays). A final form of radiation therapy we will discuss is proton particle therapy. Proton beam therapy is less widely available, currently offered at 34 institutions across the United States [35]. In spite of numerous advancements in IMRT and image guidance techniques, accurate radiation delivery in lung cancer is a challenge in large part due to lung tumors' inherent nearness to multiple OARs, all of which can suffer from significant toxicity if overdosed. This is particularly true given the tenuous nature of many lung cancer patients' pre-treatment baseline cardiopulmonary function [36]. Across different disease sites, the dose of radiation needed to achieve cure can exceed the tolerance of nearby OARs. Proton beam therapy may be dosimetrically advantageous in certain scenarios as it allows for a tighter dose distribution due to the Bragg–Peak effect, such that entry dose is lower and the majority of the dose (energy) is deposited at the tumor itself, with improved sparing of OARs distal to the tumor as there is significantly less fall-off dose 'passing through' the tumor as compared to photons. Essentially, proton beam therapy enables dose distribution to occur across a much narrower range in comparison to photon therapy where dose is delivered throughout the course of the entire beam path; see figure 5.1 of proton plan versus IMRT plan for comparison of dose distribution in a lung cancer patient.

The dose-sparing properties of proton therapy may translate to clinical improvements in the form of dose escalation to tumor targets and reduced toxicity from thoracic RT [36]. Dose-sparing of OARs may be particularly useful in the case of pediatric patients, patients who have a history of prior thoracic radiation, and those with pre-existing conditions rendering them susceptible to toxicity including interstitial lung disease or autoimmune diseases with extensive skin or lung involvement. Many retrospective studies have confirmed the benefits of proton therapy over 3D-CRT and IMRT in delivering less dose to normal tissues, however, more robust high-quality data from a randomized controlled trial is needed to prove if this translates to superiority in outcomes of toxicity, survival, and local control [37]. Chang *et al* showed in a phase II trial that proton beam therapy with concurrent chemotherapy for unresectable NSCLC had encouraging clinical outcomes and reduced toxicity compared to historical controls of photon therapy data—while such data is promising, additional phase III studies are needed to establish and clarify the benefits of proton therapy in lung cancer patients [38].

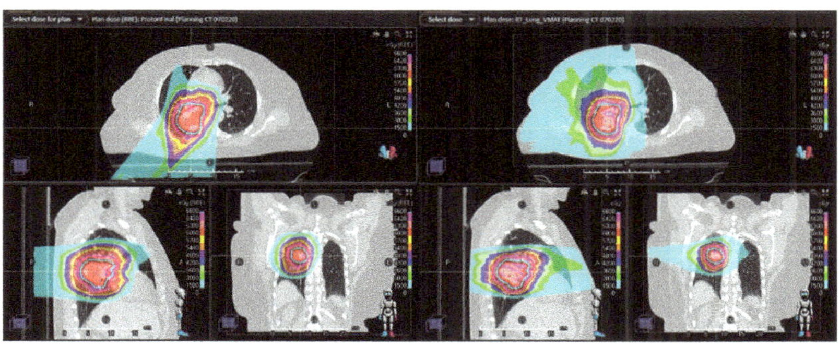

Figure 5.1. Lung cancer proton plan on left with tighter dose distribution (color wash) as compared to IMRT plan on right. Reprinted from [47], copyright (2021), with permission from Elsevier.

Managing acute and long-term side effects from radiation treatment is a central component of the clinical practice of radiation oncology. Patients are seen at least weekly while on treatment, monitored for toxicity, and are closely followed after completion of treatment for both surveillance and subacute/chronic toxicity management. For surveillance, patients are followed with serial CT scans every three months in the first six months after treatment, then twice yearly for two years, and then annually. Although PET/CT is not a standard part of the surveillance paradigm, it may be useful if needed to determine if radiographic changes represent a benign etiology—such as radiation fibrosis—versus a true recurrence [3]. The appearance of lung tissue post radiation may vary with respect to interval of time since treatment completion; radiation pneumonitis may appear as ground-glass opacities and consolidation, while subsequent changes of radiation fibrosis may present with volume loss, consolidation and bronchiectasis [39].

Possible toxicities from radiation therapy and their severity may depend on a multitude of factors including tumor location, volume treated, and total dose/fractionation selected. There is no strong data to suggest that pulmonary function tests dramatically worsen after SBRT, even in patients with poor pulmonary function prior to radiation [40]. However, special mention should be made that this does not apply to patients with pre-treatment interstitial lung disease, who have been shown to be at heightened risk of grade three radiation pneumonitis following SBRT; further, dose-constraints are observed for patients with cardiac pacemakers to prevent malfunctioning [41, 42].

SBRT tends to be very well tolerated with minimal side effects, though its high doses can result in acute toxicities ranging from mild fatigue (which is a possible side effect of virtually all radiation treatment) and esophagitis to rare but potentially fatal risks including pulmonary hemorrhage, tracheoesophageal fistula, and pneumonitis [43]. Pain in the chest wall (median onset 6–9 months post radiation) and rib fractures (median onset 13–22 months after treatment) are both considered late adverse effects, though uncommon, quoted rates vary widely from 2%–45% [44].

For conventional long-course EBRT (i.e., standard fractionation 3D-CRT, IMRT, protons), because the side effects of radiation are cumulative, acute toxicity does not manifest until the patient is several weeks into their treatment course. The most common side effects include manageable fatigue, dry cough and dermatitis as well as esophagitis. A possible subacute toxicity is radiation pneumonitis, a diagnosis of exclusion with symptoms classically including dry cough, shortness of breath, and low grade fever; this may occur in the time frame of 12 weeks—6 months following radiation therapy and tends to be self-limited however can be treated with a course of steroids [39].

Late side effects of radiation include: rib fracture (2%–3% risk) at median of 18 months following treatment, lung fibrosis, esophageal stricture (1%–2% risk) 3–4 years out from treatment, and cardiac side effects of pericarditis or coronary artery disease. In addition, patients are counseled that radiation may uncommonly cause secondary malignancies years out from treatment. Radiation induced neoplasms are extremely rare and do not usually arise in the first decade following treatment; as such, children and healthy young-adults, and patients with diseases that have long-term survivorship, are at greater risk over time given they are likely to survive for many years following their oncologic care [45, 46].

Although there have been many exciting developments in radiation technology as well as in systemic therapies in recent years, lung cancer continues to be a highly fatal malignancy and the leading cause of cancer death worldwide [36]. As such, robust prospective data is needed to answer questions of how we may continue to optimize treatment to improve outcomes of both cure and long-term disease control in these patients.

References

[1] Baker S, Dahele M, Lagerwaard F J and Senan S 2016 A critical review of recent developments in radiotherapy for non-small cell lung cancer *Radiat. Oncol.* **11** 115

[2] Roach M C, Bradley J D and Robinson C G 2018 Optimizing radiation dose and fractionation for the definitive treatment of locally advanced non-small cell lung cancer *J. Thorac. Dis.* **10** S2465–73

[3] N. C. C. Network *Non-Small Cell Lung Cancer Version 6.2020* https://nccn.org/professionals/physician_gls/pdf/nscl.pdf

[4] Zhu X, Hou R, Li X, Jiang C, Xia W and Fu X 2020 Predictive model of the first failure pattern in patients receiving definitive chemoradiotherapy for inoperable locally advanced non-small cell lung cancer (LA-NSCLC) *Radiat. Oncol.* **15** 43

[5] Ma L *et al* 2019 A current review of dose-escalated radiotherapy in locally advanced non-small cell lung cancer *Radiol. Oncol.* **53** 6–14

[6] Bradley J D *et al* 2015 Standard-dose versus high-dose conformal radiotherapy with concurrent and consolidation carboplatin plus paclitaxel with or without cetuximab for patients with stage IIIA or IIIB non-small-cell lung cancer (RTOG 0617): a randomised, two-by-two factorial phase 3 study *Lancet Oncol.* **16** 187–99

[7] *More Data Needed on Benefit of Adaptive Radiation Approaches in Locally-Advanced NSCLC* https://iaslc.org/iaslc-news/ilcn/more-data-needed-benefit-adaptive-radiation-approaches-locally-advanced-nsclc

[8] Lin A, Wood C, Hill-Kayser C, Mick R, Kaiser L and Metz J 2010 Clinical application of positron emission tomography in designing radiation fields in non-small cell lung cancer patients *Exp. Ther. Med.* **1** 1027–33

[9] Kepka L and Socha J 2015 PET-CT use and the occurrence of elective nodal failure in involved field radiotherapy for non-small cell lung cancer: A systematic review *Radiother. Oncol.* **115** 151–6

[10] Le Pechoux C *et al* 2020 LBA3_PR An international randomized trial, comparing post-operative conformal radiotherapy (PORT) to no PORT, in patients with completely resected non-small cell lung cancer (NSCLC) and mediastinal N2 involvement: primary end-point analysis of LungART (IFCT-0503, UK NCRI, SAKK) NCT00410683 *Ann. Oncol.* **31** S1178

[11] Deloch L, Derer A, Hartmann J, Frey B, Fietkau R and Gaipl U S 2016 Modern radiotherapy concepts and the impact of radiation on immune activation *Front. Oncol.* **6** 141

[12] Jaklitsch M T, Strauss G M, Healey E A, DeCamp M M Jr, Liptay M J and Sugarbaker D J 1995 An historical perspective of multi-modality treatment for resectable non-small cell lung cancer *Lung Cancer* **12** S17–32

[13] Bucci M K, Bevan A and Roach M 3rd 2005 Advances in radiation therapy: conventional to 3D, to IMRT, to 4D, and beyond *CA Cancer J. Clin.* **55** 117–34

[14] Yegya-Raman N, Zou W, Nie K, Malhotra J and Jabbour S K 2018 Advanced radiation techniques for locally advanced non-small cell lung cancer: intensity-modulated radiation therapy and proton therapy *J. Thorac. Dis.* **10** S2474–91
[15] Taylor A and Powell M E 2004 Intensity-modulated radiotherapy—what is it? *Cancer Imaging* **4** 68–73
[16] Chun S G *et al* 2017 Impact of intensity-modulated radiation therapy technique for locally advanced non-small-cell lung cancer: a secondary analysis of the NRG oncology RTOG 0617 randomized clinical trial *J. Clin. Oncol.* **35** 56–62
[17] Chan C, Lang S, Rowbottom C, Guckenberger M and Faivre-Finn C 2014 Intensity-modulated radiotherapy for lung cancer: current status and future developments *J. Thorac. Oncol.* **9** 1598–608
[18] Diwanji T P *et al* 2017 Advances in radiotherapy techniques and delivery for non-small cell lung cancer: benefits of intensity-modulated radiation therapy, proton therapy, and stereotactic body radiation therapy *Transl. Lung Cancer Res.* **6** 131–47
[19] Lin A J, Roach M, Bradley J and Robinson C 2019 Combining stereotactic body radiation therapy with immunotherapy: current data and future directions *Transl. Lung Cancer Res.* **8** 107–15
[20] Bissonnette J P *et al* 2009 Quantifying interfraction and intrafraction tumor motion in lung stereotactic body radiotherapy using respiration-correlated cone beam computed tomography *Int. J. Radiat. Oncol. Biol. Phys.* **75** 688–95
[21] Molitoris J K *et al* 2018 Advances in the use of motion management and image guidance in radiation therapy treatment for lung cancer *J. Thorac. Dis.* **10** S2437–50
[22] Muirhead R, McNee S G, Featherstone C, Moore K and Muscat S 2008 Use of Maximum Intensity Projections (MIPs) for target outlining in 4DCT radiotherapy planning *J. Thorac. Oncol.* **3** 1433–8
[23] Molitoris J K *et al* 2019 Optimizing immobilization, margins, and imaging for lung stereotactic body radiation therapy *Transl. Lung Cancer Res.* **8** 24–31
[24] Seides B J, Egan J P 3rd, French K D, Kovitz K L and Desai N R 2018 Fiducial marker placement for stereotactic body radiation therapy via convex probe endobronchial ultrasound: a case series and review of literature *J. Thorac. Dis.* **10** 1972–83
[25] Lischalk J W *et al* 2016 Long-term outcomes of stereotactic body radiation therapy (SBRT) with fiducial tracking for inoperable stage I non-small cell lung cancer (NSCLC) *J. Radiat. Oncol.* **5** 379–87
[26] Moreno A C *et al* 2020 Biologically effective dose in stereotactic body radiotherapy and survival for patients with early-stage NSCLC *J. Thorac. Oncol.* **15** 101–9
[27] Onishi H *et al* 2004 Stereotactic hypofractionated high-dose irradiation for stage I nonsmall cell lung carcinoma: clinical outcomes in 245 subjects in a Japanese multiinstitutional study *Cancer* **101** 1623–31
[28] Sebastian N T, Xu-Welliver M and Williams T M 2018 Stereotactic body radiation therapy (SBRT) for early stage non-small cell lung cancer (NSCLC): contemporary insights and advances *J. Thorac. Dis.* **10** S2451–64
[29] Timmerman R D *et al* 2018 Long-term results of stereotactic body radiation therapy in medically inoperable stage I non-small cell lung cancer *JAMA Oncol.* **4** 1287–88
[30] Breen W G, Leventakos K, Dong H and Merrell K W 2020 Radiation and immunotherapy: emerging mechanisms of synergy *J. Thorac. Dis.* **12** 7011–23

[31] Bitran J 2019 The abscopal effect exists in non-small cell lung cancer: a case report and review of the literature *Cureus* **11** e4118

[32] Chang J Y *et al* 2015 Stereotactic ablative radiotherapy versus lobectomy for operable stage I non-small-cell lung cancer: a pooled analysis of two randomised trials *Lancet Oncol.* **16** 630–7

[33] Loganadane G *et al* 2016 Stereotactic ablative radiotherapy for early stage non-small cell lung cancer: A critical literature review of predictive factors of relapse *Cancer Treat. Rev.* **50** 240–6

[34] Videtic G M M *et al* 2017 Stereotactic body radiation therapy for early-stage non-small cell lung cancer: executive summary of an ASTRO evidence-based guideline *Pract. Radiat. Oncol.* **7** 295–301

[35] T. N. A. f. P. Therapy *Map of Proton Therapy Centers in the U.S* https://proton-therapy.org/map/

[36] Vyfhuis M A L *et al* 2018 Advances in proton therapy in lung cancer *Ther. Adv. Respir. Dis.* **12** 1753466618783878

[37] Higgins K A *et al* 2017 National cancer database analysis of proton versus photon radiation therapy in non-small cell lung cancer *Int. J. Radiat. Oncol. Biol. Phys.* **97** 128–37

[38] Chang J Y *et al* 2017 Proton beam radiotherapy and concurrent chemotherapy for unresectable stage III non-small cell lung cancer: final results of a phase 2 study *JAMA Oncol.* **3** e172032

[39] Larici A R *et al* 2011 Lung abnormalities at multimodality imaging after radiation therapy for non-small cell lung cancer *Radiographics* **31** 771–89

[40] Navarro-Martin A *et al* 2016 Phase II trial of SBRT for stage I NSCLC: survival, local control, and lung function at 36 months *J. Thorac. Oncol.* **11** 1101–11

[41] Bahig H *et al* 2016 Severe radiation pneumonitis after lung stereotactic ablative radiation therapy in patients with interstitial lung disease *Pract. Radiat. Oncol.* **6** 367–74

[42] Glick D *et al* 2018 Impact of pretreatment interstitial lung disease on radiation pneumonitis and survival in patients treated with lung stereotactic body radiation therapy (SBRT) *Clin. Lung Cancer* **19** e219–26

[43] Thompson M and Rosenzweig K E 2019 The evolving toxicity profile of SBRT for lung cancer *Transl. Lung Cancer Res.* **8** 48–57

[44] Thibault I *et al* 2016 Predictors of chest wall toxicity after lung stereotactic ablative radiotherapy *Clin. Oncol. (R Coll. Radiol.)* **28** 28–35

[45] Dracham C B, Shankar A and Madan R 2018 Radiation induced secondary malignancies: a review article *Radiat. Oncol. J.* **36** 85–94

[46] Kamran S C, Berrington de Gonzalez A, Ng A, Haas-Kogan D and Viswanathan A N 2016 Therapeutic radiation and the potential risk of second malignancies *Cancer* **122** 1809–21

[47] McGunigal M, Lischalk J W, Randolph-Jackson P and Khaitan P G 2021 Radiation modalities used in lung cancer: an overview for thoracic surgeons *Semin. Thorac. Cardiovasc. Surg.* **33** 1114–21

IOP Publishing

Detection Systems in Lung Cancer and Imaging, Volume 1

Ayman El-Baz and Jasjit S Suri

Chapter 6

Application of visual sensing technology in lung cancer screening

Rongpeng Li, Yonghong Xu and Nana Xu

6.1 Introduction

Lung cancer, which originates from bronchial mucosa and alveoli, is a common malignant tumor of the respiratory tract, accounts for 11.6% of all cancers, and is the leading cause of cancer death worldwide. According to statistics, more than 1.7 million people die of lung cancer worldwide in 2018, and most of these patients are diagnosed with advanced stages [1]. Given the difficulty of screening, 75% of patients with lung cancer have missed surgery by the time they are diagnosed [2]. If lung cancer can be detected in its early stages and combined with appropriate treatment, morbidity and mortality can be remarkable reduced [3]. Therefore, early screening is the right direction and an important link to save the lives of many people at high risk of lung cancer. Blood is the preferred source of biomarkers for the early screening of lung cancer. However, sputum, bronchial lavage or suction sample, breath gas, and airway epithelial sampling may be closer to the tumor cells and their microenvironment than blood due to changes in anatomy and may provide information about molecular changes. Therefore, bronchial lavage or suction sample, breath gas, and airway epithelial sampling are considered potential biomarkers of lung cancer and other respiratory tract cancers (figure 6.1) [4]. These samples are analyzed using traditional screening methods, including radiographic testing (such as chest x-ray, CT, and magnetic resonance imaging), pathology detection (such as salivary/sputum cytology and proteomics of blood examination), and microscopy (such as bronchoscopy, microscopic examination of the chest, and mediastinum microscopy). These methods have certain limitations, such as low sensitivity, high cost, and trauma to the human body [5, 6]. In this case, the development of a highly precise, low-cost, non-invasive, and easily reproducible lung cancer diagnosis method is important.

Diagnostic methods based on the characteristics of the metabolic expiratory molecules of lung cancer (figure 6.2) have become a popular research frontier due to

doi:10.1088/978-0-7503-3355-9ch6

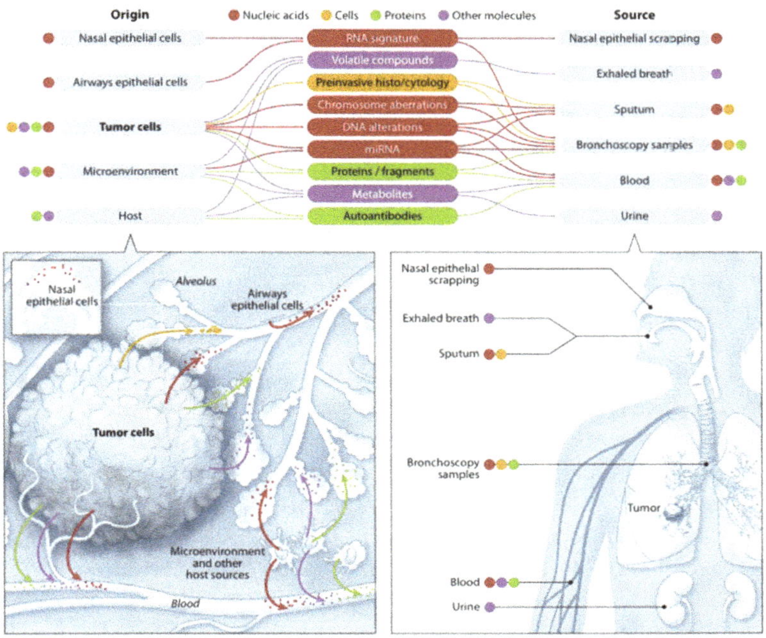

Figure 6.1. Currently explored biomarker candidates. miRNA, microRNA. Reprinted from [4], copyright (2019), with permission from Elsevier.

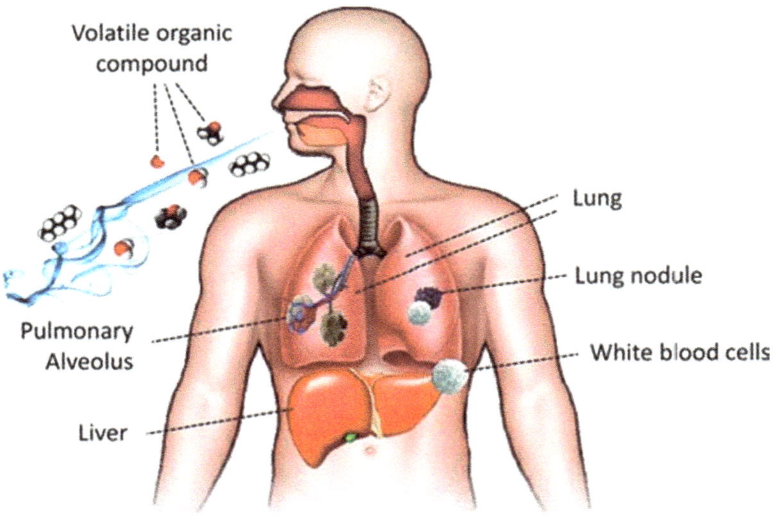

Figure 6.2. Effects of different factors in the human body on concentration and composition of VOCs of lung cancer. Changes in blood chemistry associated with cancer can be reflected in the breath, through concentration gradient that creates an instant balance between the concentration in the blood in the lungs and the air in the alveoli by the concentration gradient. Reprinted with permission from [10]. Copyright (2012) American Chemical Society.

their non-invasiveness and easy access to samples. All sorts of spectroscopic techniques have been applied to collect, detect, and analyze disease-associated volatile organic compounds (VOCs) in expiratory breath [7, 8]. Common techniques include proton transfer reaction mass, selective ion flow tube (SIFT)–mass spectrometry (MS), ion migration spectroscopy, and gas chromatography (GC) [9]. Among these techniques, GC–MS is the gold standard for the identification and quantification of single VOCs in expiratory breath [10, 11]. Despite the rapid progress over the past few decades, this method remains expensive, time-consuming, and difficult to handle in clinical settings. In recent years, the sensing technology for low-cost and easy-to-use screening applications has received a huge boost and has been widely adopted.

There are two main sensing strategies for detecting disease-related substances in exhaled air. The first is selective chemical sensor, which detects the presence of single compounds on the breath. Although quite sensitive, this method is used with non-polar targets due to the need for the complex synthesis of separated and highly selective nanomaterials to detect each VOC. In addition, no specific VOC is observed for any specific disease at present, resulting in certain drawbacks. The second approach includes a wide range of cross-responsive sensors and pattern recognition methods. Compared with the selective sensing method, the olfactory-inspired sensor array method can detect a large number of VOCs. Each sensor in this method responds to a series of VOCs, allowing the detection and analysis of individual components from the mixture. The basic mechanism of this method depends on the nature of the sensor. Among the sensors, the visual sensor is a newly developed sensing technology, stands out from many cross-response sensing strategies, and becomes an ideal method for non-invasive lung cancer screening due to its advantages (i.e., rapid, non-invasive, cheap, portable, and visualization) [12]. Visualization sensors identify different odors by detecting the chromographic information of the reaction between sensitive materials and target molecules in the array. Its working principle diagram is shown in figure 6.3. The target gas circulates through the top of the array chip and reacts chemically with the sensitive material on the array. Light source devices (low-cost white light-emitting diode, LED) combine

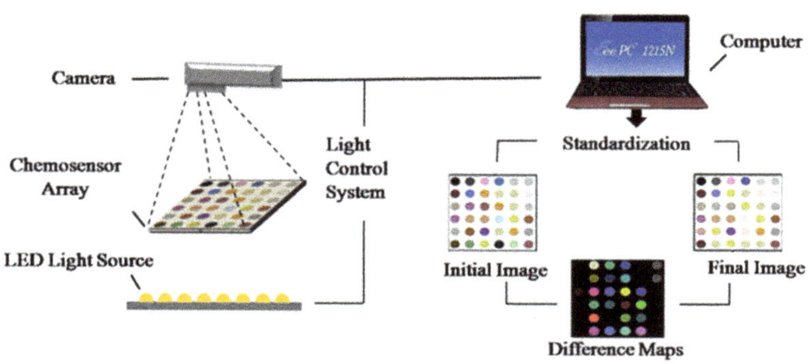

Figure 6.3. The working principle of the visual sensor.

with camera device (charge coupled device, CCD) to skillfully convert chemical reaction signals into lense focused light signals. The images are obtained by digitized, and the detailed statistical analysis of the difference spectrum is as follows: each analyte is represented by a 3N-dimensional vector (i.e., the red, green, and blue difference of N sensitive substances). A red-green-blue (RGB) difference map is generated by the absolute values of the RGB difference values of each sensitive substance point before and after reaction equilibration with the analytes. In summary, the sensor identifies gas molecules by detecting color changes in the sensitive materials in the array before and after reacting with the target gas. The working principle can be summarized into three steps. (1) The sensitive material and gas molecules get into contact and bond to cooperate. Thus, the color of the sensitive points on the surface of the array changes, and the image signal is generated. (2) The generated image signal is the output. (3) The pattern recognition system makes a judgment on the image signal.

6.2 Section 1: detection of lung cancer-related markers in exhaled breath through the visual sensing technology

6.2.1 Definition of VOCs in exhaled breath

Of the main components in N_2, O_2, CO_2, water vapor, and inert gas, some compounds with extremely low content known as VOCs are present. The composition of VOCs are complicated, and their main components include hydrocarbon, hydrocarbon oxygen, and sulfur nitrogen-containing halogen hydrocarbon, hydrocarbon and hydrocarbon. VOCs are produced by the body's cells, through biochemical processes, or by ingestion, inhalation, or skin absorption from the environment [13]. More than 500 kinds of VOCs are known to exist in human-exhaled gas and can be divided into exogenous and endogenous categories. Endogenous VOCs are derived from metabolites discharged from human blood through the lungs. Endogenous VOCs with diagnostic significance include saturated (such as ethane and pentane) and unsaturated hydrocarbons and O_2, sulfur-, and nitrogen-containing organic compounds [14]. Pauling *et al* first reported in 1971 that about 250 VOCs are present in human-exhaled gas. To date, thousands of chemicals are known to exist in human breath. However, most of these chemicals are in concentrations of pmol, and only a few are thought to be related to disease. Different groups of researchers showed that patients with lung cancer exhale VOCs at different levels than control groups [15, 16]. O'Neill *et al* proposed for the first time the detection of breathing gases to realize lung cancer diagnosis and screened 28 kinds of lung cancer-related VOCs containing alkanes, benzenes, and their derivatives. The whole study adopted large instruments, such as GC and was completed only in the laboratory. In 1999, Phillip M screened 22 kinds of VOCs, which are alkanes and their derivatives and benzene derivatives. In 2003, Phillip M and his research team selected nine VOCs from these VOCs as tumor markers for the early diagnosis or screening of lung cancer and constructed corresponding test methods and statistical models for prediction. Studies confirmed that the composition and changes in organic small molecule contents in the exhaled air of patients with lung cancer and healthy people are significantly different and can reflect the metabolic status of corresponding tissues and cells and judge the stage of the disease.

Compared with healthy people, the composition and content of trace VOCs in lung cancer patients are significantly different, which reflects the metabolic level of lung cancer cells and can determine the stage of lung cancer disease [17–20]. VOCs are markers of lung cancer, respiration detection based on VOCs is a non-invasive, convenient, and rapid method for lung cancer screening, and a variety of VOC detection methods have emerged, such as GC–MS [21], SIFT–MS [22], surface acoustic wave sensors [23, 24], quartz microbalance (QMB) gas sensors [25], ion mobility spectrometry [26], sniffer dogs [27], and electrochemical sensor [28], have been developed. Most of these methods need large, expensive, and precise instruments that require complicated operating skills and time-consuming sample pre-treatments. The SAW sensing method need to be improved in terms of sensitivity and analysis model; The QMB sensor method is susceptible to mechanical vibration, electromagnetic wave, and moisture disturbance; special sniffer dog methods require long training to develop sensitive olfactory recognition; electrochemical sensing methods still need to be improved in terms of anti-interference and selectivity. The performance of these methods is shown in table 6.1. In contrast, visual sensors [29–31] based on broad cross-reaction are ideal photochemical sensing methods for rapid disease screening because results can be obtained within minutes. Visual sensors also have the advantages of non-invasiveness; facile preparation; convenience; mild operating temperatures; and real-time, intuitive, and visual results. Visual sensors are suitable for extensive lung cancer screening of high-risk populations. The visualized sensor array is constructed to detect specific lung cancer markers in an exploratory manner, and some advances have been made in the field of lung cancer screening.

Table 6.1. Breath test performance of different methods for lung cancer detection.

Methods	T(K)	$Num._{VOC}$	Pret.	Resp. time	Sens. (%)	Spec. (%)	Acc. (%)	LOD	Ref.
GC–MS	~523	22	Yes	2 h	71.7	66.7	68.9	ppb	[21]
SIFT–MS	~543	1	Yes	Minutes	86.7	81.2	83.7	ppb	[22]
MOS-SAW	~523	11	Yes	Minutes	93.6	82.0	83.4		[23, 24]
QMB	RT		No	Minutes	92.8	85.7	88.9	ppb	[25]
IMS	573	23	Yes	15 min	71.4	99.0	79.8	ppb	[26]
Sniffer dogs	RT		Yes	Minutes	71.0	93.0	78.2		[27]
Electrochem	RT	9	No	Minutes	71.4	91.9	90.3		[28]
CS	RT		No	Minutes	70.0	86.0	75.7	ppb	[29–31]

T. temperature, Pret. pre-treatment, Resp time response time, Sens. sensitivity, Acc. accuracy, Spec. specificity, RT room temperature. CSA colorimetric sensor array, TD tunable diode, ppt parts per trillion, ppb parts per billion, Ref. Reference, Electrochem. Electrochemistry, $Num._{VOC}$. Number of VOC

6.2.2 Production mechanism of lung cancer-related VOCs in exhaled breath

When lung cancer multiplies in the body, corresponding tumor cells produce some VOCs in the blood. VOCs flow with the blood to the lungs, and finally can be expelled through exhaling. Therefore, it is a non-invasive, rapid and easily accepted feasible method to screen lung cancer in high-risk groups through exhaled gas detection. The feasibility of the method has become an important auxiliary lung examination method. Studies [32] showed that the sources of lung cancer marker VOCs in exhalation are mainly from two aspects. Exogenous VOCs are derived from respiration and skin absorption. Cytochrome P450 mixed-function oxidases, activated by these exogenous environmental factors such as smoking, promotes the transformation of oncogenic precursors, thereby increasing the risk of lung cancer. Various biochemical processes in the body, including the maintenance of cell membrane integrity, energy metabolism process, and oxidative stress, produce endogenous VOCs. Endogenous VOCs, such as alkanes generated by oxidative stress reaction, acetone produced during the decarbonylation of acetoacetate of lipid peroxidation, cholesterol produced by acetyl-CoA during biosynthesis, and isoprenodiene, are the main detection targets of disease diagnosis. In patients with lung cancer, mutations in the catalytic oxidase (cytochrome P450) of an organic compound or in the gene that encodes the enzyme can cause metabolic disorders and produce new VOCs or levels that are different from those produced in normal humans [20]. A pathophysiologic model that can account for these observations is illustrated in figure 6.4.

Given the significant difference in the VOCs in exhaled breath between patients with lung cancer and healthy subjects, the detection of VOCs in human respiratory gas composition and changes in content can reflect the status of the corresponding

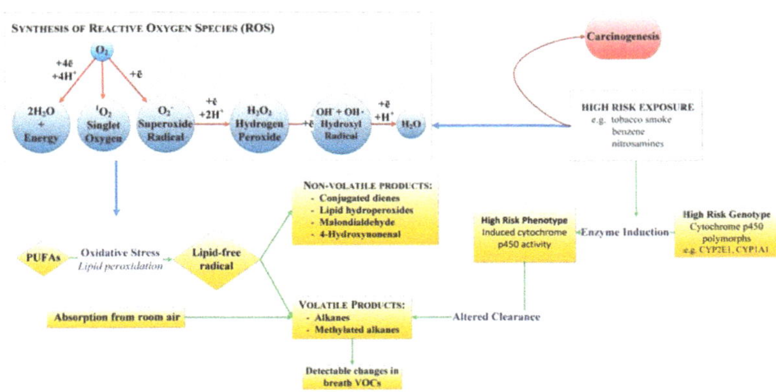

Figure 6.4. Production mechanism of lung cancer-related VOCs in exhaled breath. High-risk genotype cytochrome p450 mixed-function oxidases are activated by high-risk exposure factors such as smoking. High risk phenotype may increase the risk of lung cancer by promoting the transformation of oncogenic precursors. The activity changes of P450 mixed oxidase may regulate the catabolism of endogenous VOC products generated by oxidative stress and produce the altered pattern of respiratory VOCs. Data adapted from [10]. Reprinted with permission from [10]. Copyright (2012) American Chemical Society.

organization cell's metabolism and judge the onset of the disease stage. Therefore, the detection of exhaled breath for disease screening, as a non-invasive, rapid, and convenient screening method, has potential application value. At present, relevant research has been vigorously promoted in the screening and diagnosis of lung cancer.

6.2.3 Preparation method of sensor chip

First, a Superhydrophobic polyvinylidene fluoride (PVDF) membrane is cut into small membranes (figure 6.5(a)), which are then placed onto a transparent spot model (figure 6.5(b)). Sensitive material solution is dropped using a quartz capillary tube (figure 6.5(c)) under a N_2 protective atmosphere and smeared over the PVDF membrane until the solution spread into a uniformly sized dot (diameter = 2 mm). Micro-contact technology is used to fabricate sensor array chips so that the material adheres perfectly to the basement membrane. The prepared array chip is dried and stored in the N_2 atmosphere (figure 6.5(e)) and kept in the dark (figure 6.5(f)). The sensor chips made in the same batch and closely adjacent have a high degree of consistency. In addition, the dual-channel structure solves the field calibration problem in rapid identification for lung cancer-exhaled markers. Reversible chemical reactions, as bases of the response for array chip (figure 6.5(g)) of optical sensors, are used to detect VOCs by means of LED light source devices (low-cost white light-emitting diode) and CCD camera, and the chemical reaction signals can be perfectly transformed into the optical signals focused by lens (complementary metal–oxide semiconductor camera). The RGB difference map (figure 6.5(i)) is

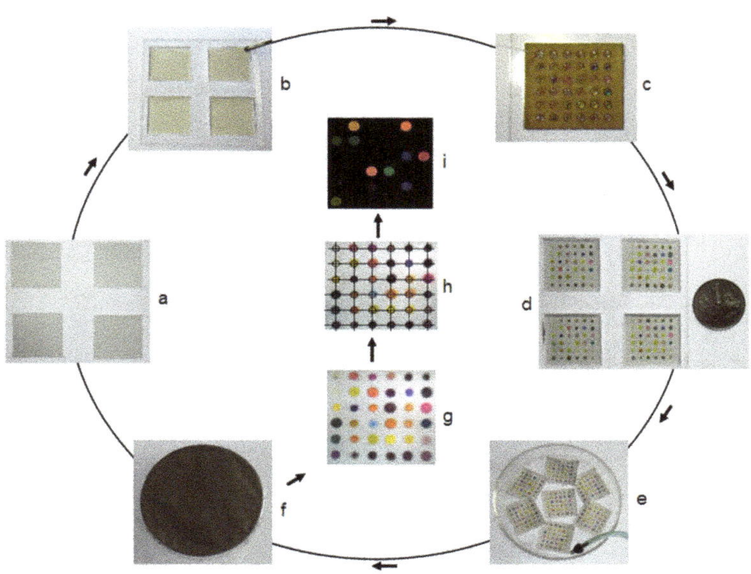

Figure 6.5. The detailed fabrication (a–d), conservation (e–f) and application (g–i) process of sensor array.

generated from the absolute values of the differences in the RGB values of each sensitive material spot before and after equilibration with analytes. In data processing, the central position of each sensitive material point is averaged to avoid the point-periphery offset (figure 6.5(h)).

6.2.4 Collection of lung cancer-related VOCs in exhaled breath

At present, a recognized standard collection method, which avoids gas leakage and pollution of external gas during operation, is not available. Commonly used methods include breath collecting apparatus or bio-voc breath sampler, which are slightly instrumental and technically demanding. The other method is to exhale directly into the sampling bag or container, and this method is easy-to-operate and does not require a special collection instrument. However, the shortcoming is that the collected gas contains dead chamber gas without blood gas exchange in the alveoli. Given the extremely low level of VOC gases in human breath, some traditional detection methods, such as GC–MS, require preconcentration and heating of samples before testing. The visual sensing technology has short response time and fast detection and does not require a complicated sample pre-treatment.

6.2.5 Analysis of VOC patterns

The color of these sensitive spots changes in accordance with the chemicals they come into contact (figure 6.6). Each colorimetric sensor array contains 36 chemically sensitive spots. The sensitivity of each point to VOCs is different. The chemicals that make up the sensitive points on the sensor array are selected as generically sensitive (i.e., not sensitive to one or two specific groups of volatiles). Given that the key volatiles that are unique to lung cancer patients' respiration are not yet established, we chose a broadly sensitive system. This type of system is sensitive to certain volatiles ranging from low parts per million to high parts per million. During the breathing acquisition process, the color change images of the array (i.e., 12 images for each study object) are captured using a camera every minute. At each collection, the color change is converted into a numeric value, representing the change in the RGB compositions of each point. This produces a 108-dimensional vector (36 points with three values for each point). Differences between expiratory and indoor air results are used in the analysis.

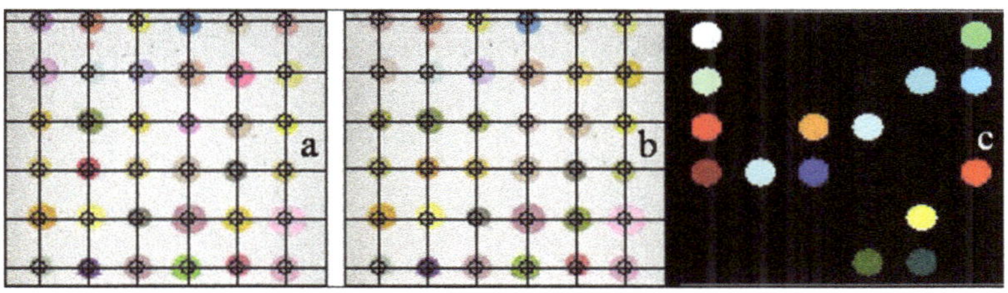

Figure 6.6. The raw image of the sensor array taken by the camera (a) and the image after the reaction with the chemical sample (e.g., breath) (b). The difference map from time a to time b. Data adapted from [35].

Figure 6.7(a) shows the specific fingerprint of VOCs at different concentrations. The initial RGB value was magnified ten-fold to clearly visualize the effectiveness of the sensor. The results show that there were significant lateral differences between different graphs of the analyte, and the analytes with similar structures had similar regional results. The results of the same analyte at different concentrations showed certain longitudinal differences, and positively correlated with the intensity of the response signal of the difference graph. A variety of lung cancer markers in expiratory sensing recognition, detection concentration can reach the level of PPB.

The data were analyzed using digital image acquisition technology, and each analyte is described using a 30-dimensional vector (RGB differences of 10 sensitive substances). The Euclidean distance (ED) is generated using equations with the following formula:

$$\mathrm{ED} = \mathrm{sqrt}[(R1 - R10)2 + (G1 - G10)2 + (B1 - B10)2 + \ldots (R10 - R100)2 + (G10 - G100)2 + (B10 - B100)2].$$

The ED–response time curve (figure 6.7(b)) represents the equilibrium time of VOCs. In addition, compared with the relatively stable analyte, the analyte containing the active group has a greater ED. For example, the ED of benzene and 1,2,4-tritoluene are greater than those of decane and undecane. As the control inert gas N2, the ED is even closer to zero, which further indicates that the system has strong anti-interference ability and high stability.

The principal component analysis (PCA) is used to visualize data, and two principal component score vectors are used to draw two-dimensional scatter plots for the five-parallel data of six VOCs. As shown in figure 6.7(c), these two

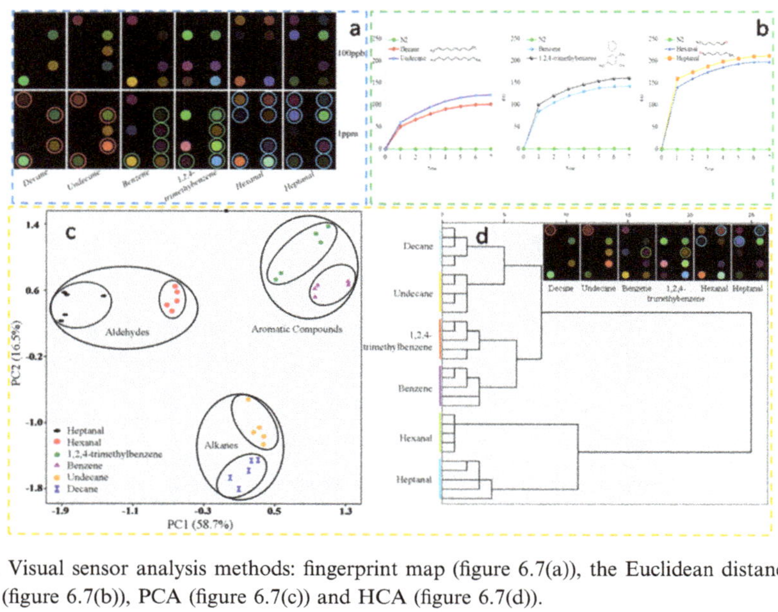

Figure 6.7. Visual sensor analysis methods: fingerprint map (figure 6.7(a)), the Euclidean distance–response time curve (figure 6.7(b)), PCA (figure 6.7(c)) and HCA (figure 6.7(d)).

Table 6.2. Computational formula of V and RSD.

Name	Computational formula
C_s	Antoine equation: $\lg P_i = A - B / (t + C)$. $C_i = P_i / RT \times 22.4 / M \times (273 + t) / 273$. $C_i \times V_i = C_s \times V_s$.
RSD	$S = \sqrt{\frac{\sum_{i=1}^{n}(x_i - \bar{x})^2}{n-1}}$ $RSD = \frac{S}{\bar{x}} \times 100\%$

components account for 75.2% of the total information and can be used to separate the analyte with no overlap between the scatter plots of all samples. When all samples were analyzed, analytes with similar structures are clustered together, while the analytes with different structures are far away. The hierarchical clustering analysis (HCA) is the process of decomposing abstract analytes into similar analytes. The response system tree obtained in this study represents the multiple distances of the analyte in the 30-dimensional RGB color space. The HCA tree diagram shows that the detection results of the parallel experiment are preliminarily clustered. The analytes are classified in accordance with the structure similarity model of VOCs. The detected objects are divided into different sets in accordance with their similarity (figure 6.7(d)). The diagram visually shows the specific reaction regions of VOCs. The visual sensing method combines the cross-response principle with the pattern recognition method to realize the characteristic fingerprint. The pattern recognition algorithm can obtain the attribute, concentration, and similarity of the target. The visualized sensor system has the advantages of rapid, low-cost, highly sensitive, and non-invasive detection and is an ideal screening method for major diseases, such as lung cancer. HCA and PCA consistently show that the classification of VOCs conforms to the law of structural similarity, which is intended to provide an important guarantee for the effective detection of clinical breath samples at a later stage.

6.2.6 Computational formulas of the relative standard deviation (RSD or %RSD) and concentrations of saturated vapor (C_s)

The computational formulas of RSD (or %RSD) and C_s are shown in table 6.2. RSD is the absolute value of the coefficient of variation and is calculated from the following formula:

$\%RSD = \frac{S}{\bar{x}} \times 100$,where S is the standard deviation, and $\bar{x}$ is the mean. A low percentage indicates low variability in the data set. The Antoine equation is used to obtain C_s. by calculating the vapor pressure and temperature

A, B, and C are Antoine parameters, C_i is the gas concentration of saturated vapor (ppm), t is the detection temperature (°C), V_i is the detected volume of saturated vapor, C_s is the detected concentration (1 ppm), V_s is 10 l, RSD is the relative standard deviation, X is the average value, and S is the standard deviation.

6.2.7 Cross-response mechanism of the visual sensor

The recognition mechanism of the visual sensor is attributed to the molecular interactions that occur between the sensitive and target materials on the sensor array (figure 6.8). Hydroxyl groups in sensitive materials may form hydrogen bonds with aldehydes. The benzene ring in sensitive substances may form π–π interaction with aromatic hydrocarbons. Porphyrins can form metal coordination with VOCs. Lewis weak acid-base reaction may occur between acid-base indicator and VOCs. The sensitive material may also have van der Waals forces and physical adsorption with the target molecule. These forces cooperate to achieve the selective cross-response of VOCs species. Compared with the electrochemical method and the mobile spectroscopy method, the proposed visualization method is simple, intuitive, accurate, fast, and anti-interference.

6.3 Section 2: detection of clinical exhaled breath of lung cancer through the visual sensing technique

6.3.1 Institutional review board approval

Studies should be reviewed and approved by the ethics committees of research and medical institutions, and all subjects should be provided with signed informed consent. The experimental data of each subject are distributed to the program implementation manager, and all of the information on each subject is encoded. Each subject has an independent serial number, and the research staff and reviewers can only view the serial number. No one else has access to the subjects' data. When the study results are published on the basis of the data of the subjects, the names of the subjects and any other data that may identify the subjects are not made public, and the ethics review committee may review study records to determine whether the study complies with relevant laws and regulations. Researchers plan to keep the

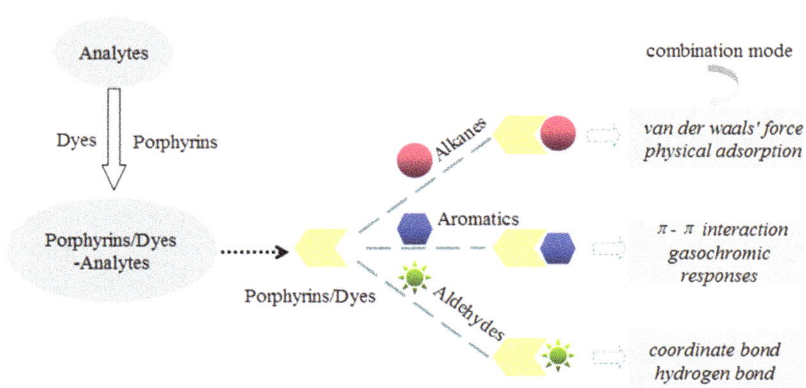

Figure 6.8. Possible visual sensor recognition mechanism for analytes.

original clinical trial data strictly conserved for many years. Thus, the ethics committee and academic integrity institutions can refer to the original data at any time to realize the traceability of original data.

6.3.2 Exhaled breath collection and analysis

The collection of exhaled breath is a simple procedure. However, several important issues should be considered (figure 6.9). First, most of the known components of exhalation are also present in the environment. Therefore, the exhaled breath signals should be distinguished from external ambient gas signals. One method is to collect VOCs in both breath and external environments to determine the alveolar gradient for each VOC. This approach is simple but ignores the complexity of the host respiratory system. Another option is to install a VOC filter at the suction inlet of a respiratory collection device to pre-filter environmental VOCs, thus increasing the purity of VOCs in exhaled sample. However, none of the methods suggest that exposure to environmental VOCs may have a lasting effect on the pattern of exhaled VOCs because VOCs are easily absorbed from ambient air into the bloodstream, where they are released along with endogenous molecules.

Second, due to the extremely low concentration of volatiles in exhaled breath, detection of exhaled VOC requires more optimized sample collection and extremely sensitive instruments. Different research groups apply widely different approaches for breath collection. For example, a non-permeable bag for VOCs is used for collection, and VOCs are captured using a solid-phase microextraction (SPME) technique from the obtained sample. In the breath analysis, the breath collection device mainly uses adsorbent materials to enrich the lung cancer markers in the breath on the collector, and then conducts GC–MS analysis. Volatiles in the oral and upper respiratory tract have an important influence on disease-related biomarkers in expiratory breath, so it can be seen that the sampling method of VOCs is very important. Some researchers collect alveolar gas by asking subjects to exhale the last portion of their lungs; other researchers asked the subjects to perform tidal breathing while the samples were being collected; to prevent nasal contamination of samples, some studies have used resistance to close the soft palate.

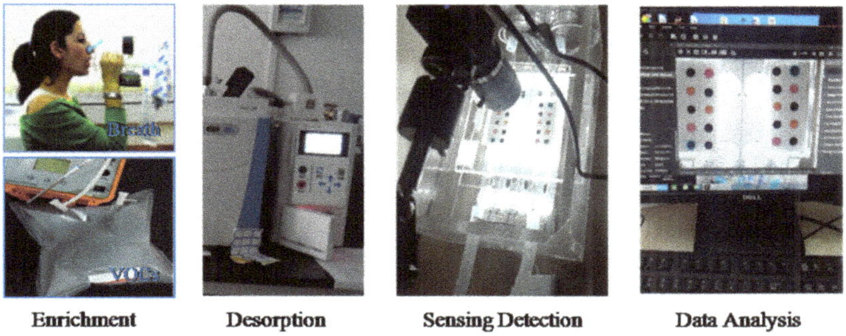

Figure 6.9. Visualized sensors detect and analyze exhaled breath of lung cancer and disease-related markers VOCs. Reprinted from [34], copyright (2009) with permission of Springer.

The modeling and double-blind detection of fingerprint of clinical samples uses clinical data processing, which includes sample feature extraction, lung cancer/healthy control group model establishment, and clinical sample double-blind detection. Most (80%) of the clinical sample test data are randomly selected as the training set for sample feature extraction and lung cancer/healthy control group model establishment. The double-blind detection is carried out on the remaining 20% of clinical samples. By comparison with the training data model library, the common-response region of the spectrum is statistically analyzed, and the decision and classification are made. The data in this study can be used for lung cancer expiratory feature spectrogram analysis. The pattern recognition data processing technology can also be used to conduct feature modeling, decision making, and classification of samples, and the results of double-blind samples can be obtained using the discriminant analysis based on the decision situation of fingerprint and pattern recognition data forms.

6.3.3 Basic data collection

The basic data collected for the lung cancer study subjects include: gender, age, smoking status, primary tumor size, primary tumor location, cancer histology, cancer stage, comorbidity, and medications. Data, including gender, age, smoking status, lung diagnosis (if any), comorbidities, and medications, are collected for non-lung cancer subjects.

6.3.4 Statistical analysis of data

Under normal circumstances, the implementer scheme is tried out in clinical samples and the basic information. The research uses the visual sensor, pattern recognition, and image processing technology analysis of clinical samples to collect data (i.e., fingerprint and Euclidean distance–response time) and PCA and HCA methods (such as feature extraction, construction of comprehensive decision-making model library). Since exhaled VOCs are a complex mixture of many different molecules, the usual goal of these studies is to distinguish lung cancer from non-lung cancer by the changes in expiratory patterns. The statistical algorithms used in the reported studies are not uniform and there is no direct comparison among these methods. In addition, the number of VOCs selected for analysis is inconsistent. Therefore, the lack of standardized sampling and statistical analysis procedures may be one of the main reasons for the different results between study groups.

The visualized sensing technology has been used in the early detection of many respiratory diseases, including lung cancer, and has achieved good results [33, 34]. The same sensor array can separate lung cancer from healthy states. Sensors and related algorithms can be tweaked to identify and classify diseases. Researchers demonstrated that sensor arrays can be used to classify patients with lung cancer and found that the visual sensing technology can well distinguish early (I and II) and late (III and IV) stages of lung cancer (accuracy = 88%), benign and malignant tumors (accuracy = 89%), small-cell lung cancer (SCLC) and non-SCLC (NSCLC, accuracy = 93%), and adenocarcinoma and squamous cell carcinoma (accuracy = 88%) [35, 36]. Many confounding factors (such as location, age, gender, race, and smoking habits) have been successfully eliminated using advanced hardware and software (algorithmic) techniques. Furthermore, in some cases, the visual sensing technology can even distinguish basic types on the basis of VOC in breath samples and identify the specific genetic variants of lung cancer (i.e., P53, K-RAS, EGFR, and ALK) to help provide personalized diagnosis and assist in customized treatment. The recent clinical study used this technique to distinguish between malignant and benign nodules with an overall accuracy of 87%. In addition, patients with EGFR mutations are successfully distinguished from 34 patients with EGFR wild-type lung cancer with an accuracy of 83%, sensitivity of 79%, and specificity of 85% [37]. As a surveillance tool, the visual sensing technology can also provide oncologists with a quick bedside method to identify the lack of response to cancer treatments. A study of patients with lung cancer showed significant differences between pre-operative and post-operative respiratory fingerprints. The visualizable sensing technology is observed with sensitivity and specificity for pre-operative and post-operative lung cancer status of 83% and 85%, respectively, thus improving the evidence for rapid identification and early detection of treatment failure [38]. A recent lung cancer clinical sample breath study classified 90 patients with lung cancer by stage through the visual sensing technology. Experimental results showed that the accuracy rate of lung cancer stage identification by visualization technique is up to 80%. Even, through sensor array combined with pattern recognition algorithm, the exhalation characteristics of smoking and other respiratory diseases can be identified and distinguished [39].

6.4 Section 3: detection of metabolic volatile products of lung cancer cells through the visual sensing technique

Lung cancer cells are divided into four main histological types, i.e., adenocarcinoma, squamous cell carcinoma, small-cell carcinoma, and large-cell carcinoma (figure 6.10). Adenocarcinomas arise from epithelial cells that secrete substances into ducts or lumens. Squamous cell carcinomas originate from epithelial cells, and their main function is to close the cavities or channels they form for the protection of the underlying cell population. SCLC, which has unclear origin, secretes bioactive peptides. Large-cell carcinoma is an excluded diagnosis with microscopic evidence of the absence of all other histological characteristics of the cells [40]. Many life activities in cells can be reflected in the metabolic level. We observe the whole metabolic process, changes in metabolites, and physiological or pathological changes in the body from the release of cell signals and energy transfer. Therefore, lung cancer-specific VOCs can also be detected from the headspace of lung cancer cells (gaseous components in the closed space above the cell line, *in vitro* method). Studying the metabolic activity of isolated cancer cells by analyzing headspace VOCs can effectively avoid body confounding factors (the patient's age, gender, lifestyle, drugs, and other chronic diseases). Cell lines provide an almost infinite number of cells with similar genotypes and phenotypes, avoiding differences

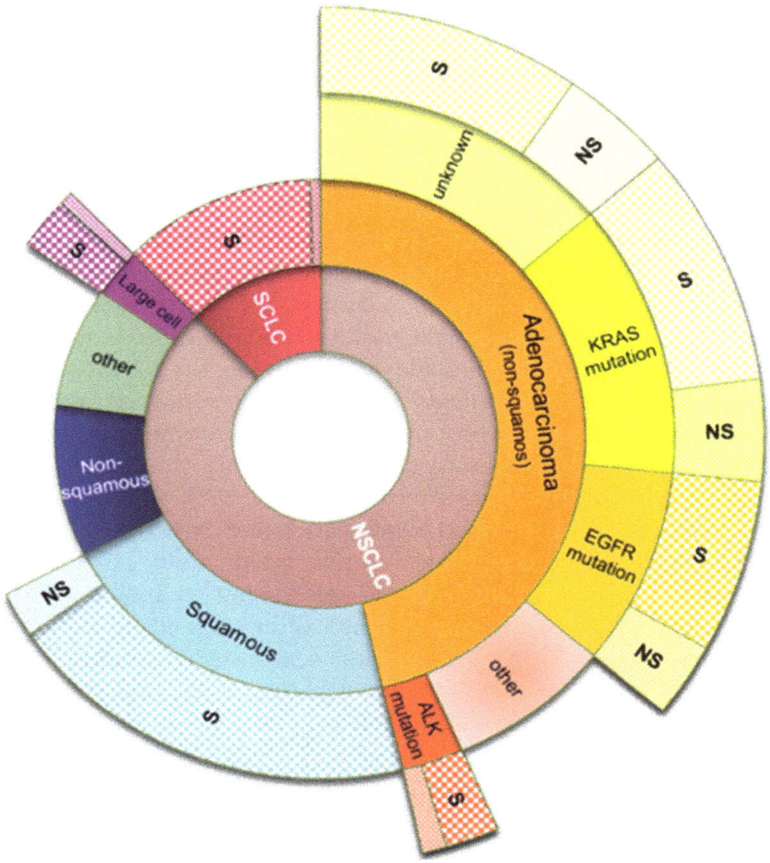

Figure 6.10. Multistep classification of lung cancer subtypes; common mutations that occur in tumors and the occurrence ratio caused by smoking tobacco for each subtype. Reprinted from [33] with permission from MDPI.

between individuals and bypassing the ethical issues associated with animal and human experiments.

At present, GC–MS and visual sensor are the most widely used rapid screening methods for detecting volatile substances in lung cancer cells. GC–MS is the most powerful tool for offline detection and has high sensitivity (sometimes below the PPB range) and high potential for identifying and quantifying unknown components from complex biological substrates. The SPME–GC detection system is used to analyze different types of cells in the culture medium, including lung cancer cells, osteoblasts, adipocytes, and bronchial epithelial cells. Through the analysis of the results, four VOCs are observed in all culture media of lung cancer cells, and the correlation between VOCs in the metabolites of lung cancer cells and in the breath of lung cancer patients is determined [41]. GC–MS was used to comprehensively analyze VOCs and their non-volatile cell metabolites released by different lung cancer cell lines [42]. The results showed that the VOC spectrum can distinguish

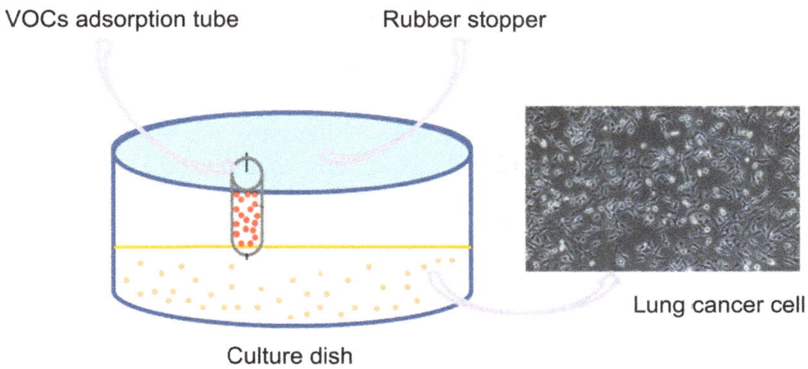

Figure 6.11. Culture of lung cancer cells and collection of VOCs.

between small- and non-small-cell carcinomas. Among non-small-cell carcinomas, large-cell carcinomas have evident VOC characteristics, mainly manifested by the increase of benzaldehyde, 2-ethylhexanol, and 2,4-decadien-1-ol in metabolites. However, GC–MS requires expensive equipment and a high level of expertise. In addition, the analysis of the results is time-consuming and labor costs. Furthermore, the sample must be dehumidified and pre-concentrated using SPME to achieve the necessary sensitivity.

The digestive subculture of lung cancer cells (A549, lung adenocarcinoma; NCIH460, large-cell lung cancer; and NCIH446, SCLC) and a self-made simple collection method of enrichment tube filled with adsorption materials are adopted to collect lung cancer-related VOCs (figure 6.11). GC–MS and sensing methods are used to detect lung cancer-related VOCs metabolized by the collected lung cancer cells, and results are compared with the detection results of the corresponding study on lung cancer breath for the purpose of correlation analysis.

Compared with GC–MS, visual sensors are generally inexpensive, easy-to-operate, and have real-time monitoring capabilities based on pattern recognition algorithms. The use of gold nanoparticle sensors can significantly differentiate lung cancer typing by metabolizing VOCs in lung cancer cells [43]. In addition, metabolic characteristics associated with specific gene mutations in lung cancer can be detected and monitored. This feature helps improve drug selection and drug resistance detection. Through safe, timely, and effective interventions, the survival and quality of life of patients can be improved, thus improving the clinical benefit of patients [44]. However, the environment of tumors *in vivo* is complex and diverse, and *in vitro* studies may not be able to replicate fully the precise cellular environment of lung tissue. Therefore, the results of the study of these cell lines can only be considered indicative. In the future, basic and clinical studies are needed to further demonstrate the feasibility of its transformation into clinical applications.

6.5 Section 4: development space of the visual sensing technology

Although the cross-sensitive visualized optical sensing method has effectively promoted the research of extensive screening for lung cancer, the sensitivity and stability of photosensitive materials remain challenging. An ideal disease screening method should be non-invasive, rapid, cheap, convenient, and intuitive and should have high sensitivity and high specificity. In addition to microarrays, sensing systems, and data processing modes, the development of new disease screening instruments depends on the development of new sensing materials with multiple active centers and easy-to-generate signals to a large extent. This finding is because the sensing material participates in the reaction as the starting material and realizes the signal control of the reaction products. Therefore, the sensing material should have multiple active centers, should be coordinated and bound, and should realize the control of reactivity and cross-selectivity. The development of new sensing materials is beneficial to the discovery of new cross-selection reactions. Therefore, the design and development of novel sensing materials with multiple active centers and easy chemical bonding has become an important task in the field of sensor research. Porphyrin compounds and pH indicators have binding sites and chromogenic groups, which are considered some of the most important optical sensing materials and have a wide range of applications in biology, medicine, materials, and other fields. However, the optical sensing method of lung cancer based on porphyrins/pH indicator composites is still in its infancy and needs to be further studied systematically. The development of other types of photosensitive materials, as new sensor materials that can be used to develop new cross-response sensing materials and build photosensitive probes, is challenging and has broad research space. The participation of composite materials as photosensitive materials in photochemical reactions and their application in optical sensors should be deeply and systematically studied. The exhaled breath contains many distractions, such as water and carbon dioxide, and remains to be further developed. Clinical sample pre-processing is used to avoid false signals and leakage. The new sensing method for lung cancer screening should be combined with efficient impurity removal-enrichment system, high sensitivity detection system and improved pattern recognition method. The differences in ethnic groups, dietary structure, living habits, and living environment of different countries may lead to slightly different exhaled gases of patients with lung cancer, leading to different research data and different lung cancer markers. The visualized sensing technology combined with GC–MS precision analysis technology is used to detect lung cancer markers and clinical breath samples and explore the relationship between lung cancer tumor formation in the host body, living habits, and external environment.

6.6 Section 5: important role and application prospect of visual sensing technology in lung cancer screening

Along with the improvement of the development of science and technology and living standards, people have rising expectations of medical technology. In the diagnosis of lung cancer, existing traditional detection methods, such as radiographic inspection and pathology, produce many false negative results, and the patient faces many unnecessary living tissue biopsies and radiographic imaging exposure. Given the rapid development of respiratory collection and analysis techniques, VOC monitoring may soon become an interesting complement or even alternative to traditional medical diagnostics. A breath test can provide an easy and safe test. However, most of the international studies on the detection of lung cancer VOCs are carried out using GC–MS and other large gas analysis instruments, which have complex structure and high cost, require professional operators, lack supporting diagnostic software, and cannot be used as a wide range of screening and diagnosis tools for lung cancer. The visualized sensing technology is a non-invasive, fast, simple, and low-cost method for early lung cancer screening. Clinical data are immediately uploaded to the cloud server for in-depth online analysis through effective comparison with the assistance of the ICT platform. Thus, this approach has the potential to reduce lung cancer mortality significantly over the next decade by improving extensive screening and compliance. Visual sensing technology is used for non-invasive early screening. Patients who test positive then undergo routine, invasive and expensive imaging tests for the confirmation of their disease and tumor location. This can effectively reduce the financial burden on patients and improve patient compliance.

In addition, the detection system must be able to deal with a variety of complex factors, such as ambient temperature, humidity, sensor element and respiratory sample instability, and these difficulties can be minimized by appropriate sampling techniques combined with ideal sensor preparation techniques.

Although visual sensing technology holds great promise for lung cancer screening, some challenges remain. These challenges include clinical, engineering, business, and ethical aspects and could take years to resolve. One of the key issues is the extensive validation of the currently available VOC profiles. The analysis of the method of respiratory gases to screen for lung cancer should be able to detect tiny traces of lung cancer-related VOCs in breath gas and standard breath samples containing nitrogen, oxygen, carbon dioxide, water vapor, and thousands of VOCs. Most of the spectral differences of VOCs among different individuals, and few cases showed that certain VOCs of exhaled gas exist only in patients but not in healthy subjects. Thus, different kinds and concentrations of VOCs are associated with disease clinical state, and few VOCs may indicate the exact state of disease. Therefore, large sample sizes and basic studies are needed worldwide to identify lung cancer-specific VOCs. In addition, the detection system must be able to deal with a variety of complex factors, such as ambient temperature, humidity, sensor element and respiratory sample instability, and these difficulties can be minimized by appropriate sampling techniques combined with ideal sensor preparation techniques. Moreover, substantial differences in methodology among different studies should be considered to establish standardized experimental methods for different databases, and the reproducibility of instruments and classifications among different sensor models must be considered to ensure the same output of results.

In conclusion, the breath test being developed for lung cancer is fast, safe, and cheap. This new diagnostic approach has real potential as a routine diagnosis and in monitoring especially in the digital age, significantly improves cure rates, and reduces the healthcare costs of society. In the future, this approach will become an important component of population-based comprehensive screening and personalized management of different types of lung cancer. However, the technology is not yet mature for immediate clinical use. Studies on different populations are needed to address the issue of reproducibility and the role of confounders.

References

[1] The Lancet 2019 Lung cancer: some progress, but still a lot more to do 2019 *Lancet* **394** 1880
[2] Siegel R L, Miller K D and Jemal A 2018 Cancer statistics, 2018 *CA Cancer J. Clin.* **68** 7–30
[3] Tota J E, Ramanakumar A V and Franco E L 2014 Lung cancer screening: review and performance comparison under different risk scenarios *Lung* **192** 55–63
[4] Seijo L M *et al* 2019 Biomarkers in lung cancer screening: achievements, promises, and challenges *J. Thorac. Oncol.* **14** 343–57
[5] Azar F E *et al* 2017 Cost-effectiveness of lung cancer screening and treatment methods: a systematic review of systematic reviews *BMC Health Serv. Res.* **17** 413
[6] Strauss G M and Dominioni L 2013 Chest x-ray screening for lung cancer: overdiagnosis, endpoints, and randomized population trials *J. Surg. Oncol.* **108** 294–300
[7] Kischkel S *et al* 2010 Breath biomarkers for lung cancer detection and assessment of smoking related effects—confounding variables, influence of normalization and statistical algorithms *Clin. Chim. Acta* **411** 1637–44
[8] Alkhouri N *et al* 2014 Analysis of breath volatile organic compounds as a noninvasive tool to diagnose nonalcoholic fatty liver disease in children *Eur. J. Gastroenterol. Hepatol.* **26** 82–7
[9] Broza Y Y and Haick H 2013 Nanomaterial-based sensors for detection of disease by volatile organic compounds *Nanomedicine (Lond)* **8** 785–806
[10] Hakim M *et al* 2012 Volatile organic compounds of lung cancer and possible biochemical pathways *Chem. Rev.* **112** 5949–66
[11] Zhou J M, Huang Z A, Kumar U and Chen D D Y 2017 Review of recent developments in determining volatile organic compounds in exhaled breath as biomarkers for lung cancer diagnosis *Anal. Chim. Acta* **996** 1–9
[12] Hashoul D and Haick H 2019 Sensors for detecting pulmonary diseases from exhaled breath *Eur. Resp. Rev.* **28** 190011
[13] Amann A, Spanel P and Smith D 2007 Breath analysis: the approach towards clinical applications *Mini-Rev. Med. Chem.* **7** 115–29
[14] Horvath I, Lazar Z, Gyulai N, Kollai M and Losonczy G 2009 Exhaled biomarkers in lung cancer *Eur. Respir. J.* **34** 261–75
[15] Chan H P, Lewis C and Thomas P S 2009 Exhaled breath analysis: novel approach for early detection of lung cancer *Lung Cancer* **63** 164–8
[16] Koureas M, Kirgou P, Amoutzias G, Hadjichristodoulou C, Gourgoulianis K and Tsakalof A 2020 Target analysis of volatile organic compounds in exhaled breath for lung cancer discrimination from other pulmonary diseases and healthy persons *Metabolites* **10** 317
[17] Bao Y, Xu P, Cai S, Yu H and Li X 2018 Detection of volatile-organic-compounds (VOCs) in solution using cantilever-based gas sensors *Talanta* **182** 148–55

[18] Gasparri R *et al* 2016 Volatile signature for the early diagnosis of lung cancer *J. Breath Res.* **10** 016007

[19] Zhou J, Huang Z A, Kumar U and Chen D D Y 2017 Review of recent developments in determining volatile organic compounds in exhaled breath as biomarkers for lung cancer diagnosis *Anal. Chim. Acta* **996** 1–9

[20] Haick H, Broza Y Y, Mochalski P, Ruzsanyi V and Amann A 2014 Assessment, origin, and implementation of breath volatile cancer markers *Chem. Soc. Rev.* **43** 1423–49

[21] Phillips M *et al* 1999 Volatile organic compounds in breath as markers of lung cancer: a cross-sectional study *Lancet* **353** 1930–3

[22] Smith D and Spanel P 2015 Pitfalls in the analysis of volatile breath biomarkers: suggested solutions and SIFT-MS quantification of single metabolites *J. Breath Res.* **9** 022001

[23] Wang D I *et al* 2012 A hybrid electronic noses' system based on mos-saw detection units intended for lung cancer diagnosis *J. Innov. Opt. Health Sci.* **05** 1150006

[24] C. X *et al* 2005 A study of an electronic nose for detection of lung cancer based on a virtual SAWgas sensors array and imaging recognition method *Meas. Sci. Technol.* **16** 1535–46

[25] Di Natale C *et al* 2003 Lung cancer identification by the analysis of breath by means of an array of non-selective gas sensors *Biosens. Bioelectron.* **18** 1209–18

[26] Westhoff M, Litterst P, Freitag L, Urfer W, Bader S and Baumbach J I 2009 Ion mobility spectrometry for the detection of volatile organic compounds in exhaled breath of patients with lung cancer: results of a pilot study *Thorax* **64** 744–8

[27] Ehmann R *et al* 2012 Canine scent detection in the diagnosis of lung cancer: revisiting a puzzling phenomenon *Eur. Respir. J.* **39** 669–76

[28] Peng G *et al* 2009 Diagnosing lung cancer in exhaled breath using gold nanoparticles *Nat. Nanotechnol.* **4** 669–73

[29] Machado R F *et al* 2005 Detection of lung cancer by sensor array analyses of exhaled breath *Am. J. Respir. Crit. Care Med.* **171** 1286–91

[30] Rakow N A and Suslick K S 2000 A colorimetric sensor array for odour visualization *Nature* **406** 710–3

[31] Mazzone P J *et al* 2012 Exhaled breath analysis with a colorimetric sensor array for the identification and characterization of lung cancer *J. Thorac. Oncol.* **7** 137–42

[32] Amann A *et al* 2014 The human volatilome: volatile organic compounds (VOCs) in exhaled breath, skin emanations, urine, feces and saliva *J. Breath Res.* **8** 034001

[33] Ratiu I A, Ligor T, Bocos-Bintintan V, Mayhew C A and Buszewski B 2021 Volatile organic compounds in exhaled breath as fingerprints of lung cancer, asthma and COPD *J. Clin. Med.* **10** 32

[34] Peng G *et al* 2009 Diagnosing lung cancer in exhaled breath using gold nanoparticles *Nat. Nanotechnol.* **4** 669–73

[35] Mazzone P J *et al* 2007 Diagnosis of lung cancer by the analysis of exhaled breath with a colorimetric sensor array *Thorax* **62** 565–8

[36] Chang J E *et al* 2018 Analysis of volatile organic compounds in exhaled breath for lung cancer diagnosis using a sensor system *Sens. Actuators B-Chem.* **255** 800–7

[37] Shlomi D *et al* 2017 Detection of lung cancer and EGFR mutation by electronic nose system *J. Thorac. Oncol.* **12** 1544–51

[38] Haick H and Hashoul D 2019 Lung cancer breath tests *Expert. Rev. Respir. Med.* **13** 597–9

[39] C. K *et al* 2021 Recognizing lung cancer and stages using a self-developed electronic nose system *Comput. Biol. Med.* **131** 104294

[40] Weinberg R A 2014 *The Biology of Cancer* Second edition (New York: Garland Science, Taylor & Francis Group) pp. xx, 876, A 6, G 30, I 28
[41] Chen X *et al* 2007 A study of the volatile organic compounds exhaled by lung cancer cells *in vitro* for breath diagnosis *Cancer* **110** 835–44
[42] Jia Z *et al* 2018 Detection of lung cancer: concomitant volatile organic compounds and metabolomic profiling of six cancer cell lines of different histological origins *ACS Omega* **3** 5131–40
[43] Barash O, Peled N, Tisch U, Bunn P A Jr, Hirsch F R and Haick H 2012 Classification of lung cancer histology by gold nanoparticle sensors *Nanomedicine* **8** 580–9
[44] Peled N *et al* 2013 Volatile fingerprints of cancer specific genetic mutations *Nanomedicine* **9** 758–66

IOP Publishing

Detection Systems in Lung Cancer and Imaging, Volume 1

Ayman El-Baz and Jasjit S Suri

Chapter 7

Precision molecular imaging can perhaps be enhanced for lung cancer management via integrated analysis of general parameters such as age, gender, genetics, and lifestyle

Kshitish K Acharya[1]

7.1 Multiple molecular imaging modalities have been beneficial in the clinical management of various cancer types, including different types of lung cancer

Computed tomography (CT), magnetic resonance imaging (MRI) and positron emission tomography (PET) have been commonly applied to various cancer applications. The clinical applications involve diagnostics, prognostics and other clinical decision making, including those related to response-adapted therapies. A list of examples of reviews in this regard has been compiled in table 7.1 using PubMed and Google Scholar. The literature review approach followed to prepare this write-up was based on our previous work on search engine comparisons [1].

PET is considered to be a more accurate technique than CT for predicting survival post radiation therapy (RT), whereas MRI could have better accuracy for soft tissue imaging with potential applications in online monitoring and treatment decisions [2].

Molecular imaging provides an opportunity to quantitatively assess biological processes within the body, particularly the metabolic activities and proliferation of cells and tissues, non-invasively [3]. Several technological advancements in molecular imaging, combined with molecular biology research related to cancer, have contributed to personalized assessments during diagnosis and prognosis, and more rational treatment approaches. A combined application of functional parameters with MRI and PET and molecular imaging could improve detection, characterization, staging and monitoring of

[1] Correspondence: juneindia@gmail.com.

Table 7.1. Examples of recent reviews on progress in imaging applications for lung cancer

Imaging modality	Main focus of the review	PMID
PET	Multiple testing, cut-point optimization, and signs of publication bias prognostic FDG-PET imaging	33271785 [83]
PET	18F-FDG-PET for SCLC	30465520 [17]
PET	Radiotherapy planning	32913277 [84]
PET	FDG-PET Imaging for NSCLC	32764429 [85]
CT	Imaging and comorbidities in chronic obstructive pulmonary disease (COPD)	32835707 [86]
CT	Interpretation pitfalls and limitations	31295144 [87]
CT	CT for NSCLC with anaplastic lymphoma kinase rearrangements	31164317 [88]
PET/CT	Radiopharmaceuticals for lung cancer imaging	33062275 [89]
PET/CT	Evaluation of multimodal treatment efficacy and toxicity in NSCLC	33760957 [90]
PET/CT	Imaging therapy	32723523 [91]
MRI	NSCLC staging	29803524 [92]

specific types of cancer, and expand the possibilities of personalized medicine [4]. PET/CT is considered to be important for planning radiotherapy for lung cancer as it helps in assessing staging and re-staging of disease, detecting recurrent or residual disease, evaluating response to therapy, and providing prognostic information—especially by functional tumour volume assessment in cases of non-small cell lung carcinoma (NSCLC), the major type (80%) of lung cancer [5, 6]. Rapid developments have occurred in the specialization of molecular imaging, identifying new targets and imaging probes, and their role in lung disorder management [7, 8]. Several molecular imaging probes have undergone, or are currently undergoing, either clinical use or studies under pre-clinical or clinical settings. A recent multi-institutional clinical trial (phase II) on intraoperative molecular imaging tested a near-infrared (NIR), folate-receptor targeted contrast agent, OTL38 [9]. The study showed improved ability of surgeons to identify hard-to-find nodules, occult cancers, and positive margins, in the case of 26% of patients with lung adenocarcinomas, the major histological subtype of the NSCLC type of lung cancer. The intraoperative molecular imaging found additional nodules in these patients, nine of which were cancerous and undetected pre-operatively. The imaging also located lesions in 12% cases, which were not detected earlier by the surgeon. Interesting observations were made during the margin checks as well. The imaging revealed positive margins in 9% of cases that were missed by the surgeon. The advantages of intraoperative molecular imaging were more obvious in the cases of sublobar pulmonary resections and in patients with ground-glass opacities. Such research on molecular probes is needed to enhance our ability to visualize cellular and molecular actions in specific regions. Different types of probe molecules can enhance the imaging outcomes via their ability to bind cancer-specific membrane proteins or receptor molecules, or molecules in adjacent tissues during various stages of development of specific types of cancer, including metastases. For example, radiolabeled analogues of choline, acetate, glucose, amino acids, and nucleotides can be used to evaluate increased metabolism and vascular changes in cancerous tissues [10]. An evaluation of the correlation of non-Gaussian diffusion kurtosis imaging found strong correlation of the imaging parameters with differential expression of epidermal growth factor receptor [EGFR], anaplastic lymphoma kinase [ALK], and Ki-67 protein in advanced lung adenocarcinoma [11]. Two homologous types of fluorescent probes (CH1055-PEG-PT and CH1055-PEG-Affibody) also seem to be attractive due to a higher uptake and better (spatial and temporal) resolution, and may be worth exploring for their use in imaging in the context of lung metastasis of osteosarcoma [12]. Several such explorations have been on the rise in recent decades, focusing on specific types of disorders, including several pleural disorders and lung cancer [7, 13–15].

7.2 There have been constant efforts for development of new probes for molecular imaging

Along with the research and progress in multiple molecular imaging modalities, developments in the probe varieties have also transformed diagnostic and prognostic nuclear medicine, which has become one of the main strategies for cancer management. For example, knowledge of the role of Cu in cell proliferation and angiogenesis has prompted researchers to explore studies on 64Cu as PET-probes using animal models in various tumors, including lung cancer [16]. Even with small cell lung cancer (SCLC), a relatively small proportion of all lung cancers, Sager *et al* [17] have recently reviewed the utility of PET imaging using 2-deoxy-2-[fluorine-18] fluoro-D-glucose PET (18F-FDG-PET), and summarized the efforts for improved staging, re-staging, selecting patients for curative/palliative intent, locating target regions, identifying suitable treatment options, detecting any residual disease or its recurrence, and assessing responses and predicting the treatment efficiency. The PET or PET/CT imaging applications for lung cancer, particularly using 18F-FDG, have been drawing significant attention in the recent years [18–21]. However, a specific probe cannot be relied on completely as there could be specific types of disadvantages with each type of probe [5]. Another probe of significance in the context of lung cancer is MHI-148—a type of heptamethine cyanine dye with the potential to be an effective imaging agent for clinical analysis of tumors. *In vivo* imaging with MHI-148 seems promising because it can cross the cytoplasmic membrane of lung cancer cells and a nude-mice-model study has suggested low cytotoxicity. The *ex vivo* fluorescence imaging in this study also suggested a higher uptake of MHI-148 in tumour cells than in other selected organs. Another fluorine-18 labeled probe, N-[18F]fluoroacetylcrizotinib, which is a derivative of crizotinib—an FDA approved tyrosine kinase inhibitor for the treatment of a type of NSCLC (anaplastic lymphoma kinase rearranged), seems to be useful as a PET ligand with applications in NSCLC imaging. This molecule has been shown to inhibit kinase activity as well as tumour growth [22, 23] proposed a new multifunctional drug-loaded nanosystem for MRI-guided diagnostics and therapeutics.

But there is more work to be done. While reviewing the progress of imaging-derived biomarkers that could predict genetic alterations and immunotherapy targets in lung cancer, Ninatti *et al* [24] conclude: 'Despite the promising results in terms of predictive performance, image-based models, suffering from methodological bias, require further validation before replacing traditional molecular pathology testing'. The progress and positive impact of research efforts towards better molecular probes and their imaging applications, for lung cancer and other cancer types, are expected to continue in the years to come as well. Similarly, research needs to continue for identifying novel target molecules as well!

7.3 Identifying novel biological molecules as targets for molecular imaging: research often starts with an exploration of gene expression patterns and mutations in the DNA, particularly those within the genes

Optical probe designs used for imaging are generally based on (endogenous or exogenous) fluorophores. Organic fluorophore probes that emit fluorescence only upon binding to targets are being engineered more frequently to target specific tissues in recent years. In this context, comparative studies on gene expression patterns across cancer conditions [25] and genetic variation association studies (see figure 7.1) can provide useful leads of molecules that could eventually be useful as markers for molecular imaging by direct-labelling or labelling of their antibodies. Using molecular markers to analyze cancer diagnosis, progress and exploring their use as potential target candidates have been common practice. But most of such analysis would involve collecting blood, other peripheral body fluids, pleural body fluids or biopsied cancer tissues followed by laboratory tests using sequencing or other molecular biology techniques. Next-generation sequencing (NGS) and microarrays have formed two primary techniques that serve as gateways for screening potential biomarkers. In almost all studies using such mass-scale techniques or 'omics' approaches, however, further studies have to be carried out eventually with detailed attention to specific genes and other molecules to short-list the candidate biomarkers for further research towards applications such as probe designing for molecular imaging.

Molecular imaging provides certain advantages in making better use of such markers, compared to the other molecular biology techniques such as PCR, RT-PCR, ELISA and FISH. The advantage of molecular imaging technology lies in its ability to visualize and enable the assessment of the spatial distribution of specific molecules within the cancerous tissue and its neighbourhood. The androgen receptor, prostate-specific membrane antigen-based PET radiotracers (e.g., N-[N-[(S)−1,3-dicarboxypropyl]carbamoyl]−4−^{18}F-fluorobenzyl-l-cysteine, ^{89}Zr-DFO-J591, and ^{68}Ga [HBED-CC]), and gastrin-releasing peptide receptor form good examples that may be targeted by specific radiolabeled imaging probes to explore prostate cancer [26, 27], Improved renal cell cancer detection with carbonic anhydrase IX (CAIX)-based antibody (^{124}I-girentuximab) and radioimmunotherapy targeting with ^{177}Lu-cG250 have been suggested too [26, 27]. Zhou *et al* [28] have

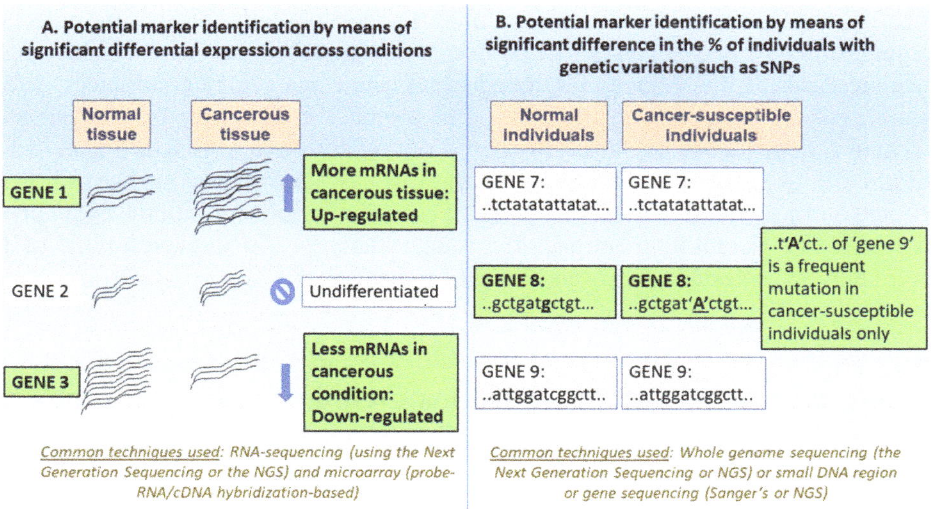

Figure 7.1. Two common approaches for large scale analysis and identification of genes and proteins that may play a key role in disease conditions. Even though these methods can help to short-list some genes among all human genes, further research is required to confirm even the candidature of these molecules for their biomarker potential. Additional studies are necessary first to short-list some of them to explore their use in applications as targets for diagnostics, prognostics, therapeutics, theranostics or molecular imaging. Hypothetical gene names/numbers are used in the figure. (a) A few hundreds of genes or even specific mRNA or non-coding RNA (ncRNA) molecules may be identified as differentially expressed in the disease condition in the disease-affected tissue or other peripheral body fluids. (b) A few protein-coding or non-protein-coding (coding for ncRNAs) genes may have SNPs occurring predominantly among one group of individuals. Similarly, indels or CNVs could also occur at a significantly different frequency among individuals with specific clinical characteristics such as susceptibility to disease and better or poor survival rates. These variations are observed in germ-line (basically, cells from any tissue) or somatic DNA (usually referring to DNA from cells that do not pass on the DNA to the next generation, such as the cancerous cells in most tissues). Depending on the type of source, they have a different biological significance

suggested an association of image characteristics from NSCLC patients with a selected set of genes chosen from specific molecular pathways.

NSCLC has been researched even better in terms of imaging applications. The epidermal growth factor receptor (EGFR)-mediated signalling pathway has been paid significant attention as this pathway is closely associated with NSCLC. Many drugs developed as inhibitors to target epidermal growth factor receptor tyrosine kinase have been very promising for NSCLC treatment. EGFR-tyrosine kinase inhibitors (EGFR-TKI) have been used in the clinical treatment of NSCLC. 18F-FDG-PET/CT imaging can be useful for monitoring of EGFR mutation and EGFR-TKI treatment efficacy. Several large scales of studies have shown that people with EGFR-sensitive mutation can specifically benefit from such EGF-kinase inhibitors. The variations of EGFR mutations within the cancer tissue can be crucial, and combinatorial use of EGFR-targeted molecular probes in PET-CT has enabled us to explore *in vivo* and analyze the diversity of the EGFR mutations in lung cancer tissues. Many genes, proteins and even non-coding RNAs such as the microRNAs [29, 30] still need to be explored for their potential utilities in molecular imaging.

But research in the above-mentioned areas alone may not be sufficient. Many research efforts (e.g., [31]) in the context of biomarker discovery or analysis have indicated a dependence or variations based on general factors that are likely to be brushed off as insignificant. Such observations, as summarized in the following sections, on these types of metadata seem to be more important than thought earlier. They have the potential to impact the image analysis and interpretations of the image features in terms of various clinical applications.

7.4 Combinatorial analysis of metadata on age, gender, lifestyle, etc, has not received enough attention even though this approach has great potential to enhance precision medicine in the area of molecular imaging

The notion that management may have to be different across people with a similar or identical clinical condition is not new. Recently this concept is referred to first as 'personalized medicine' and later as 'precision medicine'. In Ayurveda, the ancient Indian medicine system, people have been identified under seven types based on their behavioural and physiological nature, and treated differently [32–34]. We now know of single nucleotide polymorphisms (SNPs), insertions and deletions (InDels), and copy number variations (CNVs) that can help us identify the genetic basis of differences in the people in each clinical context. There are also multiple reports to suggest, or even clearly demonstrate, that many general parameters or confounding variables could influence the overall anatomical, physiological and metabolic details of normal individuals (see table 7.2). These parameters include gender, age, exercises, diet, ethnicity, comorbidities, sexuality, smoking habits, alcohol consumption, and pollution. And such details could, in turn, influence their disease susceptibility, the rate of progress and the extent of the severity of diseases. Hence, the confounding variables such as those listed above, could also potentially influence the outcome of the imaging. More importantly, considering these parameters while interpreting the imaging results may be beneficial in further decision making for various clinical applications. Currently, the role of such aspects may only be evident at some level in many cases. But studies with specific attention to such factors may reveal new associations. For example, colorectal cancer seems to be more frequent in industrialized countries compared to anal cancer. But an increase in the latter type of cancer may be associated with HIV infections, male homosexuality, and younger age of the first sexual encounter, particularly in high-income nations [35]. The table 7.2 summarizes some of such known influences of general biological and non-biological factors on health conditions, particularly on cancer of multiple types. It should be noted that some studies already indicate possible combinatorial influences by these parameters on the particulars of cancer. Genetic and molecular aspects may play a central role in the mechanism of such influences.

Table 7.2. Examples of general parameters that may be confounding variables potentially influencing the image characters, along with examples of reports on possible influence in recent times.

Parameter	Focus of the study/review	PubMed ID of the article(s)
Gender	Molecular basis of gender differences in cancer	33358908 [31], 27165743 [65]
Age	Thyroid cancer: age, gender and race, and neck CT imaging	3403709 [93]
Age	Imaging in aging males with bladder cancer	32401117 [94]
Age	MRI before biopsy in age-based screening for prostate cancer	33704474 [95]
Exercises	Breathing exercises in lung cancer patients	31007262 [96], 30357997 [97]
Exercises	Postoperative inspiratory muscle training and breathing exercises	26489835 [98]
Exercises	Aerobic, resistance, and mixed exercises on quality of life in cancer patients	33360071 [99]
Exercises	Spinal stabilization exercises for patients with spinal metastasis	33429892 [100]
Diet	Ketogenic diet influence on FDG-PET imaging (lung cancer mouse model)	29968182 [101]
Diet	Cancer and nutrition: MRI	24626110 [102]
Pollution	Air pollution and lung cancer	33974841 [103], 33752019 [104]
Pollution	Air pollution, microRNA and lung cancer	33477935 [105]
Lifestyle and nutrigenomics	Breast and colon cancer progression	33797366 [106]
Lifestyle and stress	Breast cancer development	29292669 [107]
Lifestyle and SNPs	Prostate cancer progression	28993831 [108]
Lifestyle, SNPs and diet	Breast and colorectal cancer	28968965 [109]; 26109419 [110]
Lifestyle, systemic inflammation	Pre-chemotherapy for breast cancer	25097833 [111]

Various genetic aspects are well-known to influence the anatomical and physiological aspects of humans. In many cases, specific genes and mutations that influence image features have been identified. For example, mutations in the CHRNG gene are known to be associated with autosomal recessive multiple pterygium syndrome (MPS) and they can influence muscle imaging features [36]. Cases with aneurysmal bone cysts present in soft tissue locations belong to a spectrum of tumours with USP6 gene rearrangements and MRI along with examinations of the samples with histopathology and molecular biology techniques may be helpful [37]. Smoking is an obvious candidate for in-depth analysis in the context of any lung disorder. Hence, many researchers have explored the impact of smoking on specific clinical phenotypes. Billatos *et al* [38] have recently explored whether quantitative CT can be used to analyze the smoking-related lung pathogenesis in conditions with a potential association of differential expression of genes in bronchial epithelium. They classified the smokers in three groups (preserved, interstitial predominant and emphysema predominant) and, based on gene expression variations across these groups, suggested enhanced inflammation in severe clinical phenotype possibly mediated by the tumor necrosis factor-α and interferon-β pathways.

Such changes at the level of DNA sequence or gene expression often have a strong dependence on multiple general parameters, as described below in the case of one such parameter (gender). Hence, a combinatorial analysis of data from molecular images along with different biological and non-biological parameters that can affect the health in general, may facilitate tailor-making medical decisions and pave the way to personalized diagnostic and prognostic decisions as well as preventive or therapeutic interventions. Such efforts towards individualized medicine can also help to avoid unnecessary expenses, toxicity of futile treatments and mental trauma to patients and relatives by offering treatments selectively to only those who respond. Lung cancer is a particularly heterogeneous disease functionally and morphologically. It is likely to be influenced by multiple general health conditions and external factors. Hence, exploring the potential influence of such general factors in the context of a specific type of lung cancer and various clinical procedures, including imaging, would be helpful.

However, enough attention is often not being paid to collect sufficient metadata related to the general parameters neither during the routine clinical image analysis nor during extensive research efforts while studying specific aspects of imaging applications. It would have been ideal if most clinical studies, including imaging and image analysis studies, reported as many associated general parameters as possible. It may then be possible to explore a potential influence of various confounding variables or factors associated with the clinical aspects and image features. Age and gender could also be some such basic aspects. For example, Rafiee F *et al* [39] reviewed the value of the potential role of molecular imaging, PET/CT in particular, in the detection and management of coronavirus disease 2019. They found that the mean age of 52 patients, across 30 publications was 60 ± 12.74, while the range was 27–87 years, with 28 (53.8%) men, and 19 (36.5%) women. The study also found an underlying malignancy among a good number of patients, including 18 different types of primary cancers and six metastatic cancer disease. Whereas the main focus of this review was on different aspects, gathering such a variety of metadata will have a long term value. Even if nothing seems important in individual studies, it is critical to collect data for later cumulative analysis—even to establish the lack of significance of each specific biological and non-biological parameter. Many of the metadata components may make more sense during large scale cumulative analysis, as indicated in the case study below where smoking and gender disparities have been discussed as an example of combinatorial analysis with gene expression patterns.

7.5 Gender as a special case of a general parameter that has the potential to contribute to precision medicine in the area of molecular imaging

The prevalence of lung cancer, and fatalities due to this disease, seem to vary depending on geographical location, gender, socioeconomic status, and other factors. Many of such differential influences may be because of the differences in smoking patterns [40]. Smoking is a well-known risk factor for lung cancer development. The risk seems to increase with the number of cigarettes smoked and the duration of smoking [41].

General anatomical and physiological differences in men versus women are obvious. But, while addressing possible factors associated with differences in lung cancer prevalence, progress and mortality, gender has not been an obvious candidate parameter for most researchers and clinicians. In men, lung cancer forms a leading cause of cancer deaths in the US and worldwide, and it is also the leading cause of cancer death among women in more developed countries [42, 43]. The gender-based variations in diseases, including cancer, have drawn the attention of researchers, particularly over the past decade. In fact, several studies have indicated the importance of gender bias and its consistency in multiple contexts of cancer [44–46]. As per a 2018 report [42], lung and bronchus cancer cases in males declined from the 1980s, while the trend increased from 1975 to 2005 [47]. Though lung cancer is generally more prevalent in men than women, the gender-wise proportions of people diagnosed with the disease seem to be changing with time [42, 48]. Several studies have indicated a possible higher chance of lung cancer detection or prevalence in women with different cigarette/tobacco smoke exposure levels than men with similar smoking history or exposure [49–54]. Lung cancer prevalence in non-smokers may also be higher among women than men [55, 56]. Lung adenocarcinoma is also reported to be more common in women than men, irrespective of smoking history [57, 58]. But a few studies [59–62] have shown a reverse trend. The correlations of any type seem to be debatable [63, 64].

Gender associated genes may help in exploring the gender-based susceptibility, diagnosis and responses to treatment, etc. Listing genes that may have gender association in terms of disease susceptibility and progress may help to explore the molecular basis of gender-biased physiological responses in lung cancer, as well as several aspects of this disorder. There have been efforts to explore the differences in male versus female cancer patients at the molecular level [65–67]. The frequency of some of the mutations in EGFR and KRAS may be higher in women than in men [68, 69]. It is possible that the type of gender difference, or such a possibility, is influenced by other factors.

The possibilities of gender differences to the susceptibility and prognosis of lung cancer were explained through the variations in processing of carcinogens, hormonal effects [70, 71], DNA adduct levels [72], etc. Possible gender-biased trends in such cases could be better studied if genes expressed differently across the genders are identified. With the availability of enormous data from mass-scale studies, it is possible to obtain valuable insights by revisiting the molecular signatures of several male and female lung cancer patients. Meta-analysis of high-throughput gene expression data from various techniques has been widely used to identify functional association of genes in normal tissues [73, 74] as well as diseases including cancer [75–77]. There were also studies reporting meta-analysis of gene expression signatures to identify candidate genes in lung cancer [7, 79, 80], but not in the context of smoking-associated gender differences.

Understanding any gender bias at a molecular level is important to establish the gender differences associated with lung cancer. Such an understanding may open new approaches while addressing diagnostics, prognostics and therapeutics. A meta-analysis of TCGA-RNA-seq data reported gender-biased genes from multiple cancer types, and stressed the significance of developing sex-specific targets in certain cancer types, including lung cancer [65]. We had earlier found such a gender-specific molecular profile via meta-analysis of microarray datasets [81, 82] by performing a focused analysis of gene expression patterns showing gender bias in the lungs of lung cancer patients who smoked. We recently reported this work where we had selected multiple, mass-scale gene expression datasets and performed a meta-analysis of these datasets to identify differential gene expressions in the lung tissue across the genders among the smoking and non-smoking patients of lung cancer [31]. After selecting 13 microarray studies and 1100 samples from these studies, we identified 1159 genes that showed sexual dimorphism in their expression among lung cancer patients who were smokers. Of these, 400 and 474 genes showed differential expression in the cancerous lung compared to the normal lung of women and men, respectively. The expression pattern of the genes that showed expression-based association with lung cancer specific to female smokers (LCFS) and to male smokers (LCMS) was compared with an independent microarray-report as well as TCGA-RNA-sequencing data. Although a smaller number of genes showed a sexual dimorphism in the differential expression pattern consistently in four or five studies, a combination of some of these genes can be perhaps explored for the generation of a panel of potential biomarker genes for further analysis in the context of gender-based prognosis and therapeutics of NCSLC among smokers. A similar analysis found a gender bias of 904 genes in the adenocarcinoma subtype of NSCLC. It should be noted that very few genes consistently showed gender bias across studies or samples. The number of genes that showed over- or under-expression across any two studies was higher than those differentially expressed across any three, and so on. The genes SNX20, GIMAP6, MTMR2, FAM171B, IDH1, MOBP, FBXO17, LPXN and WIPF1 showed consistent differential expressed across genders in smoking in at least four studies. Among these SNX20, MTMR2, LPXN and WIPF1 genes were particularly interesting as their quantity of expression was significantly different between the male and female lung cancer patients across five studies. There were no genes showing such consistency beyond 5 of the 14 studies considered. However, a combinatorial analysis of expression of these genes with other variables such as age, lifestyle, ethnicity etc might reveal better consistency within small groups of patients.

Genes expressed in higher quantities, specifically in the lungs of female lung cancer patients who smoked, were notably involved in immune-responses and cell-adhesion, while those upregulated in comparable male patients were associated with other processes namely, signal-transduction, gene expression, and cell-cycle. Our analysis [31] found specific immune-related processes and pathways, including lymphocyte activation, endocytosis, to be enriched among the genes expressed in higher quantity in the lung tissues of smoking female lung cancer patients compared to male lungs, under similar conditions. This study also identified four mitochondrial ribosomal genes namely, MRPL24, MRPL35, MRPS34 and MRPS10 that were expressed significantly less in female lung cancer smokers than similar male patients.

The approach in our study [31] was unique for many reasons: (a) we used a very select set of gene expression datasets; the number of samples analysed for the lung cancer was considerably less in other similar meta-analysis reports. (b) We obtained gender-biased genes having consistent differential regulation between male and female smokers of lung cancer, but separated those with a gender-biased expression in the normal lung tissue of smokers as well as non-smokers. We had also filtered out those expressed differently among lung cancer patients who did not smoke. Such filtering was not considered in the other studies reporting gender-specific genes across multiple cancers, and it is essential to make a difference to focus on specific types of confounding variables this way.

7.6 Conclusion

Multiple factors are known to influence different aspects of cancer initiation, progress and survival. Logically, they would also influence the image features and could be useful in imaging outcome. There are already indications that support such possibilities. Hence, it is essential to consider seemingly insignificant general parameters, while studying or developing different imaging modalities, target biological molecules and molecular probes. Even when there is no significant attention paid during individual studies on such parameters, inclusion of all such metadata in the research reports is essential for assessing the potential impact of these confounding variables on image characters, analysis and the following clinical decisions, via meta-analysis. Clustering the individuals based on combination of information about the general parameters is a better research approach for precision medicine. Such approaches are likely to enhance the quality of clinical decisions, including those for molecular image analysis and interpretations in lung cancer.

7.7 Funding and conflict of interest

This research did not receive any specific grant from funding agencies in the public, commercial, or not-for-profit sectors. IBAB is supported by the IT, BT and ST department of the Government of Karnataka. The author received financial support only from IBAB, even though he is a scientific adviser for Shodhaka LS Pvt. Ltd., and founded this company. This company supports basic research, and the affiliation with this company in no way alters the pure academic nature of the work being reported.

References

[1] Bajpai A, Davuluri S, Haridas H *et al* 2011 In search of the right literature search engine(s) *Nat. Prec.* https://doi.org/10.1038/npre.2011.2101.3
[2] MacManus M *et al* 2017 Anatomic, functional and molecular imaging in lung cancer precision radiation therapy: treatment response assessment and radiation therapy personalization *Transl. Lung Cancer Res.* **6** 670–88
[3] Wibmer A G *et al* 2016 Molecular imaging of prostate cancer *Radiographics.* **36** 142–59
[4] Pinker K *et al* 2016 'Multiparametrische und molekulare Bildgebung von Brusttumoren mit MRT *und* PET-MRT' [Multiparametric and molecular imaging of breast tumors with MRI and PET/MRI] *Radiologe* **56** 612–21
[5] Filice A *et al* 2020 Radiotherapy planning and molecular imaging in lung cancer *Curr. Radiopharm.* **13** 204–17
[6] Greenspan B S 2017 Role of PET/CT for precision medicine in lung cancer: perspective of the Society of Nuclear Medicine and Molecular Imaging *Transl. Lung Cancer Res.* **6** 617–20
[7] Francis R *et al* 2011 Novel molecular imaging in lung and pleural diseases *Respirology* **16** 1173–88
[8] MacManus M *et al* 2015 The evolving role of molecular imaging in non-small cell lung cancer radiotherapy *Semin. Radiat. Oncol.* **25** 133–42
[9] Gangadharan S *et al* 2020 Multi-institutional phase 2 clinical trial of intraoperative molecular imaging of lung cancer *Ann. Thorac. Surg* **112** 1150–9
[10] Wibmer A G *et al* 2016 Molecular imaging of prostate cancer *Radiographics.* **36** 142–59
[11] Peng Q *et al* 2020 Diffusion kurtosis imaging: correlation analysis of quantitative model parameters with molecular features in advanced lung adenocarcinoma *Chin. Med. J.* **133** 2403–9
[12] Zhou H *et al* 2020 Specific small-molecule NIR-II fluorescence imaging of osteosarcoma and lung metastasis *Adv. Healthcare Mater.* **9** e1901224
[13] Nishino M *et al* 2011 Imaging of lung cancer in the era of molecular medicine *Acad. Radiol.* **18** 424–36
[14] Dharmarajan S and Daniel P S 2005 Molecular imaging of the lungs *Acad. Radiol.* **12** 1394–405
[15] McWilliams A *et al* 2002 Innovative molecular and imaging approaches for the detection of lung cancer and its precursor lesions *Oncogene* **21** 6949–59
[16] Chakravarty R *et al* 2016 $^{64}Cu^{2+}$ ions as PET probe: an emerging paradigm in molecular imaging of cancer *Mol. Pharm.* **13** 3601–12
[17] Sager O *et al* 2019 Utility of molecular imaging with 2-Deoxy-2-[Fluorine-18] Fluoro-DGlucose positron emission tomography (^{18}F-FDG PET) for small cell lung cancer (SCLC): a radiation oncology perspective *Curr. Radiopharm.* **12** 4–10
[18] Zukotynski K A and Gerbaudo V H 2017 Molecular imaging and precision medicine in lung cancer *PET Clin.* **12** 53–62
[19] Jiménez-Bonilla J F *et al* 30 Sep. 2016 The role of PET/CT molecular imaging in the diagnosis of recurrence and surveillance of patients treated for non-small cell lung cancer *Diagnostics* **6** 36

[20] Novello S *et al* 2012 Functional imaging in predicting response to antineoplastic agents and molecular targeted therapies in lung cancer: a review of existing evidence *Crit. Rev. Oncol. Hematol* **83** 208–15

[21] van Loon J *et al* 2011 Therapeutic implications of molecular imaging with PET in the combined modality treatment of lung cancer *Cancer Treat. Rev.* **375** 331–43

[22] Buck J R *et al* 2020 N-[^{18}F]-Fluoroacetylcrizotinib: a potentially potent and selective PET tracer for molecular imaging of non-small cell lung cancer *Bioorganic Med. Chem. Lett.* **30** 127257

[23] Gao P *et al* 2018 Designing multifunctional cancer-targeted nanosystem for magnetic resonance molecular imaging-guided theranostics of lung cancer *Drug Deliv.* **25** 1811–25

[24] Ninatti G *et al* 2020 Imaging-based prediction of molecular therapy targets in NSCLC by radiogenomics and AI approaches: a systematic review *Diagnostics* **10** 359

[25] Grimm J *et al* 2005 Use of gene expression profiling to direct *in vivo* molecular imaging of lung cancer *Proc. Natl. Acad. Sci. U.S.A.* **102** 14404–9

[26] Wibmer A G *et al* 2016 Molecular imaging of prostate cancer *Radiographics.* **36** 142–59

[27] Cho S Y and Szabo Z 2014 Molecular imaging of urogenital diseases *Semin. Nucl. Med.* **44** 93–109

[28] Zhou M *et al* 2018 Non-small cell lung cancer radiogenomics map identifies relationships between molecular and imaging phenotypes with prognostic implications *Radiology* **286** 307–15

[29] Boeri M *et al* 2015 Recent advances of microRNA-based molecular diagnostics to reduce false-positive lung cancer imaging *Expert Rev. Mol. Diagn.* **15** 801–13

[30] Zhu H-Z *et al* 2018 Identification and imaging of miR-155 in the early screening of lung cancer by targeted delivery of octreotide-conjugated chitosan-molecular beacon nanoparticles *Drug Deliv.* **25** 1974–83

[31] Davuluri S *et al* 2021 The molecular basis of gender disparities in smoking lung cancer patients *Life Sci.* **267** 118927

[32] Sharma P V editor. Ch. 1. Varanasi: Chowkambha Sanskrit Series *Chaukambha Orientalia; 1981–86* 4th edn Caraka Samhita

[33] Hankey A 2005 The scientific value of Ayurveda *J. Altern. Complement. Med.* **11** 221–5

[34] Dey S and Pahwa P 2014 Prakriti and its associations with metabolism, chronic diseases, and genotypes: possibilities of new born screening and a lifetime of personalized prevention *J. Ayurveda Integr. Med.* **5** 15–24

[35] Sandach P *et al* 2020 Molecular imaging and therapy of colorectal and anal cancer *Semin. Nucl. Med.* **50** 465–70

[36] Carrera-García L *et al* 2019 CHRNG-related nonlethal multiple pterygium syndrome: muscle imaging pattern and clinical, histopathological, and molecular genetic findings *Am. J. Med. Genet.* A **179** 915–26

[37] Song W *et al* 2019 Soft tissue aneurysmal bone cyst: six new cases with imaging details, molecular pathology, and review of the literature *Skelet. Radiol.* **487** 1059–67

[38] Billatos E *et al* 2021 Distinguishing smoking-related lung disease phenotypes via imaging and molecular features *Chest* **1592** 549–63

[39] Rafiee F *et al* 2021 Coronavirus disease 2019 (COVID-19) in molecular imaging: a systematic review of incidental detection of SARS-CoV-2 pneumonia on PET studies *Semin. Nucl. Med.* **51** 178–91

[40] Torre L A *et al* 2016 Lung cancer statistics *Adv. Exp. Med. Biol.* **893** 1–19

[41] Dela Cruz C S *et al* 2011 Lung cancer: epidemiology, etiology, and prevention *Clin. Chest Med.* **324** 605–44
[42] Siegel R L *et al* 2018 Cancer statistics, 2018 *CA: Cancer J. Clin.* **68** 7–30
[43] Torre L A *et al* 2015 Global cancer statistics, 2012 *CA: Cancer J. Clin.* **65** 87–108
[44] Dorak M T and Karpuzoglu E 28 Nov. 2012 Gender differences in cancer susceptibility: an inadequately addressed issue *Front. Genet.* **3** 268
[45] Wessels H *et al* 2010 Gender-related needs and preferences in cancer care indicate the need for an individualized approach to cancer patients *Oncologist* **15** 648–55
[46] Gabriele L *et al* 2016 The gender perspective in cancer research and therapy: novel insights and on-going hypotheses *Ann. Ist. Super. Sanita* **52** 213–22
[47] Boloker G *et al* 2018 Updated statistics of lung and bronchus cancer in United States (2018) *J. Thorac. Dis.* **10** 1158–61
[48] Barrera-Rodriguez R and Morales-Fuentes J 15 Dec. 2012 Lung cancer in women *Lung Cancer* **3** 79–89
[49] Kabat G C 1996 Aspects of the epidemiology of lung cancer in smokers and nonsmokers in the United States *Lung Cancer* **15** 1–20
[50] Zang E A and Wynder E L 1996 Differences in lung cancer risk between men and women: examination of the evidence *J. Natl. Cancer Inst.* **88** 183–92
[51] Risch H A *et al* 1993 Are female smokers at higher risk for lung cancer than male smokers? A case-control analysis by histologic type *Am. J. Epidemiol.* **138** 281–93
[52] Osann K E *et al* 1993 Sex differences in lung-cancer risk associated with cigarette smoking *Int. J. Cancer* **54** 44–8
[53] Int. Early Lung Cancer Action Program Investigators *et al* 2006 Women's susceptibility to tobacco carcinogens and survival after diagnosis of lung cancer *JAMA* **296** 180–4
[54] Hansen M S *et al* 2018 Sex differences in risk of smoking-associated lung cancer: results from a cohort of 600,000 Norwegians *Am. J. Epidemiol.* **187** 971–81
[55] Sun S *et al* 2007 Lung cancer in never smokers–a different disease *Nat. Rev. Cancer* **7** 778–90
[56] Subramanian J and Govindan R 2007 Lung cancer in never smokers: a review *J. Clin. Oncol.* **25** 561–70
[57] Radzikowska E *et al* 2002 Lung cancer in women: age, smoking, histology, performance status, stage, initial treatment and survival. Population-based study of 20 561 cases *Ann. Oncol.* **13** 1087–93
[58] de Perrot M *et al* 2000 Sex differences in presentation, management, and prognosis of patients with non-small cell lung carcinoma *J. Thorac. Cardiovasc. Surg.* **119** 21–6
[59] Prescott E *et al* 1998 Gender and smoking-related risk of lung cancer. The Copenhagen Center for Prospective Population Studies *Epidemiology* **9** 79–83
[60] Kreuzer M *et al* 2000 Gender differences in lung cancer risk by smoking: a multicentre case-control study in Germany and Italy *Br. J. Cancer* **82** 227–33
[61] De Matteis S *et al* 2013 Are women who smoke at higher risk for lung cancer than men who smoke *Am. J. Epidemiol.* **177** 601–12
[62] Yu Y *et al* 2014 Gender susceptibility for cigarette smoking-attributable lung cancer: a systematic review and meta-analysis *Lung Cancer* **85** 351–60
[63] Twombly R 2004 New studies fan controversy over gender risk in lung cancer *J. Natl. Cancer Inst.* **96** 898–900
[64] Kligerman S and White C 2011 Epidemiology of lung cancer in women: risk factors, survival, and screening *AJR Am. J. Roentgenol.* **196** 287–95

[65] Yuan Y *et al* 2016 Comprehensive characterization of molecular differences in cancer between male and female patients *Cancer Cell* **29** 711–22
[66] Cheng F 2016 Gender dimorphism creates divergent cancer susceptibilities *Trends Cancer* **2** 325–26
[67] Mukhtar F *et al* 2018 Disparities by race, age, and sex in the improvement of survival for lymphoma: findings from a population-based study *PLoS One* **13** e0199745
[68] Zhang Y-L *et al* 2016 The prevalence of EGFR mutation in patients with non-small cell lung cancer: a systematic review and meta-analysis *Oncotarget* **7** 78985–93
[69] Kim H R *et al* 2012 Distinct clinical features and outcomes in never-smokers with nonsmall cell lung cancer who harbor EGFR or KRAS mutations or ALK rearrangement *Cancer* **118** 729–39
[70] Gasperino J and William N R 2004 Gender and lung cancer *Clin. Lung Cancer* **5** 353–9
[71] Cote M L *et al* 2009 Tobacco and estrogen metabolic polymorphisms and risk of non-small cell lung cancer in women *Carcinogenesis* **30** 626–35
[72] Olak J and Colson Y 2004 Gender differences in lung cancer: have we really come a long way, baby? *J. Thorac. Cardiovasc. Surg.* **128** 346–51
[73] Thakur A *et al* 2005 The role of X-linked genes in breast cancer *Breast Cancer Res. Treat.* **93** 135–43
[74] Neubauer H *et al* 2013 Possible role of PGRMC1 in breast cancer development *Climacteric* **16** 509–13
[75] Li Y *et al* 26 Oct. 2018 Transcriptomic and functional network features of lung squamous cell carcinoma through integrative analysis of GEO and TCGA data *Sci. Rep.* **8** 15834
[76] Waldron L and Riester M 2016 Meta-analysis in gene expression studies *Methods Mol. Biol* **1418** 161–76
[77] Fehrmann R S N *et al* 2015 Gene expression analysis identifies global gene dosage sensitivity in cancer *Nat. Genet.* **47** 115–25
[78] Chen R *et al* 2014 A meta-analysis of lung cancer gene expression identifies PTK7 as a survival gene in lung adenocarcinoma *Cancer Res.* **74** 2892–902
[79] Kim J *et al* 6 Aug. 2018 Relative efficacy of checkpoint inhibitors for advanced NSCLC according to programmed death-ligand-1 expression: a systematic review and network meta-analysis *Sci. Rep.* **8** 11738
[80] Tang M *et al* 2018 Prognostic significance of CIP2A expression in solid tumors: a meta-analysis *PLoS One* **13** e0199675
[81] Davuluri S, Bajpai AK, Thirumurugan K and Acharya K K 2015 Integrated analysis of microarray and RNA-Seq data identified novel genes associated with lung cancer, particularly with female smokers *Indo-French Seminar on 'Women in Science' through CEFIPRA, 3rd–5th February Indian Institute of Science, Bengaluru, India*
[82] Nov 2015 *Int. Conf. on cancer Research: New Horizons* conducted by NCCS, Pune
[83] Clausen M M *et al* 1 Dec. 2020 Multiple testing, cut-point optimization, and signs of publication bias in prognostic FDG-PET imaging studies of head and neck and lung cancer: a review and meta-analysis *Diagnostics* **10** 1030
[84] Lee S J and Park H J 10 Sep. 2020 Single photon emission computed tomography (SPECT) or positron emission tomography (PET) imaging for radiotherapy planning in patients with lung cancer: a meta-analysis *Sci. Rep.* **10** 14864
[85] Kaseda K 5 Aug. 2020 Recent and current advances in FDG-PET imaging within the field of clinical oncology in NSCLC: a review of the literature *Diagnostics* **10** 561

[86] Singhvi D and Bon J 2021 CT imaging and comorbidities in COPD: beyond lung cancer screening *Chest* **159** 147–53
[87] Feng S H and Su-Tso Y 2019 The new 8th TNM staging system of lung cancer and its potential imaging interpretation pitfalls and limitations with CT image demonstrations *Diagn. Interv. Radiol.* **25** 270–79
[88] Mendoza D P *et al* 2019 Computed tomography imaging characteristics of non-small-cell lung cancer with anaplastic lymphoma kinase rearrangements: a systematic review and meta-analysis *Clin. Lung Cancer* **20** 339–49
[89] Theodoropoulos A S *et al* 2020 Modern radiopharmaceuticals for lung cancer imaging with positron emission tomography/computed tomography scan: a systematic review *SAGE Open Med.* **8** 2050312120961594
[90] Eze C *et al* 2021 PET/CT imaging for evaluation of multimodal treatment efficacy and toxicity in advanced NSCLC-current state and future directions *Eur. J. Nucl. Med. Mol. Imaging* **48** 3975–89
[91] Sheikhbahaei S *et al* 2020 Imaging in therapy response assessment and surveillance of lung cancer: evidenced-based review with focus on the utility of ^{18}F-FDG PET/CT *Clin. Lung Cancer* **21** 485–97
[92] Brea T P *et al* 2019 Use of magnetic resonance imaging for n-staging in patients with non-small cell lung cancer. a systematic review *Arch. Bronconeumol.* **55** 9–16
[93] Ma G M Y *et al* 2021 Neck CT imaging and correlation with thyroid cancer incidence across age, gender and race *Clin. Endocrinol.* **94** 872–9
[94] Kutluhan M A *et al* 2020 How reliable are imaging techniques in aging males with bladder cancer? *Aging Male* **23** 1339–45
[95] Callender T *et al* 2021 Benefit, harm, and cost-effectiveness associated with magnetic resonance imaging before biopsy in age-based and risk-stratified screening for prostate cancer *JAMA Network Open* **4** e2037657
[96] Liu X *et al* 2019 Effects of breathing exercises on patients with lung cancer *Oncol. Nurs. Forum* **46** 303–17
[97] Wang Y-Q *et al* 2019 Impact of breathing exercises in subjects with lung cancer undergoing surgical resection: a systematic review and meta-analysis *J. Clin. Nurs.* **28** 717–32
[98] Brocki B C *et al* 2016 Postoperative inspiratory muscle training in addition to breathing exercises and early mobilization improves oxygenation in high-risk patients after lung cancer surgery: a randomized controlled trial *Eur. J. Cardiothorac. Surg.* **49** 1483–91
[99] Fukushima T *et al* 2021 Effects of aerobic, resistance, and mixed exercises on quality of life in patients with cancer: a systematic review and meta-analysis *Complement. Ther. Clin. Pract.* **42** 101290
[100] Rosenberger F *et al* 2021 Spinal stabilization exercises for cancer patients with spinal metastases of high fracture risk: feasibility of the DISPO-II training program *Cancers* **13** 201
[101] Cussó L *et al* 2019 Effects of a ketogenic diet on [^{18}F]FDG-PET imaging in a mouse model of lung cancer *Mol. Imaging Biol.* **21** 279–85
[102] Neamat-Allah J *et al* 2014 Validation of anthropometric indices of adiposity against whole-body magnetic resonance imaging–a study within the German European Prospective Investigation into Cancer and Nutrition (EPIC) cohorts *PLoS One* **9** e91586
[103] Yang S *et al* 2021 Association between long-term exposure to high levels of ambient air pollution and incidence of lung cancer in a population-based cohort *Environ. Res.* **198** 111214

[104] Chung C Y *et al* 2021 An investigation into the impact of variations of ambient air pollution and meteorological factors on lung cancer mortality in Yangtze River Delta *Sci. Total Environ.* **779** 146427

[105] Sima M *et al* The impact of air pollution exposure on the MicroRNA machinery and lung cancer development *J. Pers. Med.* **11** 60

[106] Ray S, Kumar and Mukherjee S 31 Mar. 2021 Nutrigenomics and life style facet- a modulatory molecular evidence in progression of breast and colon cancer with emerging importance *Curr. Mol. Med.* https://doi.org/10.2174/1566524021666210331151323

[107] Yıldırım N K *et al* 2018 Possible role of stress, coping strategies, and life style in the development of breast cancer *Int. J. Psychiatry Med.* **53** 207–20

[108] Bandil K *et al* 2017 Association of SNPs/haplotypes in promoter of TNF A and IL-10 gene together with life style factors in prostate cancer progression in Indian population *Inflamm. Res.* **66** 1085–97

[109] Kopp T I *et al* 2017 Association between single nucleotide polymorphisms in the antioxidant genes *CAT*, *GR* and *SOD1*, erythrocyte enzyme activities, dietary and life style factors and breast cancer risk in a Danish, prospective cohort study *Oncotarget* **8** 62984–97

[110] Kopp T I *et al* 2015 Polymorphisms in ATP-binding cassette transporter genes and interaction with diet and life style factors in relation to colorectal cancer in a Danish prospective case-cohort study *Scand. J. Gastroenterol.* **50** 1469–81

[111] Debra E L *et al* 2014 Health promoting life-style behaviors and systemic inflammation in African American and Caucasian women prior to chemo-therapy for breast cancer *Health Promot. Perspect.* **4** 18–26

IOP Publishing

Detection Systems in Lung Cancer and Imaging, Volume 1

Ayman El-Baz and Jasjit S Suri

Chapter 8

Computed tomography ventilation imaging in lung cancer: theory, validation and application

Bilal A Tahir

8.1 Introduction

Worldwide, lung cancer is the leading cause of cancer-related deaths [1], with the majority (> 87%) of patients dying within five years of their initial diagnosis [2]. Despite significant improvements in alternative treatment techniques, surgical resection remains the standard of care for early-stage non-small cell lung cancer (NSCLC) and a component of the multimodality approach to stage IIIA disease, offering cancer control, improved overall survival and quality of life. However, a majority of lung cancer patients smoke, and smoking is a significant risk factor for developing other pulmonary co-morbidities, including chronic obstructive pulmonary disease (COPD), which is present in around 75% of patients [3]. Such pre-existing lung function impairment means patients are at higher risk of post-operative morbidity and mortality, and pulmonary complications have been shown to be the most costly post-operative complication, resulting in more extended hospital stays [4]. A significant proportion of patients with NSCLC are unable to tolerate the further loss in lung function from resection and are thus unsuitable for potentially curative surgery. Thoracic radiotherapy provides an alternative, potentially curative, treatment modality. However, its efficacy is limited by the incidence of radiation-induced lung injury for cancer patients who already tend to suffer from reduced pre-treatment pulmonary function [5].

The current paradigm in thoracic radiotherapy is to assume homogenous function throughout the lungs [6]. However, lung cancer patients have been shown to have regional alterations in lung function, owing to other pulmonary co-morbidities [3]. Consequently, it is highly desirable to acquire regional measures of lung function to spatially assist in preferential sparing of functional lung during the treatment planning process. This ‘functional lung avoidance treatment planning’ concept has been applied to several functional lung imaging modalities, including single-photon emission computed tomography (SPECT) [7, 8] and hyperpolarised gas magnetic resonance imaging (MRI) [9, 10]. However, current regional lung function modalities suffer from some or all of the following: poor spatial and temporal resolution, requirement of a contrast agent and highly specialised equipment inaccessible to most clinical radiotherapy centres.

Computed tomography (CT) images of the lungs are routinely utilised in the clinic for the diagnosis, treatment planning, monitoring and treatment assessment of patients with lung cancer. CT-based surrogates of regional ventilation, sometimes referred to as 'CT ventilation images (CTVIs)', which are derived from thoracic CT images acquired at different inflation levels without exogenous contrast, have been proposed as alternatives to clinically established lung function modalities [11, 12]. However, prior to widespread clinical use, the physiological accuracy must be validated to provide confidence that the computed image is a true reflection of regional ventilation.

This chapter reviews the underlying theory of CTVI techniques, previous validation studies and clinical applications in lung cancer. Limitations for clinical adoption and a roadmap for future research are also detailed.

8.2 Theory

8.2.1 Overview

Computation of conventional CTVI is a three-step process. Firstly, CT images are acquired either at multiple breath-holds at different respiratory states (most commonly inspiration and expiration) or during tidal breathing via respiratory-correlated 4D-CT. Secondly, a deformation field is created, which spatially maps one of the acquired images (e.g., inspiration) to another (e.g., expiration) through non-rigid image registration. Finally, a ventilation metric is either computed directly on the deformation field by quantifying the local volume change or on the aligned images by quantifying intensity change on a voxel by voxel basis. Several methods have been proposed to compute CTVIs, the most prevalent being the intensity [11] and Jacobian [12] metrics. Figure 8.1 shows the workflow to generate conventional CTVIs.

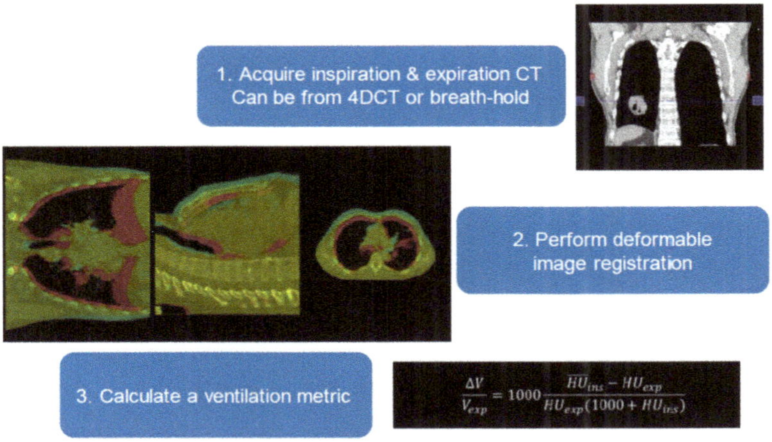

Figure 8.1. Workflow to generate conventional CT-based surrogates of ventilation.

8.2.2 Intensity metric

The intensity-based metric originates from theory proposed by Simon *et al* [13]. Guerrero *et al* first used it to derive a ventilation metric from multi-inflation breath-hold CT images deformably registered using an optical flow algorithm [11]. The underlying assumption of this theory is that the fraction of air in a pulmonary parenchymal voxel located in a CT image with an associated Hounsfield unit (HU) is equal to:

$$F_{\text{air}} = -\frac{\text{HU}}{1000} \tag{8.1}$$

Any voxel in the lung parenchyma is comprised of both air and tissue, each with an associated HU [13]. If it can be assumed that uniform air distribution exists in the volume and that the change in volume between respiratory phases is attributable to changes in air volume only as shown in figure 8.2 (i.e. tissue is incompressible and there is no change in the volume of tissue between inspiration and expiration) [13], then the fractional volume change between inspiration and expiration can be calculated as follows [11]:

$$\frac{\Delta V}{V_{\text{air}}^{\text{exp}}} = \frac{F_{\text{ins}} - F_{\text{exp}}}{F_{\text{exp}}(1 - F_{\text{ins}})} \tag{8.2}$$

where ΔV is the local air volume change between inspiration and expiration, $V_{\text{air}}^{\text{exp}}$ is the local air volume at expiration and F_{ins} and F_{exp} are the voxel fractions of air in the inspiration and expiration images, respectively. This measure is assumed to be a surrogate for specific ventilation, which is defined as the ratio of fresh gas (including oxygen) volume delivered to the alveoli following inspiration over the expiratory volume [14, 15] and can be calculated directly from the aligned inspiratory and expiratory CT images by the following equation [11, 16–18]:

$$\frac{\Delta V}{V_{\text{air}}^{\text{exp}}} = 1000\frac{\overline{\text{HU}}_{\text{ins}} - \text{HU}_{\text{exp}}}{\text{HU}_{\text{exp}}(1000 + \overline{\text{HU}}_{\text{ins}})} \tag{8.3}$$

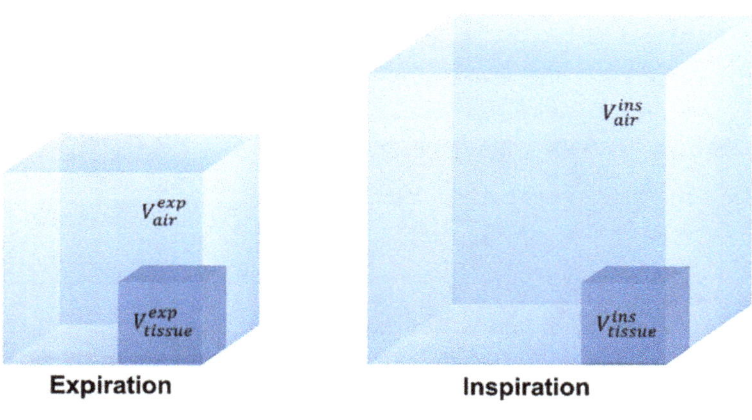

Figure 8.2. Example parenchymal region at expiration (left) and inspiration (right), demonstrating the fundamental assumption of the intensity metric in terms of constant tissue volume between inflation levels.

where $\overline{\text{HU}}_{\text{ins}}$ is the interpolated HU value of the voxels in the deformed inspiratory CT image, which spatially correspond to the voxel in the expiratory CT image, and HU_{exp} is the HU of the expiratory voxel. Thus, the intensity metric is effectively a measure of change in fractional content of air per voxel between respiratory phases.

8.2.3 Jacobian metric

The Jacobian metric is independent of the image intensity value. This metric was introduced to circumvent uncertainties introduced into the CT image by noise and reconstruction artefacts [12]. This metric calculates local volume change between the two respiratory phase images by computing the Jacobian determinant (J) directly on the deformable image registration-defined deformation vector field $h(x,y,z)$ as follows:

$$J(h(x, y, z)) = \begin{vmatrix} 1 + \dfrac{\partial h_x(x, y, z)}{\partial x} & \dfrac{\partial h_x(x, y, z)}{\partial y} & \dfrac{\partial h_x(x, y, z)}{\partial z} \\ \dfrac{\partial h_y(x, y, z)}{\partial x} & 1 + \dfrac{\partial h_y(x, y, z)}{\partial y} & \dfrac{\partial h_y(x, y, z)}{\partial z} \\ \dfrac{\partial h_z(x, y, z)}{\partial x} & \dfrac{\partial h_z(x, y, z)}{\partial y} & 1 + \dfrac{\partial h_z(x, y, z)}{\partial z} \end{vmatrix} \tag{8.4}$$

The Jacobian determinant provides a measure of volume change such that a voxel value of one represents the preservation of local volume. In contrast, values less than and greater than one correspond to contraction and expansion of local volume, respectively. Values less than zero are indicative of singularities in the deformation vector field.

Strictly speaking, the Jacobian metric computes an image of regional volume change and is not equivalent to specific ventilation, which is a direct physiological measure of the fractional volume of fresh gas delivered to the lung volume unit [14, 15]. In addition, as shown in figure 8.3, it is based on the assumption that no

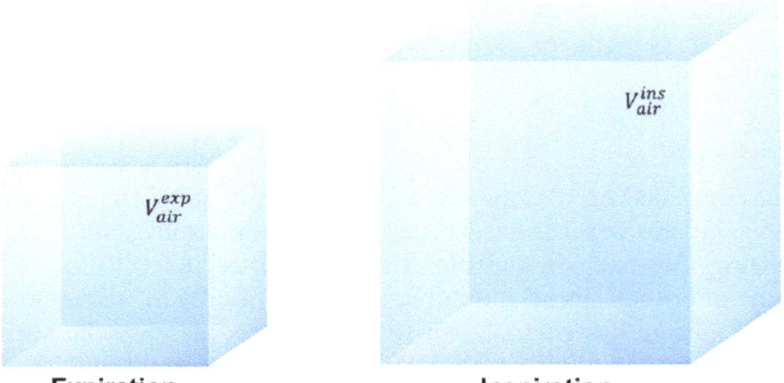

Figure 8.3. Example parenchymal region at expiration (left) and inspiration (right), demonstrating the fundamental assumption of the Jacobian metric in terms of zero tissue volume between inflation states.

tissue volume exists in the inspiratory and expiratory images and volume changes are solely due to changes in air volume [12, 19].

8.2.4 Specific gas volume

A recent metric to be proposed is based on inflation-induced changes in specific gas volume [20]. This metric computes surrogates of ventilation from HU differences between aligned inhale and exhale images similar to the intensity metric. It differs, however, in the way that it models ventilation. Specific gas volume (SGV) was initially proposed by Coxson *et al* [21] and is defined in units of millilitres of gas volume per gram of tissue (ml/g). It is calculated for each inhalation level via the following equation:

$$\text{SGV} = \text{specific} \quad \text{volume}_{\text{gas+tissue}} - \text{specific} \quad \text{volume}_{\text{tissue}} \tag{8.5}$$

The specific volume of tissue is assumed to be constant, regardless of inflation level, and is equivalent to 0.94 ml g^{-1} [22]. The specific volume of gas and tissue is computed directly from thoracic CT images as follows:

$$\text{specific} \quad \text{volume}_{\text{gas+tissue}} = \frac{1024}{\text{HU} + 1024} \tag{8.6}$$

8.2.5 Other metrics

Several non-conventional metrics to model ventilation have also been proposed. These include a geometric method first proposed by Zhang *et al* [23], which computes volume change by partitioning cubic voxels into six independent tetrahedrons defined by the positions of eight voxel vertices at expiration which are deformed at inspiration [23, 24]. The volumetric sum of these tetrahedrons yields the surrogate of specific ventilation [18, 23, 24]. Ding *et al* [19] have devised a hybrid metric comprising of both intensity and Jacobian based metrics, which purports to account for both air and tissue volume changes. Kipritidis *et al* proposed to use the 4D-CT time-averaged regional product of air and tissue densities as a surrogate of ventilation [25]. It is pertinent to note that this metric does not rely on deformable registration.

8.2.6 Discussion

The metrics computed on the raw HU values are susceptible to registration errors and CT noise at the voxel level. To account for these uncertainties, a common post-processing approach in the literature is to filter the CTVIs [11, 18], thus providing a smoothed local measure of ventilation with some loss of data complexity. Filtering has been shown to significantly increase the correlation of the ventilation images against more established modalities [26, 27]. Although metrics computed directly on the deformation field such as the Jacobian metric are independent of CT noise and thus only affected by registration error [28], their numerical stability has been questioned; small variations in deformation vectors fields with similar registration accuracies have been shown to lead to significantly larger changes in the underlying distributions of the computed ventilation images [29]. To circumvent the problems asscotiated with the intensity and Jacobian metrics, Castillo *et al* have recently proposed two novel robust numerical methods, namely, the mass conserving volume change [30] and integrated Jacobian formulation [31] methods, respectively.

The fundamental assumption inherent in most ventilation metrics is that changes in lung density and volume between inflation levels are due solely to the influx of air whilst regional tissue and blood volume remain constant [19]. Previous 4D-CT work has shown lung mass to vary cyclically with respiratory phase, perhaps due to the distention of the vasculature and inflation-related differences in cardiac output [16]. More recent investigations with dual-energy CT have confirmed that the regional distribution of pulmonary blood volume is sensitive to inflation level with marked variations observed in dependant and non-dependant regions [32]. The hybrid metric purports to account for the effects of inflation-induced regional perfusion variations. However, as it is based on both the intensity and Jacobian metrics, it suffers from the aforementioned limitations of both metrics.

8.3 Validation

For CTVI to be used in the clinic, its physiological accuracy must be validated against established clinical imaging modalities. This includes determining the best ventilation metric and the most robust deformable registration algorithm. Initial studies were limited to global measures [11, 16]. Currently, there is a growing body of literature evaluating the technique with comparisons against assumed ground truth or gold standard ventilation imaging modalities such as nuclear medicine imaging, hyperpolarised gas MRI and Xenon (Xe)-CT. This section reviews the studies relating to each validation technique and identifies limitations and gaps in the literature. Table 8.1 summarises previous studies validating CTVIs against other pulmonary functional imaging modalities.

8.3.1 Comparisons with global measures

Early studies were limited to validation of the ventilation information by a self-consistency check involving the comparison of segmented lung from the ventilation images with the tidal volumes calculated from the difference between the segmented lung masks at inspiration and expiration [11, 16, 18]. Guerrero *et al* [11] compared breath-hold CT ventilation volumes derived from the intensity metric with CT-dervied tidal volumes and demonstrated high correlation via linear regression ($R^2 = 0.985$). A similar result was shown for 4D-CT ventilation with $R^2 = 0.984$. Castillo *et al* [18] compared left and right lung tidal volumes with ventilation volumes derived from three metrics: intensity, Jacobian and geometric. They demonstrated high correlation with R^2 values of 0.99, 0.94 and 0.94, respectively.

Yamamoto *et al* [33] evaluated the effect of thresholding on the tidal volume comparison method. Lung ventilation contours derived from the intensity and Jacobian based metrics were segmented and compared against CT derived tidal

Table 8.1. Summary of previous pre-clinical and clinical studies validating non-contrast CT-based surrogates of ventilation against contrast-based functional lung imaging modalities. Where multiple metrics were studied, the value for the highest performing metric is quoted.

Study	Reference Modality	Subjects	Time interval between CT and reference	CT breathing manoeuvre	Reference breathing manoeuvre	CT ventilation metric	Comparison method	Key finding(s)†
Nuclear Medicine:								
[18]	^{99m}Tc-DTPA SPECT ventilation	7 humans	Same day	4D-CT	Free breathing	Intensity and Jacobian	DSC of five percentile bands, ranging from 0–20% up to 81–100%	Low DSCs with highest correlation for lowest percentile band (<0.4).
[36]	^{99m}Tc-DTPA/^{99m}Tc-MAA SPECT ventilation/ perfusion	1 human	Same day	4D-CT	Free breathing	Intensity and Jacobian	Voxel-wise SCC	Low/moderate SCCs for V/Q (0.18/0.48)
[37]	^{99m}Tc-DTPA SPECT ventilation	6 humans	⩽ 24 hours	Breath-hold (FRC and TLC)	Free breathing	Lobar expansion	Absolutes differences in percent lobar ventilation	Low differences (2.1%)
[38]	^{99m}Tc-MAA SPECT perfusion	10 humans	One week	4D-CT	Free breathing	Intensity	DSC of defect regions	High DSCs (0.78)
[35]	^{99m}Tc-DTPA SPECT ventilation	16 humans	9 days	4D-CT	Free breathing	Intensity and Jacobian	DSC of defect regions	Low DSCs (0.39)

(Continued)

Table 8.1. *(Continued)*

Study	Reference Modality	Subjects	Time interval between CT and reference	CT breathing manoeuvre	Reference breathing manoeuvre	CT ventilation metric	Comparison method	Key finding(s)†
[39]	^{99m}Tc-DTPA planar ventilation	15 humans	$\leqslant$ 62 days	4D-CT	Free breathing	Intensity	Correlation of percent ventilation in each lung and lung third.	Good and moderate correlation for each lung (0.65) and lung third (0.45).
[40]	^{99m}Tc-DTPA SPECT ventilation	8 humans	4 days	4D-CT	Free breathing	Intensity and Jacobian	Voxel-wise SCC	Moderate SCC (0.47).
[41]	Technegas SPECT ventilation	11 humans	33 days	4D-CT	Free breathing	Intensity, Jacobian and time-averaged regional product of air and tissue densities	Voxel-wise SCC and DSC	Weak SCC (0.26) and moderate DSCs for defect (0.39) and non-defect (0.69) regions.
[42]	^{99m}Tc-DTPA SPECT ventilation	15 humans	N/R (both pre-RT)	4D-CT	Free breathing	IJF and MCVC	Voxel-wise SCC	High SSC for IJF (0.82) and moderate SSC for MCVC (0.48)
[26]	^{68}Ga-aerosol PET ventilation	12 humans	Same session	4D-CT	Free breathing	Intensity and Jacobian	Voxel-wise SCC and DSC	Moderate SCC (0.42); moderate and strong DSCs for low

								function (0.52) and good function (0.88) regions.
[43]	^{68}Ga-aerosol PET ventilation	11 humans	Same session	Breath-hold (End-expiration and inhalation)	Free breathing	Intensity	Correlation for percent lobar ventilation	Excellent correlation (0.96)
[25]	^{68}Ga-aerosol PET ventilation	25 humans (25 pre-RT, 22 mid-RT and 18 post-RT)	Same session	4D-CT	Free breathing	Intensity, Jacobian and time-averaged regional product of air and tissue densities	Voxel-wise SCC	Moderate SCC (0.50)
Xenon CT:								
[17]	Xe-CT specific ventilation	4 sheep	Same session	4D-CT	Mechanically ventilated	Intensity	Correlation for manually defined ROIs with varying size (average: 1.6 ml)	Increasing correlation for increasing ROI size (small: 0.59; medium: 0.71; large: 0.76)
[12]	Xe-CT specific ventilation	5 sheep	Same session	4D-CT	Mechanically ventilated	Jacobian	Correlation for 4 mm thick ROIs	High correlation (0.73)
[19]	Xe-CT specific ventilation	4 sheep	Same session	4D-CT	Mechanically ventilated			High correlation (0.82)

(*Continued*)

Table 8.1. *(Continued)*

Study	Reference Modality	Subjects	Time interval between CT and reference	CT breathing manoeuvre	Reference breathing manoeuvre	CT ventilation metric	Comparison method	Key finding(s)†
						Intensity, Jacobian and Hybrid	Correlation for 20×20×20 mm^3 ROIs	
[44]	Xe-CT specific ventilation	4 sheep	Same session	4D-CT	Mechanically ventilated	Intensity, Jacobian and Geometric	Voxel-wise SCC and DSC	Moderate SCC (0.44) and DSC for lower 30% ventilated volumes (0.55)
MRI:								
[45]	^{3}He-MRI static ventilation	11 humans	1.5 weeks	4D-CT	Breath-hold (FRC+1L)	Intensity	DSC of ventilated volume of each individual lung	High DSCs (0.87)
[46]	^{3}He-MRI static ventilation	30 humans	1.5 days	Breath-hold (FRC and TLC)	Breath-hold (FRC+1L)	Lobar expansion	Absolutes differences in percent lobar ventilation	Low differences (4.0%)
[27]	^{3}He- and ^{129}Xe-MRI static ventilation	11 humans	Same day	Breath-hold (FRC and FRC+1L)	Breath-hold (FRC+1L)	Intensity, Jacobian and specific gas volume	Voxel-wise and ROI SCC	Voxel level: 0.1–0.8;ROI 20x20 voxels: 0.2–0.9
[47]	^{3}He-MRI static ventilation	7 humans	1.5 days	Breath-hold (FRC and TLC)	Breath-hold (FRC+1L)	Intensity	DSC of percentage ventilated volumes	High DSCs (0.93)

Abbreviations: DTPA = diethylenetriamine-pentaacetic acid; MAA = macroaggregated albumin; DSC = Dice similarity coefficient; SCC = Spearman's correlation coefficient; ROI = region of interest; RT = radiotherapy; FRC = functional residual capacity; TLC = total lung capacity; IJF = integrated Jacobian formulation; MCVC = mass conserving volume change; N/R = not reported. † Highest value given.

volumes with a threshold at -250 HU and -600 HU. They showed that the -600 HU threshold method yielded higher correlation values, suggesting that the higher contrast features such as small vessels in the -250 threshold mask could have led to inaccuracies in the HU values [33].

CTVI has also been validated against global measures of emphysema. Yamamato *et al* [33] investigated the correlation of 4D-CT derived ventilation for 12 patients with emphysema. They hypothesised that as lung regions not affected by emphysema are significantly more ventilated than emphysematous regions, 4D-CT ventilation would demonstrate higher ventilation in non-emphysematous regions. They tested this hypothesis for ventilation derived from the intensity and Jacobian metrics. Voxels with HU values lower than -910 were identified as emphysematous. Statistically significant differences were demonstrated only for the intensity metric, indicating that it could be a better surrogate of ventilation than the Jacobian metric.

Comparing CT ventilation-derived metrics such as defective lung volumes and coefficients of variation with global measurements of spirometry, moderate correlations between FEV_1 and FEV/FVC, ranging from 0.43 to 0.73 ($n = 15$) and 0.38 to 0.73 ($n = 98$) for the intensity and Jacobian metrics have been reported, respectively, in lung cancer [34, 35].

Given the regional nature of ventilation heterogeneity, the major limitation of these studies is that they only compare global measures and do not physiologically validate the local/regional ventilation information against clinically established functional lung imaging techniques.

8.3.2 Comparisons with nuclear medicine imaging

Nuclear medicine imaging is the most common method for imaging regional lung function. It employs radioactive tracers that are either inhaled or administered intravenously to image ventilation and perfusion, respectively. Common tracers for imaging ventilation include technetium-99m (^{99m}Tc) diethylenetriamine-pentaacetic acid (DTPA) and xenon-133 (^{133}Xe) gas. Pulmonary perfusion is normally imaged by ^{99m}Tc macroaggregated albumin (MAA). Once in the body, the radioactive tracer emits gamma photons that a gamma camera can detect and can yield superimposed planar images of the distribution of the radiotracer by a technique referred to as planar scintigraphy. By acquiring images at multiple angles around the patient and subsequently performing image reconstruction, 3D images of lung function can be computed. The SPECT technique typically requires 10–30 minutes for a volumetric acquisition [48].

Castillo *et al* performed the first physiological validation of CTVI against SPECT [18]. They compared the spatial overlap of 5% intervals of 20% up to 100% by the dice similarity coefficient (DSC) between 4D-CT ventilation computed from the intensity, Jacobian and geometric metrics with that of ^{99m}Tc-DTPA SPECT ventilation imaging for seven patients. They found statistically significant differences in the coefficients in favour of the intensity metric over the Jacobian and geometric metrics, with the highest correlation observed in the lowest percentile band. However, the reported DSCs for each percentile were low (< 0.4), possibly due to the susceptibility of ^{99m}Tc-DTPA to airway deposition artefacts.

In a methodological study of one patient, 4D-CT ventilation images derived from both intensity and Jacobian based metrics were compared with both SPECT ventilation and perfusion imaging, resulting in poor correlation coefficients of 0.030/0.357 and 0.184/0.479 for each metric, respectively [49]. This was consistent with the findings of Castillo *et al* [18], who also reported weak correlations. Surprisingly, the correlation of SPECT perfusion was slightly higher despite the ventilation signal being compared. The higher correlation for perfusion could be attributable to the severe COPD disease progression of the patient in the study; ^{99m}Tc-DTPA SPECT ventilation images commonly exhibit false ventilation due to central airway deposition [50, 51].

Although the study had the advantage that images for both modalities were acquired on the same day, similar to Castillo *et al* [18], there were some differences in the breathing manoeuvre and patient positioning. The SPECT scans were acquired during free breathing without respiratory coaching to improve patient breathing and reduce artefacts. This contrasts with the 4D-CT acquisition, which employed audio-visual biofeedback [52] to control breathing. Furthermore, the 4D-CT ventilation images were derived from the end-inspiration and end-expiration images only, while the SPECT images were averaged over many breathing cycles. An improvement to this methodology would be to compare 4D-CT ventilation derived from all phases in the respiratory cycle [49] and, in conjunction, use breathing coaching to ensure similar breathing techniques for both imaging modalities.

Another limitation of the SPECT validation method relates to the inherent low resolution of SPECT images (around 10 mm slick thickness). The high-resolution 4D-CT ventilation image has to be downsampled to match the SPECT resolution, thus losing local ventilation information. This provides a more regional ventilation comparison which would not validate the local ventilation represented by each voxel in the CT ventilation image. Perhaps the major limitation of this study is the limited clinical conclusions that can be drawn from it because there was only one patient in the cohort.

^{99m}Tc-MAA SPECT perfusion has also been compared to 4D-CT ventilation derived from the intensity metric for ten patients with malignant airway stenosis [38]. Moderately high spatial coincidence was shown (mean DSC = 0.78) in non-functional regions distal to lesion obstruction [38]. From a methodological view, the major limitation of this study was the validation of the ventilation information against a non-ventilation perfusion measurement assumed to be ground truth; Castillo *et al* [38] assumed matched ventilation and perfusion defects for the cohort of patients in this study. However, in a recent study comparing SPECT ventilation and perfusion defects for 51 lung cancer patients, Yuan *et al* [53] showed 39% of patients in their cohort to have discrepancies between ventilation and perfusion, with 8% of patients with higher ventilation than perfusion and 31% showing the opposite. Their own conclusions are that perfusion is insufficient to provide a complete picture of lung function and additional ventilation information is needed [53].

Another limitation of this study is that SPECT scans were acquired one week after the 4D-CT scans [38]. Although both were acquired before treatment, thus ensuring that radiation-induced changes did not affect the underlying ventilation distribution, some physiological changes may have occurred during the time interval between scans. A further drawback of this study and potential cause of error relates to the multi-modal image registration between the SPECT and 4D-CT ventilation images. An affine registration was employed which does not account for the postural differences in imaged physiological states due to different breathing manoeuvres. Furthermore, registration validation only consisted of a visual inspection. An improvement would be to use a more objective validation method such as measuring Euclidean distances between anatomical landmarks.

Although regional lung function has traditionally been assessed by nuclear imaging, conventional planar and tomographic techniques suffer from poor accuracy, spatial and temporal resolution and aerosol depositions in defect regions [48]. This may reduce correlation against CTVI. The efficacy of ventilation-based nuclear imaging can be improved by position emission tomography (PET) by inhalation of Gallium-68 (^{68}Ga) carbon nanoparticles, commonly referred to as Galligas, and has shown moderate vowel-wise correlations with 4D-CT derived ventilation [25, 26]. However, although the imaging data of these studies were acquired to enable improvements over the CTVI versus SPECT studies with 4D-CT acquired at the same session and couch as PET, inherent discrepancies in image acquisition settings remained. In general, the PET Galligas ventilation images were acquired over a minimum time scale of 10 minutes to ensure sufficient tracer accumulation, increasing for poor inhalations or low administered doses [54]. Conversely, 4D-CT was acquired over a single tidal breath. Such differences may reduce spatial correlations between the two modalities.

Given the uncertainties in the HU values due to image noise and registration errors, several investigators have compared CT-based ventilation models with nuclear medicine imaging at the lobar level. In previous work by De Backer *et al* [37], a CT model of lobar ventilation computed from two breath-hold CT scans based on the volume expansion between lobes was compared to SPECT lobar ventilation in a cohort of six mildly asthmatic patients. As this ventilation model utilized lobar segmentations only, it has the advantage of being independent of image registration. More recently, Eslick *et al* [43] compared ventilation derived from the intensity metric with PET Galligas for 11 lung cancer surgical resection candidates. Both studies have observed high correlations, indicating that correlation may be improved at courser levels. However, the same aforementioned limitations in comparisons with nuclear imaging apply.

8.3.3 Comparisons with xenon-enhanced CT

Ventilation can also be imaged and quantified by xenon-enhanced CT (Xe-CT). This technique employs radio-dense Xe gas as an inhaled contrast agent to increase the HU values of the pulmonary airspaces. The rate of gas wash-in and wash-out can be estimated from serial Xe-CT images, providing a direct and quantifiable measure of regional specific ventilation [15].

Several studies have validated non-contrast CT surrogates of ventilation against Xe-CT specific ventilation. The first published study compared ventilation CT derived from the Jacobian metric in 4 mm thick regions equally spaced along the ventral–dorsal direction for the lungs of five healthy sheep at constant pressure [12]. Using linear regression, moderately high correlation (mean $R^2 = 0.73$) was demonstrated.

In a follow-up study, intensity, Jacobian and hybrid Jacobian metrics of ventilation were compared with Xe-CT ventilation for four sheep [19]. Using linear regression, spatial correspondence was evaluated for 20×20×20 mm^3 cubes with average correlation coefficients of $R^2 = 0.58$, $R^2 = 0.75$ and $R^2 = 0.82$ demonstrated for each measure, respectively. Statistically significant differences between the hybrid and intensity measurements were observed for all animals in the study. Figure 8.4 shows the comparison for a sheep representative of their study cohort.

Ding *et al* [19] also evaluated the spatial correspondence for 150×8×40 mm^3 regions of interests and demonstrated higher correlation for intensity ($R^2 = 0.87$), Jacobian ($R^2 = 0.88$) and hybrid metrics ($R^2 = 0.92$). Furthermore, statistically significant differences between the metrics were not demonstrated for most animals for the larger 150×8×40 mm^3 regions of interests, suggesting that local and regional evaluation is preferred over global measures for improved assessment of the most sensitive ventilation metric [19]. Both studies [12, 19] reported limited clinical findings due to the small cohort and the use of non-human subjects. Zhang *et al* [44] employed the same dataset and performed voxel-wise correlations for the intensity, Jacobian and geometric metrics, observing moderate Spearman correlations of 0.44.

Although Xe-CT is considered the gold standard in ventilation imaging and provides superior resolution to other modalities, it suffers from limited axial coverage of up to 3 cm [12], due to the requirement of high temporal resolution, thus not allowing for full volumetric validation of CTVI. This also poses significant challenges in performing viable spatial correlations, owing to the difficulties in accurately registering the selected Xe-CT slabs to the volumetric CT images.

8.3.4 Comparisons with hyperpolarised gas MRI

Conventional MRI provides images of the hydrogen protons in water molecules. However, it suffers from several drawbacks for the lungs. These include the low proton density in the lungs, the millions of air–tissue interfaces which give rise to magnetic susceptibility artefacts and the negligible signal from the airspaces. These limitations can be overcome with hyperpolarised gas MRI, a technique that requires inhalation of discreet volumes of magnetised noble gases such as helium-3 (^{3}He) or xenon-129 (^{129}Xe). [55, 56] The technique provides images of the noble gas distribution in the pulmonary airspaces with high spatial and temporal resolution. Regions of hyposignal are indicative of ventilation defects [56].

Mathew *et al* [45] first evaluated the spatial correspondence of 4D-CT ventilation derived from the intensity metric with ^{3}He-MRI for eleven lung cancer patients. Using DSCs, they demonstrated a high degree of spatial overlap for both ipsilateral (0.86±0.12) and contralateral (0.88±0.12) lung.

However, this work had several methodological limitations. Firstly, the image acquisition protocol was not optimised to minimise potential discrepancies between the two modalities; the two different scans were acquired at a mean interval of

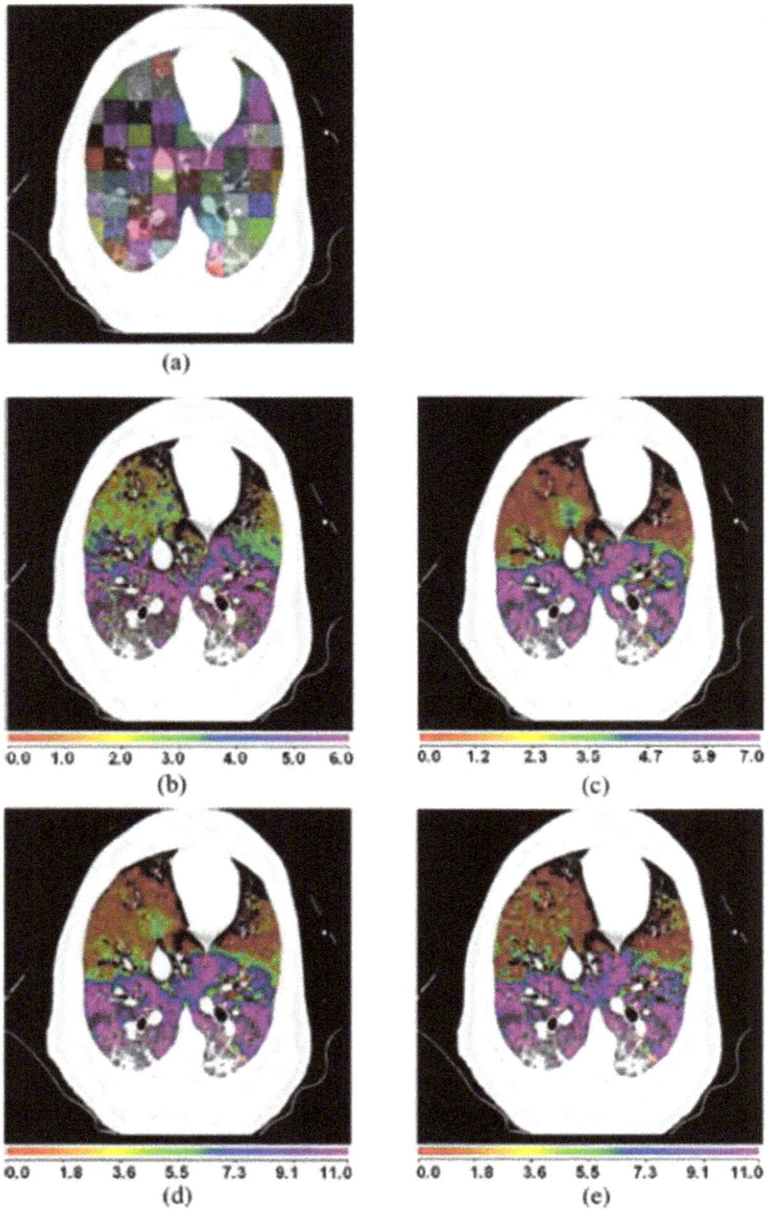

Figure 8.4. Example sheep comparison of (b) Xe-CT ventilation with 4D-CT ventilation derived from (c) Jacobian, (d) hybrid and (e) intensity metrics. (a) Colour coded cubes representing regions of interests. Reproduced with permission from [19], copyright (2012) John Wiley & Sons.

1.5 weeks for each patient and, thus, some of the regional ventilation differences in their study could be attributable to disease progression. Furthermore, differences in patient positioning (treatment planning couch versus diagnostic MRI couch) and

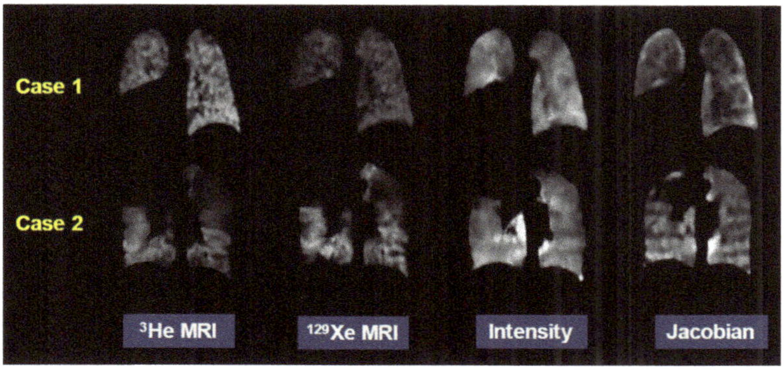

Figure 8.5. Example coronal slices of ^{3}He and ^{129}Xe-MRI and CT ventilation images derived from the intensity and Jacobian metrics for two lung cancer patients. Adapted with permission from [27], copyright (2018) with permission from Elsevier.

breathing manoeuvre (inspiratory breath-hold versus tidal breathing) were not explicitly accounted for, potentially leading to differences in the imaged physiologic states and registration errors; Ireland *et al* [57] demonstrated significant improvements in rigid registration by reproducing the same breath-hold and body positions during image acquisition of CT and ^{3}He-MRI. Secondly, only fiducial anatomical landmark affine registration was used to ensure the CT ventilation and HP gas images were in the same spatial domain without accounting for deformable differences between the two images, owing to postural differences. Thirdly, only ventilation derived from an intensity metric was evaluated in this study with no reference to other prominent metrics such as the Jacobian metric. Fourthly, the assessment of spatial correlation was limited to comparing the spatial overlap of binary thresholded images from both modalities by DSCs. Such overlap measures provide a more global comparison. Thus voxel-wise and region of interest analysis may improve the comparison by assessing the correlation of the intensity distribution of corresponding regions within the binary segmentations.

An alternative gas to ^{3}He for hyperpolarised gas MRI is ^{129}Xe. ^{129}Xe has begun to play a more important role in recent years, owing to global depletions in ^{3}He [55]. ^{129}Xe-MRI exhibits some differences in ventilation distributions compared with ^{3}He-MRI [58, 59].

Tahir *et al* investigated the spatial correlation of CT-based ventilation techniques against both ^{3}He and ^{129}Xe-MRI using an improved image acquisition and analysis strategy to minimize differences between imaging modalities, thus enhancing the accuracy of spatial correlation analysis [27]. They observed that the spatial correlation between MRI and CT was significantly less than between both noble gases, indicating that CTVIs may not be solely measuring lung ventilation. Figure 8.5 shows example hyperpolarised gas MRI and CTVIs derived from the intensity and Jacobian metrics for two representative patients in their study.

8.3.5 Reproducibility

Reproducibility of CTVI derived from 4D-CT images has been investigated by Du *et al* [28] and Yamamoto *et al* [60]. In the former, the intra-session ventilation reproducibility of two consecutive 4D-CT scans was investigated for three sheep and nine human patients [28]. The scans were acquired within 10 minutes of each other. The ventilation metric used was the Jacobian metric and the spatial correspondence between scans was compared by computing the average voxel by voxel ratio of the CTVIs. Although strong correlations were shown for the sheep cohort, the human cohort demonstrated moderately weak correlations, attributable perhaps to the fact that the sheep were mechanically ventilated while under anaesthesia without being moved during image acquisition while the humans breathed via audio coaching [28].

The results demonstrated for the human cohort in Du *et al* [28] are in agreement with those of Yamamoto *et al* [60], who evaluated the reproducibility for both intra- and inter-session 4D-CT image acquisition. For the intra-session patients, 4D-CT image acquisition was repeated for six lung cancer patients with a five-minute interval. The inter-session cohort consisted of another six patients imaged by 4D-CT repeated at an interval of fifteen days. Using the Spearman's correlation analysis, they demonstrated only moderate correlations with coefficients of 0.53±0.20 and 0.48±0.11 for intra- and inter-session scans, respectively [60]. Figure 8.6 shows a comparison between scans for the weakest correlated inter-session patient in the study.

One factor which could have caused the ventilation discrepancies between scans is the possible presence of artefacts in the 4D-CT images, which has been shown to affect 90% of scans [61]. Another factor relates to the degree of respiratory variation between scans. Recently, Mistry *et al* [62] evaluated the effects of different breathing manoeuvres during CT imaging and observed marked differences in the distribution of CTVIs. Gated image acquisition and breathing training could improve the reproducibility of the tidal breathing procedure [60].

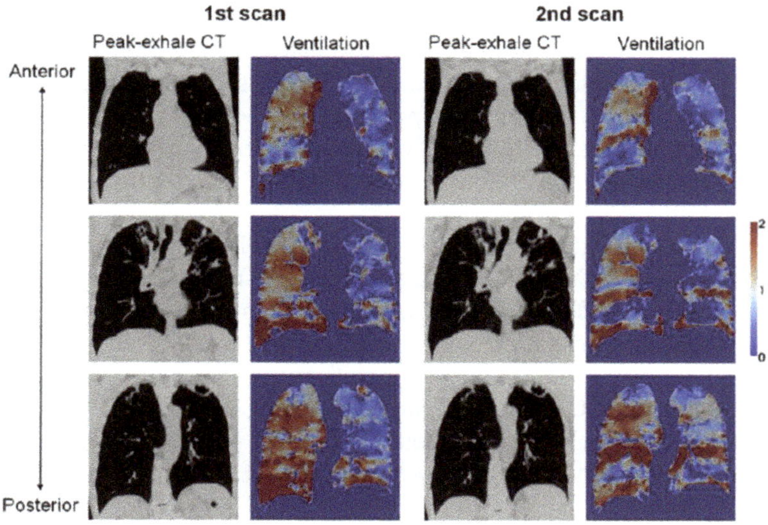

Figure 8.6. Comparison of baseline scan with follow-up for an inter-session patient with weakest spatial correlation (Spearman coefficient = 0.36) in study. Reproduced with permission from [60], copyright (2012) with permission from Elsevier.

The inferior reproducibility for the inter-session cohort could be due to several factors including differences in patient positioning and underlying physiological changes occurring during the fifteen-day interval [60]. A drawback of this study was that the repeat scans were acquired with different arm positions (arms down versus up). Differences in ventilation and respiratory measures have been shown to be sensitive to arm position [63]. An improved follow-up study would thus ensure the same imaging protocol be used for repeat scans.

To date, only 4D-CT ventilation reproducibility has been investigated in the literature. However, no published work exists evaluating the reproducibility of breath-hold CT ventilation. Such a study would be of clinical relevance to the radiotherapy community as breath-holds are integrated into several motion mitigation strategies to reduce safety margins in thoracic radiotherapy.

8.4 Clinical applications in lung cancer

8.4.1 Functional lung avoidance radiotherapy treatment planning

One of the major driving forces behind the development of CTVI is its potential for functional lung avoidance radiotherapy treatment planning [6]. This is due to its potential advantages over alternative functional lung imaging modalities in terms of superior spatial resolution, not requiring a contrast agent and its widespread availability in radiotherapy clinics. In fact, in many centres worldwide, breath-holds or 4D-CT are a pre-treatment requirement and would thus not require additional scanner time, ionising radiation or patient inconvenience. Hence, the ventilation information is referred to as 'freely available' [64] as only image processing is required.

In an initial feasibility study, Yaremko *et al* [65] evaluated the dosimetric impact of incorporating intensity-based 4D-CTVI in intensity-modulated radiotherapy (IMRT) for 21 lung cancer patients. Nine equidistant fields were used and a functionally-guided approach to treatment planning was employed to test the hypothesis that the incorporation of the ventilation information results in statistically significant reductions in dose to functional lung. The study demonstrated a reduction in several functional dosimetric parameters, including the mean dose to functional lung, which was shown to reduce by 2.9 Gy.

In another retrospective study, Yamamoto *et al* [66] evaluated the dosimetric effects of incorporating 4D-CTVI in volumetric modulated arc therapy (VMAT) in addition to IMRT planning for 15 lung cancer patients. Six fixed-field coplanar IMRT and single arc VMAT treatment plans, with and without ventilation information, were created for each patient. Field arrangements were the same for paired plans incorporating anatomical information only and those incorporating the additional functional information. However, optimization constraints differed, where plans incorporating functional informational had constraints chosen to minimise dose to functional lung while only dose to the total lung parenchyma volumes were minimised for anatomical plans [66]. Statistically significant reductions in mean dose to functional lung of 1.8 Gy and 2.0 Gy for IMRT and VMAT were demonstrated, respectively. However, this was to the detriment of the target volume dose conformity and homogeneity.

Caution should be exercised when drawing conclusions from the results of the two aforementioned CTVI treatment planning studies. Careful examination of their methodology indicates that the reductions observed could be attributable to their ventilation segmentation methodology, where functional lung parameters were reported as percentile ventilation masks. Yaremko *et al* [65] used a threshold mask to delineate the 10% of ventilated lung with the highest value. The method proposed by Yamamoto *et al* [66] differed slightly in that the ventilated lung volumes were divided equally into three volumes referred to as low, moderate and highly ventilated lung. The optimisation constraints of the inverse algorithm were prioritised to preferentially reduce the dose to highly ventilated regions. This may explain why a lower reduction in mean dose to functional lung of 1.8 Gy was demonstrated in Yamamoto *et al* [66] for IMRT, compared with the 2.7 Gy value in Yaremko *et al* [65], as the 90% percentile would inevitably lead to smaller ventilated lung volumes.

Neither study presents a physiological basis for selecting their respective threshold segmentation methods. Furthermore, their methods do not conform to published validation studies evaluating the physiological accuracy against established pulmonary functional imaging modalities.

So far, the clinical efficacy of functional lung avoidance treatment planning has not been proven. Ultimately, randomised clinical trials are needed to ensure widespread clinical use of the technique. To this end, three clinical trials are currently investigating the clinical utility of CTVI for functional lung avoidance treatment planning (ClinicalTrials.gov: NCT02528942, NCT02308709, NCT02843568).

8.4.2 Post-radiotherapy functional lung assessment

Several CTVI studies have also investigated the effects of radiotherapy on pulmonary ventilation. Similar to previous SPECT perfusion and ventilation studies [67, 68], a general trend in regional function decline post-RT has been observed with CTVI measurements for the intensity [69] and Jacobian metrics [70, 71]. These effects tend to occur at doses greater than 20 Gy [69, 70].

Whilst the SPECT studies have investigated lung function changes for more conventional dose fractionation schemes, the CT ventilation studies provide the only functional imaging evidence for ventilation decline after stereotactic body radiotherapy (SBRT), where greater ventilation decline has been observed in SBRT compared with conventional RT, perhaps attributable to the larger biological effect of SBRT.

Despite this general trend in post-RT function decline, pulmonary function recovery has also been observed in the CTVI literature. Vinogradskiy *et al* [72] studied weekly ventilatory changes using the intensity metric during the course of radiotherapy and noted re-ventilation in some patients. This phenomenon was observed mainly in lobes containing tumours, which could be due to airway opening as tumour volume reduces. This was supported by statistically significant reductions in pre-treatment ventilation for lobes containing tumours. Whereas other CT-based studies have chiefly focussed on post-RT effects, with the largest patient study to date (n=30) using data with a median time interval of 1.2 years (range: 0.3–3.3 years) between pre- and post-RT imaging, the study of Vinogradskiy *et al* is the only systematic analysis of CT-based regional lung ventilation over the course of treatment. However, their results could be masked by limited patient numbers ($n = 6$) and uncertainties in ventilation computation; thus caution should be exercised when extrapolating their results and more research is required before making firm conclusions.

The recovery of ventilated lung could limit the ability of functional lung avoidance strategies to preserve functional regions as the technique is premised on the assumption that the snapshot of functional defects pre-radiotherapy remains constant throughout treatment [6]. To mitigate these problems, greater personalisation of the technique may be needed via adaptive functional treatment planning by modifying treatment plans throughout treatment according to lung function changes rather than relying solely on a baseline CTVI.

8.5 Discussion and future research directions

8.5.1 Multi-institutional validation studies

Since the emergence of CTVI, no consensus exists as to the most accurate algorithm to use. Whilst numerous single institutional attempts have been made to validate the modality against established contrast-based ventilation imaging modalities, there are several possible CT acquisition protocols and numerous algorithms to generate the regional ventilation surrogates. As such, there is a need for a comprehensive multi-institutional validation study. To date, only one preliminary multi-institutional study has attempted a cross-modality validation of CT ventilation imaging [73]. Whilst that study demonstrated worldwide interest and the feasibility of running a major grand challenge in CT ventilation imaging validation, there were several notable limitations: (i) no validation was performed against pulmonary function tests; (ii) all CT scans were acquired during tidal breathing (4D-CT) with no breath-hold data included despite it being shown to exhibit greater physiological accuracy [74]; (iii) despite the potential applications for non-oncological respiratory diseases, human data consisted only of lung cancer patients; (iv) only three imaging datasets were included, two of which were from human subjects with nuclear imaging as the reference modality despite significant improvements in spatial and temporal resolution and aerosol deposition artefacts with hyperpolarised gas ventilation MRI [6]; accordingly, a thorough multi-institutional validation of CT ventilation imaging via a comprehensive dataset is critical to the translation of this modality into the clinic. To this end, the author and several CT ventilation researchers worldwide recently launched the CT ventilation imaging evaluation (CTVIE) grand challenge (https://www.aapm.org/GrandChallenge/CTVIE/). It is hoped that the insight this study will provide in understanding algorithmic differences and correlation to other more established measures of ventilation will be a crucial step towards the translation of the technique into the clinic.

8.5.2 Alveolar ventilation versus lung expansion

It may be argued that the term ‘ventilation’ applied to CTVI is, in fact, a misnomer as it is not identical to the pulmonary physiologist’s definition of specific ventilation, which is the fractional volume of fresh gas (rather than dead space gas) exchanged at the alveoli per unit time [14, 15]. Simon *et al* [15] note that although dead space gas may have an equivalent composition to alveoli gas, its redistribution at the alveoli is not considered 'fresh gas' exchange. Consequently, it plays no part in the removal of carbon dioxide from the body [15]. The so-called ventilation surrogate image comprises both fresh and dead space gas and does not explicitly differentiate between the two. Therefore, although CTVI may be related to specific ventilation, it is not equivalent; rather, it provides information on local lung expansion.

8.5.3 Ventilation versus perfusion

One major drawback in the clinical translation of CT-based surrogates of ventilation is their inability to provide a complete representation of lung function; the lung's function of gas exchange comprises both ventilation and perfusion [75]. Moreover, it has been suggested that perfusion is more relevant than ventilation because hypoperfused lung with viable ventilation is more widespread than the reverse [76]. If it is assumed that CTVI is a true surrogate for ventilation, there is the risk that a higher dose is received by perfused lung identified as non-ventilated [6]. An improved approach would be to incorporate perfusion information in addition to the ventilation information for truly pulmonary functionally-guided treatment. Recently, Castillo *et al* have proposed a novel method to model regional perfusion information from multi-inflation non-contrast CT [77]. Preliminary correlations of this technique against SPECT perfusion are promising but further validation studies are warranted.

8.6 Conclusion

Prior to clinical use, the physiological accuracy of CTVIs need to be established. A growing body of literature devoted to validation of the modality is emerging. Whilst preliminary studies were limited to global validations, more recent work has shown an increased interest in local and regional validations against pulmonary functional imaging modalities. Although considerable efforts have been made towards this goal, previous studies suffer from a number of methodological limitations which may have led to an erroneous evaluation of the modality's physiological accuracy. These include discrepancies in acquisition settings between scans such as different breathing manoeuvres, prolonged time intervals, limited volumetric coverage of the reference modality, inaccurate registration of CT and the reference modality and unsophisticated methods of comparison. Although several methods have been proposed to compute CTVIs, conflicting results are reported and it is not clear which, if any, of the methods is a suitable surrogate for pulmonary ventilation. A concerted effort, therefore, is warranted to develop and evaluate methods to address these limitations.

References

[1] Sung H, Ferlay J, Siegel R L, Laversanne M, Soerjomataram I and Jemal A *et al* 2021 Global cancer statistics 2020: GLOBOCAN estimates of incidence and mortality worldwide for 36 cancers in 185 countries *CA Cancer J. Clin.* **71** 209–49

[2] Gibson G J, Loddenkemper R, Lundback B and Sibille Y 2013 Respiratory health and disease in Europe: the new European Lung White Book. *Eur Respir. J.* **42** 559–63
[3] Papi A, Casoni G, Caramori G, Guzzinati I, Boschetto P and Ravenna F *et al* 2004 COPD increases the risk of squamous histological subtype in smokers who develop non-small cell lung carcinoma *Thorax.* **59** 679–81
[4] Dimick J B, Chen S L, Taheri P A, Henderson W G, Khuri S F and Campbell D A Jr 2004 Hospital costs associated with surgical complications: A report from the private-sector National Surgical Quality Improvement Program *J. Am. Coll. Surg.* **199** 531–7
[5] Rodrigues G, Lock M, D'Souza D, Yu E and Van Dyk J 2004 Prediction of radiation pneumonitis by dose-volume histogram parameters in lung cancer - a systematic review *Radiother. Oncol.* **71** 127–38
[6] Ireland R H, Tahir B A, Wild J M, Lee C E and Hatton M Q 2016 Functional image-guided radiotherapy planning for normal lung avoidance *Clin. Oncol. (R. Coll. Radiol.)* **28** 695–707
[7] Seppenwoolde Y, Engelsman M, De Jaeger K, Muller S, Belderbos J and Boersma L *et al* 2000 Optimising radiation treatment plans for lung cancer using functional information *Radiother. Oncol* **56**
[8] Christian J A, Partridge M, Nioutsikou E, Cook G, McNair H A and Cronin B *et al* 2005 The incorporation of SPECT functional lung imaging into inverse radictherapy planning for non-small cell lung cancer *Radiother. Oncol.* **77** 271–7
[9] Ireland R H, Bragg C M, McJury M, Woodhouse N, Fichele S and van Beek E J *et al* 2007 Feasibility of image registration and intensity-modulated radiotherapy planning with hyperpolarized helium-3 magnetic resonance imaging for non-small-cell lung cancer *Int. J. Radiat. Oncol., Biol., Phys.* **68** 273–81
[10] Tahir B A, Bragg C M, Wild J M, Swinscoe J A, Lawless S E and Hart K A *et al* 2017 Impact of field number and beam angle on functional image-guided lung cancer radiotherapy planning *Phys. Med. Biol.* **62** 7114–30.
[11] Guerrero T, Sanders K, Noyola-Martinez J, Castillo E, Zhang Y and Tapia R *et al* 2005 Quantification of regional ventilation from treatment planning CT *Int. J. Radiat. Oncol., Biol. Phys.* **62** 630–4
[12] Reinhardt J M, Ding K, Cao K, Christensen G E, Hoffman E A and Bodas S V 2008 Registration-based estimates of local lung tissue expansion compared to xenon CT measures of specific ventilation *Med. Image Anal.* **12** 752–63
[13] Simon B A 2000 Non-invasive imaging of regional lung function using x-ray computed tomography *J. Clin. Monitor. Comput.* **16** 433–42
[14] Simon B A 2005 Regional ventilation and lung mechanics using x-ray CT *Acad. Radiol* **12** 1414–22
[15] Simon B A, Kaczka D W, Bankier A A and Parraga G 2012 What can computed tomography and magnetic resonance imaging tell us about ventilation? *J. Appl. Physiol* **113** 647–57
[16] Guerrero T, Sanders K, Castillo E, Zhang Y, Bidaut L and Pan T *et al* 2006 Dynamic ventilation imaging from four-dimensional computed tomography *Phys. Med. Biol.* **51** 777–91
[17] Fuld M K, Easley R B, Saba O I, Chon D, Reinhardt J M and Hoffman E A *et al* 2008 CT-measured regional specific volume change reflects regional ventilation in supine sheep *J. Appl. Physiol.* **104** 1177–84
[18] Castillo R, Castillo E, Martinez J and Guerrero T 2010 Ventilation from four-dimensional computed tomography: density versus Jacobian methods *Phys. Med. Biol.* **55** 4661–85

[19] Ding K, Cao K, Fuld M K, Du K, Christensen G E and Hoffman E A *et al* 2012 Comparison of image registration based measures of regional lung ventilation from dynamic spiral CT with Xe-CT *Med. Phys.* **39** 5084–98
[20] Aliverti A, Pennati F, Salito C and Woods J C 2013 Regional lung function and heterogeneity of specific gas volume in healthy and emphysematous subjects. *Eur. Respir. J.* **41** 1179–88
[21] Coxson H O, Mayo J R, Behzad H, Moore B J, Verburgt L M and Staples C A *et al* 1995 Measurement of lung expansion with computed tomography and comparison with quantitative histology *J. Appl. Physiol.* **79** 1525–30
[22] Hogg J C and Nepszy S 1969 Regional lung volume and pleural pressure gradient estimated from lung density in dogs *J. Appl. Physiol.* **27** 198–203
[23] Zhang G G, Huang T C, Dilling T, Stevens C and Forster K M Derivation of high-resolution pulmonary ventilation using local volume change in four-dimensional CT data ed O Dössel and W Schlegel 2010 *World Congress on Medical Physics and Biomedical Engineering, September 7–12, 2009, Munich, Germany. IFMBE Proc. 25/4* (Berlin: Springer) 1834–7
[24] Zhang G, Huang T C, Dilling T, Stevens C and Forster K 2011 Comments on 'Ventilation from four-dimensional computed tomography: density versus Jacobian methods' *Phys. Med. Biol* **56** 3445–6
[25] Kipritidis J, Hofman M S, Siva S, Callahan J, Le Roux P Y and Woodruff H C *et al* 2016 Estimating lung ventilation directly from 4D CT Hounsfield unit values *Med. Phys.* **43** 33
[26] Kipritidis J, Siva S, Hofman M S, Callahan J, Hicks R J and Keall P J 2014 Validating and improving CT ventilation imaging by correlating with ventilation 4D-PET/CT using 68Ga-labeled nanoparticles *Med. Phys.* **41** 011910
[27] Tahir B A, Hughes P J C, Robinson S D, Marshall H, Stewart N J and Norquay G *et al* 2018 Spatial comparison of CT-based surrogates of lung ventilation with hyperpolarized Helium-3 and Xenon-129 gas MRI in patients undergoing radiation therapy *Int. J. Radiat. Oncol. Biol. Phys.* **102** 1276–86
[28] Du K, Bayouth J E, Cao K, Christensen G E, Ding K and Reinhardt J M 2012 Reproducibility of registration-based measures of lung tissue expansion *Med. Phys.* **39** 1595–608
[29] Castillo E, Castillo R, Vinogradskiy Y and Guerrero T 2017 The numerical stability of transformation-based CT ventilation *Int. J. Comput. Assist. Radiol. Surg* **12** 569–80
[30] Castillo E, Vinogradskiy Y and Castillo R 2019 Robust and HU-based CT ventilation from an integrated mass conservation formulation *Med. Phys.* **46** 5036–46
[31] Castillo E, Castillo R, Vinogradskiy Y, Dougherty M, Solis D and Myziuk N *et al* 2019 Robust CT ventilation from the integral formulation of the Jacobian *Med. Phys.* **46** 2115–25
[32] Fuld M K, Halaweish A F, Haynes S E, Divekar A A, Guo J and Hoffman E A 2013 Pulmonary perfused blood volume with dual-energy CT as surrogate for pulmonary perfusion assessed with dynamic multidetector CT *Radiology.* **267** 747–56
[33] Yamamoto T, Kabus S, Klinder T, Lorenz C, von Berg J and Blaffert T *et al* 2011 Investigation of four-dimensional computed tomography-based pulmonary ventilation imaging in patients with emphysematous lung regions *Phys. Med. Biol.* **56** 2279–98
[34] Brennan D, Schubert L, Diot Q, Castillo R, Castillo E and Guerrero T *et al* 2015 Clinical validation of 4-dimensional computed tomography ventilation with pulmonary function test data *Int. J. Radiat. Oncol. Biol. Phys.* **92** 423–9

[35] Yamamoto T, Kabus S, Lorenz C, Mittra E, Hong J C and Chung M *et al* 2014 Pulmonary ventilation imaging based on 4-dimensional computed tomography: comparison with pulmonary function tests and SPECT ventilation images *Int. J. Radiat. Oncol. Biol. Phys.* **90** 414–22
[36] Tokihiro Y, Sven K, Jens V B, Cristian L, GM L and LB W *et al* 2010 Evaluation of four-dimensional (4D) computed tomography (CT) pulmonary ventilation imaging by comparison with single photon emission computed tomography (SPECT) scans for a lung cancer patient *Proc. 3rd Int. Workshop on Pulmonary Image Analysis*
[37] De Backer J W, Vos W G, Vinchurkar S C, Claes R, Drollmann A and Wulfrank D *et al* 2010 Validation of computational fluid dynamics in CT-based airway models with SPECT/CT *Radiology.* **257** 854–62
[38] Castillo R, Castillo E, McCurdy M, Gomez D R, Block A M and Bergsma D *et al* 2012 Spatial correspondence of 4D CT ventilation and SPECT pulmonary perfusion defects in patients with malignant airway stenosis *Phys. Med. Biol* **57** 1855–71
[39] Vinogradskiy Y, Koo P J, Castillo R, Castillo E, Guerrero T and Gaspar L E *et al* 2014 Comparison of 4-dimensional computed tomography ventilation with nuclear medicine ventilation-perfusion imaging: a clinical validation study *Int. J. Radiat. Oncol. Biol. Phys.* **89** 199–205
[40] Kida S, Bal M, Kabus S, Negahdar M, Shan X and Loo B W Jr *et al* 2016 CT ventilation functional image-based IMRT treatment plans are comparable to SPECT ventilation functional image-based plans *Radiother. Oncol.* **118** 521–7
[41] Hegi-Johnson F, Keall P, Barber J, Bui C and Kipritidis J 2017 Evaluating the accuracy of 4D-CT ventilation imaging: first comparison with Technegas SPECT ventilation *Med. Phys.* **44** 4045–55
[42] Castillo E, Castillo R, Vinogradskiy Y, Nair G, Grills I and Guerrero T *et al* 2020 Technical Note: On the spatial correlation between robust CT-ventilation methods and SPECT ventilation *Med. Phys.* **47** 5731–8
[43] Eslick E M, Bailey D L, Harris B, Kipritidis J, Stevens M and Li B T *et al* 2016 Measurement of preoperative lobar lung function with computed tomography ventilation imaging: progress towards rapid stratification of lung cancer lobectomy patients with abnormal lung function *Eur. J. Cardiothorac. Surg.* **49** 1075–82
[44] Zhang G G, Latifi K, Du K, Reinhardt J M, Christensen G E and Ding K *et al* 2016 Evaluation of the DeltaV 4D CT ventilation calculation method using *in vivo* xenon CT ventilation data and comparison to other methods *J. Appl. Clin. Med. Phys.* **17** 5985
[45] Mathew L, Wheatley A, Castillo R, Castillo E, Rodrigues G and Guerrero T *et al* 2012 Hyperpolarized (3)He magnetic resonance imaging: comparison with four-dimensional x-ray computed tomography imaging in lung cancer *Acad. Radiol.* **19** 1546–53
[46] Tahir B A, Van Holsbeke C, Ireland R H, Swift A J, Horn F C and Marshall H *et al* 2016 Comparison of CT-based Lobar Ventilation with ^{3}He MR Imaging Ventilation Measurements *Radiology.* **278** 585–92
[47] Tahir B A, Marshall H, Hughes P J C, Brightling C E, Collier G and Ireland R H *et al* 2019 Comparison of CT ventilation imaging and hyperpolarised gas MRI: effects of breathing manoeuvre *Phys. Med. Biol.* **64** 055013
[48] Petersson J, Sanchez-Crespo A, Larsson S A and Mure M 2007 Physiological imaging of the lung: single-photon-emission computed tomography (SPECT) *J. Appl. Physiol.* **102** 468–76
[49] Yamamoto T, Kabus S, Berg J, Lorenz C, Loo M L G W and Keall P J 2010 Evaluation of four-dimensional (4D) computed tomography (CT) pulmonary ventilation imaging by

comparison with single photon emission computed tomography (SPECT) scans for a lung cancer patient. *Proc. 3rd Int. Workshop on Pulmonary Image Analysis*

[50] Magnant J, Vecellio L, De Monte M, Grimbert D, Valat C and Boissinot E *et al* 2006 Comparative analysis of different scintigraphic approaches to assess pulmonary ventilation *J. Aerosol Med.-Deposit. Clear. Effect Lung* **19** 2

[51] Jogi J, Jonson B, Ekberg M and Bajc M 2010 Ventilation-perfusion SPECT with (99m)Tc-DTPA versus technegas: a head-to-head study in obstructive and nonobstructive disease *J. Nucl. Med.* **51** 735–41

[52] Venkat R B, Sawant A, Suh Y, George R and Keall P J 2008 Development and preliminary evaluation of a prototype audiovisual biofeedback device incorporating a patient-specific guiding waveform *Phys. Med. Biol.* **53** N197

[53] Yuan S, Frey K A, Gross M D, Hayman J A, Arenberg D and Curtis J L *et al* 2011 Semiquantification and classification of local pulmonary function by V/Q single photon emission computed tomography in patients with non-small cell lung cancer potential indication for radiotherapy planning *J. Thorac. Oncol.* **6** P71–8

[54] Callahan J, Hofman M S, Siva S, Kron T, Schneider M E and Binns D *et al* 2014 High-resolution imaging of pulmonary ventilation and perfusion with 68Ga-VQ respiratory gated (4-D) PET/CT *Eur. J. Nucl. Med. Mol. Imag.* **41** 343–9

[55] Patz S, Hersman F W, Muradian I, Hrovat M I, Ruset I C and Ketel S *et al* 2007 Hyperpolarized (129)Xe MRI: a viable functional lung imaging modality? *Eur. J. Radiol.* **64** 335–44

[56] van Beek E J, Wild J M, Kauczor H U, Schreiber W, Mugler J P 3rd and de Lange E E 2004 Functional MRI of the lung using hyperpolarized 3-helium gas *J. Magnet. Reson. Imag.* **20** 540–54

[57] Ireland R H, Woodhouse N, Hoggard N, Swinscoe J A, Foran B H and Hatton M Q *et al* 2008 An image acquisition and registration strategy for the fusion of hyperpolarized helium-3 MRI and x-ray CT images of the lung *Phys. Med. Biol.* **53** 6055–63

[58] Svenningsen S, Kirby M, Starr D, Leary D, Wheatley A and Maksym G N *et al* 2013 Hyperpolarized (3) He and (129) Xe MRI: differences in asthma before bronchodilation *J. Magnet. Reson. Imag.* **38** 1521–30

[59] Kirby M, Svenningsen S, Kanhere N, Owrangi A, Wheatley A and Coxson H O *et al* 2013 Pulmonary ventilation visualized using hyperpolarized helium-3 and xenon-129 magnetic resonance imaging: differences in COPD and relationship to emphysema *J. Appl. Physiol.* **114** 707–15

[60] Yamamoto T, Kabus S, von Berg J, Lorenz C, Chung M P and Hong J C *et al* 2012 Reproducibility of four-dimensional computed tomography-based lung ventilation imaging *Acad. Radiol.* **19** 1554–65

[61] Yamamoto T, Langner U, Loo B W Jr, Shen J and Keall P J 2008 Retrospective analysis of artifacts in four-dimensional CT images of 50 abdominal and thoracic radiotherapy patients *Int. J. Radiat. Oncol. Biol. Phys.* **72** P1250–8

[62] Mistry N N, Diwanji T, Shi X, Pokharel S, Feigenberg S and Scharf S M *et al* 2013 Evaluation of fractional regional ventilation using 4D-CT and effects of breathing maneuvers on ventilation *Int. J. Radiat. Oncol. Biol. Phys.* **87** 825–31

[63] Couser J I, Martinez F J, Celli B R and Rassulo J 1992 Respiratory response and ventilatory muscle recruitment during arm elevation in normal subjects *Chest* **101** P336–40

[64] Partridge M, Yamamoto T, Grau C, Hoyer M and Muren L P 2010 Imaging of normal lung, liver and parotid gland function for radiotherapy *Acta Oncol* **49** 997–1011

[65] Yaremko B P, Guerrero T M, Noyola-Martinez J, Guerra R, Lege D G and Nguyen L T *et al* 2007 Reduction of normal lung irradiation in locally advanced non-small-cell lung cancer patients, using ventilation images for functional avoidance *Int. J. Radiat. Oncol. Biol. Phys.* **68** 562–71

[66] Yamamoto T, Kabus S, von Berg J, Lorenz C and Keall P J 2011 Impact of four-dimensional computed tomography pulmonary ventilation imaging-based functional avoidance for lung cancer radiotherapy *Int. J. Radiat. Oncol. Biol. Phys.* **79** 279–88

[67] Marks L B, Munley M T, Spencer D P, Sherouse G W, Bentel G C and Hoppenworth J *et al* 1997 Quantification of radiation-induced regional lung injury with perfusion imaging *Int. J. Radiat. Oncol. Biol. Phys.* **38** 399–409

[68] Theuws J C M, Kwa S L S, Wagenaar A C, Boersma L J, Damen E M F and Muller S H *et al* 1998 Dose–effect relations for early local pulmonary injury after irradiation for malignant lymphoma and breast cancer *Radiother. Oncol.* **48** 33–43

[69] King M T, Maxim P G, Diehn M, Loo B W Jr and Xing L 2015 Analysis of long-term 4-dimensional computed tomography regional ventilation after radiation therapy *Int. J. Radiat. Oncol. Biol. Phys.* **92** 683–90

[70] Ding K, Bayouth J E, Buatti J M, Christensen G E and Reinhardt J M 2010 4DCT-based measurement of changes in pulmonary function following a course of radiation therapy *Med. Phys.* **37** 1261

[71] Latifi K, Feygelman V, Moros E G, Dilling T J, Stevens C W and Zhang G G 2013 Normalization of ventilation data from 4D-CT to facilitate comparison between datasets acquired at different times *PLoS One* **8** e84083

[72] Vinogradskiy Y Y, Castillo R, Castillo E, Chandler A, Martel M K and Guerrero T 2012 Use of weekly 4DCT-based ventilation maps to quantify changes in lung function for patients undergoing radiation therapy *Med. Phys.* **39** 289–98

[73] Kipritidis J *et al* 2019 The VAMPIRE challenge: preliminary results from a multi-institutional study of CT ventilation image accuracy *Med. Phys.* **46** 1198–217

[74] Eslick E M, Kipritidis J, Gradinscak D, Stevens M J, Bailey D L and Harris B *et al* 2018 CT ventilation imaging derived from breath hold CT exhibits good regional accuracy with Galligas PET *Radiother. Oncol.* **127** 267–73

[75] Zhang G, Dilling T J, Stevens C W and Forster K M 2008 Functional lung imaging in thoracic cancer radiotherapy *Cancer Control* **15** 112–9

[76] Marks L B, Sherouse G W, Munley M T, Bentel G C and Spencer D P 1999 Incorporation of functional status into dose-volume analysis *Med. Phys.* **26** 196–9

[77] Castillo E, Nair G, Turner-Lawrence D, Myziuk N, Emerson S and Al-Katib S *et al* 2021 Quantifying pulmonary perfusion from noncontrast computed tomography *Med. Phys.* **48** 1804–14

IOP Publishing

Detection Systems in Lung Cancer and Imaging, Volume 1

Ayman El-Baz and Jasjit S Suri

Chapter 9

Novel non-invasive methods used in the early detection of lung cancer: from biomarkers to nanosystems

Özlem Çoban and Yeşim Kaya Yaşar

9.1 Introduction

Lung cancer is both one of the most frequently diagnosed cancers and the leading cause of cancer-related death, worldwide. It is reported that it causes an estimated 2.20 million new cases and 1.79 million deaths annually. Lung cancer is often classified as non-small cell lung carcinoma (NSCLC, 85% of diagnoses) or small cell lung carcinoma (SCLC, 15% of diagnoses) [1]. The NSCLC class includes squamous cell carcinoma (SqCC), adenocarcinoma (ADC), and large cell carcinoma species [2]. Of these, ADC and SqCC are responsible for 80% of all lung cancer cases (ADC and SqCC are the most common and second common subtypes of lung cancer, respectively) [1, 2]. Large cell carcinoma, also called undifferentiated, constitutes 5%–10% of lung cancers. It is usually diagnosed by eliminating other species, as they do not show squamous or glandular maturation at diagnosis [3]. Approximately 50% of NSCLC patients have metastatic disease at presentation (stage IV) [4].

SCLC is an aggressive and fatal form of lung cancer characterized by rapid growth, early metastasis, and acquired therapeutic resistance [5]. Two subtypes are in the current classification of SCLC: pure SCLC and combined SCLC. The combined one is determined by the presence of features that include a distinct histologic carcinoma, non-small cell lung carcinoma, variant, or at least 10% large cell carcinoma component. Approximately 28% of surgically removed SCLC tumors are combined SCLC, and 16% of these belong to the large cell carcinoma variant [6].

Smoking is one of the main risk factors for this disease [7]. In fact, the lifetime cumulative risk of lung cancer may be less than 1% in non-smokers and up to 30% in heavy smokers. As the amount of cigarette consumption increases, the risk of lung cancer also increases. The number of cigarettes smoked per day, the age to start smoking, the level of breathing in, the amount of tar and nicotine in cigarettes, and

doi:10.1088/978-0-7503-3355-9ch9

the use of unfiltered cigarettes also have an effect on this increase in smoking-related risk. More than 80% of lung cancer cases occur in people exposed to tobacco. However, less than 20% of smokers develop lung cancer. It can be suggested that genetic predisposition and environmental factors are responsible for the variability in the effect of smoking on the lung cancer incidence [8]. However, passive smoking is one of the factors involved in the etiology of lung cancer in non-smokers. In accordance with the US Surgeon General, when a non-smoker lives with a smoker, their possibility of catching lung cancer may increase by about 20%–30% [3]. Apart from these risk factors for non-smokers, conditions such as burning wood or coal, air pollution, radioactive substances like uranium, radium and radon, occupational exposures like asbestos, arsenic, beryllium, cadmium, chromium, nickel, silica, and diesel fumes can also cause lung cancer [3, 8–10]. Due to around 3 billion people worldwide using solid fuels such as wood and coal as their primary source of domestic energy, there is growing evidence indicating that utilisation of solid fuels to obtain domestic energy increases the lung cancer prevalence. For example, a positive correlation between utilization of coal as a source of domestic energy and lung cancer incidence has been observed in China. Another study which took into account smoking status and adjusted the results accordingly reported that using coal and untreated biomass (product scraps, wood, sticks, and twigs) increases the risk of lung cancer. The International Agency for Research on Cancer classified domestic emissions from coal-burning in homes as carcinogenic and emissions from biomass fuel, particularly wood, as possible carcinogens [8]. Infections (*Mycobacterium tuberculosis*, human immunodeficiency virus and human papilloma virus) and inflammatory diseases can also predispose to lung cancer. For example, the results obtained from meta-analysis studies, indicated that the risk of lung cancer increases in people with inflammatory diseases such as asthma and sarcoidosis [9].

Various approaches, with or without surgery, are used in the treatment of lung cancer. The basic mechanism of surgical procedures is the removal of cancerous tissues from the area. Lung resection is also a common treatment for lung cancer. It can increase the survival rate up to 75% in stages I and II in lung cancer [11]. Pneumonectomy (removal of the entire lung), pulmonary lobectomy (removal of whole lung lobe together with regional lymph nodes) and sublobar resection (wedge resection and segmentectomy) are used as surgical approaches. Wedge resection is the operation to remove a pulmonary tumor along with a surrounding margin of normal lung tissue, while segmentectomy is an anatomical resection in which most of the lung is removed, although not the entire lobe of the lung, including one or more pulmonary parenchymatous segments, segmental bronchovascular elements, and intraparenchymal, hilar, and mediastinal lymph nodes. However, removal of the whole lung shows high rates of complications that can cause respiratory failure and even death in the post-operative period [12]. Non-surgical therapy approaches of lung cancer are chemotherapy, radiotherapy, stereotactic body radiotherapy, targeted drug therapy, immunotherapy and palliative care [13–17]. Early generation chemotherapeutic agents such as methotrexate and doxorubicin were used in the treatment of lung cancer in the 1970s, but therapeutic efficacies of these agents have been limited. In the 1980s and 1990s, increased survival rates were observed with the development of platinum and new generation chemotherapeutic agents such as taxane, vinorelbine and gemcitabine [18]. In addition, traditional Chinese medicine such as acupuncture, herbal medicine, moxibustion, food therapy, and physical exercise is thought to give successful results in the treatment of lung cancer due to its mechanisms of inhibiting NSCLC cells growth, invasion, and migration, inducing apoptosis of NSCLC cells [13].

Lung cancer is the second most commonly diagnosed cancer both in men and women. Because lung cancer is asymptomatic at an early stage, most new cases are detected at an advanced stage. However, patients with advanced lung cancer have a poor prognosis and a 5-year survival rate of about 5.2%. Therefore, along with strategies aimed at reducing smoking rates, early detection is an important strategy to reduce the prevalence of lung cancer [19, 20]. Although various methods such as low-dose computed tomography (CT), positron emission tomography (PET), magnetic resonance imaging (MRI) are used for diagnosis of lung cancer [21], the main purpose here is to diagnose the disease at an earlier stage, which allows the success of treatment to be increased and to reduce mortality [19]. Both invasive and non-invasive methods are used in diagnosis of lung cancer. However, the method which is used in diagnosis depends on the type of lung cancer (NSCLC or SCLC), the size and location of the primary tumor, the presence of metastases, and the patient's general clinical condition [22].

In this chapter, methods (invasive and non-invasive) used in the diagnosis of lung cancer, the place of nanosystems in these methods and the success of the methods in the early stages will be discussed.

9.2 Diagnostic methods for lung cancer

Lung cancer is suspected in people who present abnormal chest radiograph findings or symptoms caused by the local or systemic effects of the tumor. Therefore, it should be detected using various diagnostic methods [22]. Various methods, invasive or non-invasive, are used in diagnosis of lung cancer. CT-guided lung biopsy, bronchoscopic-guided procedures, extrathoracic biopsy, mediastinoscopy, thoracentesis and pericardiocentesis are examples of invasive methods [23] (figure 9.1). Non-invasive methods are as follows: low-dose CT, MRI, PET and PET-CT

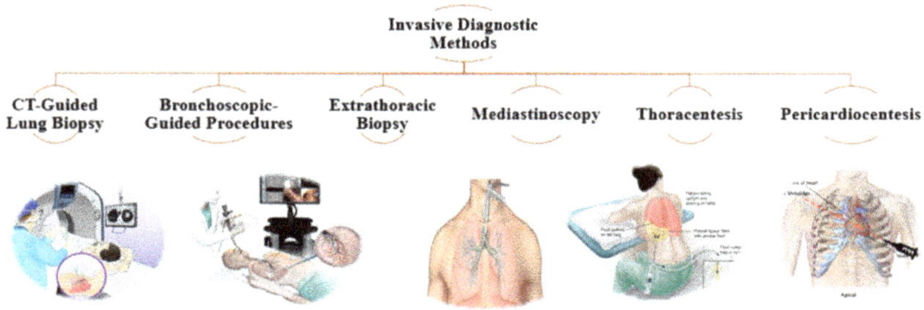

Figure 9.1. Schematic image of invasive methods used in the diagnosis of lung cancer.

[23, 24]. Since the stage of the cancer determines the effectiveness of the diagnostic applications, diagnosis and staging of the disease are usually done together at this stage. In order to provide effective treatment in these patients, the reliability of diagnostic methods must be carefully discussed to maximize the sensitivity of the diagnostic process and avoid multiple or unnecessary invasive procedures [22].

It is crucial to determine the stage of disease in diagnosis, due to the treatment strategies for lung cancer differing according to the stage of disease. Lung nodules 5 mm to 25 mm in size are the smallest ones that grow in the lung. Malignant nodules are larger in size than the others and have a greater growth rate. In segmentation, the nodule is detected, and the stages of lung cancer can be identified depending on its features and measure of the extent to which it has spread throughout the body. Lung cancer is generally staged from I to IV. Features of these phases; the cancer is confined to the lung in stage I, the cancer is confined to the chest in stage II and III, and cancer has spread from the chest to other parts of the body in stage IV [25].

9.2.1 Invasive diagnostic methods

According to The National Cancer Institute data, the 5-year survival in lung cancer increased from 15.4% in 2000 to 20.5% in 2020. This low level of improvement over 20 years is usually due to late diagnosis with limited treatment options. Because it has been seen that recovery rates of more than 80% can be achieved with early diagnosis and treatment [23].

We can divide invasive techniques into two groups: surgical open biopsy or needle biopsy. Surgical open biopsy is a more 'invasive' procedure than needle biopsy, as it requires general anesthesia, although in this method larger specimens can usually be obtained than with needle biopsy. Standard cervical or extended cervical mediastinoscopy, anterior mediastinotomy, or video-assisted thoracoscopic surgery (VATS) as surgical open biopsy. As needle biopsy, transbronchial needle aspiration (TBNA), transthoracic needle aspiration (TTNA), endoscopic ultrasound-guided fine-needle aspiration (EUS-FNA) and endobronchial ultrasound-guided transbronchial needle aspiration (EBUS-TBNA) techniques are used [24].

Minimally invasive methods, in which the invasion process is reduced, are also used. Because, although computed tomography (CT) has been used recently in the detection of early peripheral lung cancer, since the rate of misdiagnosis is high in this method, biopsy is often required to confirm the diagnosis. However, biopsy complicates intervention and requires more time, especially for small peripheral lung cancer. Therefore, it the aim is to develop new and appropriate early lung cancer diagnosis and treatment strategies. A minimally invasive multimodal image-guided (MIMIG) intervention system was developed by He and coworkers to diagnose lesions, verify small peripheral lung cancer, and probably provide guidance for *in situ* cure at an early stage. In this study, CT imaging and electromagnetic (EM) monitoring were used together so that interventional radiologists can reach out to the lesion effectively. After targeting the lesion, a fiber optic probe combined with optical molecular imaging contrast agents was used to obtain images of cancerous tissues at microscopic level. With the software developed in this system, pulmonary vessels, airways, and nodules were subdivided, then the divisions were converted to in-procedural CT for use in EM monitoring, and endomicroscopy was performed via an IntegriSense 680 fiber optic probe with fluorescent contrast agent to visualize tumor tissues. Finally, confirmed cancers were treated *in situ* using radio frequency ablation (RFA). This developed system was evaluated using rabbit VX2 lung cancer models and found to be successful [26].

9.2.2 Non-invasive diagnostic methods

One of the methods used in diagnosis is low-dose computed tomography (CT). Recent large, randomized studies with centers such as the National Lung Screening Trial (NLST) and the Dutch–Belgian Lung Cancer Screening Trial have confirmed that lung cancer screening with this method provides significant mortality benefits [23, 27]. So much so that in 2013 the US Preventive Services Task Force (USPSTF) suggested annual screening for lung cancer with low-dose computed tomography (LDCT) in adults aged 55–80 who smoke 30 packs a year and either currently smoke or have quit within the last 15 years. However, screening high-risk individuals with LDCT can result in false positive results due to unnecessary tests and invasive procedures, overdiagnosis, accidental findings and increases in stress, and rarely, cancer induction due to radiation. Therefore, existing nodule assessment protocols which can reduce invasive procedures for false positive results should be used [28].

Unidentified non-calcified lung nodules are commonly observed when low-dose spiral computed tomography (LDCT) is used. Therefore, 5201 high-risk individuals were screened in a study which used this method. They monitored the individuals for 1 year by applying re-LDCT after 1 year and 3 months later in ⩽5 and 5.1–8 mm nodules, respectively, and combined CT-PET in >8 mm nodules. As a result of the study, at least one non-calcified nodule was observed in 53% of the volunteers. A total of 92 lung cancers were diagnosed, 55 at the initial stage and 37 during annual screening; 66% of them were in stage I. These results show that LDCT scanning reduces the invasive diagnostic process and its applicability in lung cancer screening in high-risk individuals, however, causes a delay in diagnosis in a small number of patients [29].

9.2.2.1 Biomarker-based diagnostic methods

Apart from these methods, one of the more sensitive and specific test methods for the detection of the disease at an early stage, as a promising approach, is the determination of lung cancer-specific biomarkers and the detection of these biomarkers by non-invasive methods [30]. Therefore, there is increasing interest in non-invasive techniques and methods based on molecular, cellular or volatile biomarkers to diagnose lung cancer. At the same time, some specific genetic changes such as epidermal growth factor receptor, anaplastic lymphoma kinase and *BRAF* genes observed in lung cancer are used for a potential therapeutic target as well as diagnosis. However, there is a need to develop new techniques which are faster and more efficient in order to identify different biomarkers for use in diagnosis [31].

The LDCT method often causes unnecessary biopsy, especially in cases where nodules are ⩽ 10 mm, since its specificity is low. Therefore, lung cancer can be differentiated from benign lung disease using circulating genetically aberrant cells (CACs). To evaluate this, CACs values were determined by fluorescent *in situ* hybridization in 125 patients with malignant pulmonary nodules 10 mm and below between January 2019 and January 2020. Subsequently, histopathological examination of the nodules in the patients was performed to confirm the status of lung cancer or benign disease. In conclusion, multivariable logistic regression models were constructed to determine the efficacy of CACs in the diagnosis of lung cancer. When the cut-off value for CACs was >2, the sensitivity and specificity values of the method were obtained as 70.5% and 86.4%, respectively. In addition, evaluation of bisected CACs (>2 versus ⩽2) and other clinical factors together in this method gave more successful results in accordance with the evaluation of them alone. Thus, it can be said that CACs is an important diagnostic method for lung cancer in patients with pulmonary nodules ⩽10 mm [32].

Volatile organic compounds (VOCs) such as hydrocarbon, alcohol, aldehyde (also branched aldehyde), ketone, ester, nitrile and aromatic, which contain metabolic information about human tissues, are present in different amounts in different tissues in the body. After gene-specific VOC biomarkers are metabolized, they are transported to the lungs through the bloodstream and excreted from the alveoli [31]. Because exhaled breath analysis is one of the non-invasive methods that can be used in the diagnosis of lung cancer and can be mentioned as an ideal diagnostic method because it is completely painless. The method is based on the difference in the amount of some compounds such as isoprene, acetone and methanol in the breath of people with lung cancer and healthy people. In this study, as a result of gas chromatography–mass spectrometry (GC–MS) analysis of exhaled breath, the amounts of more than 50 compounds were found to be different in healthy and cancerous individuals. However, since the sensitivity of the method is different for each compound (for some, it is lower), four compounds with high discrimination (alcohols, aldehydes, ketones and hydrocarbons) were identified as potential markers [33]. In a study conducted by Jia *et al* using GC quadrupole time of flight/MS (GC-Q-TOF/MS), for six different lung cancer cells the combination of benzaldehyde, 2-ethylhexanol, and 2,4-decadiene-1-ol as potential volatile organic compounds biomarkers [34]. Images from a single computed tomography scan and breath biomarkers from a single breath have been combined to develop a non-invasive, automated, and clinical diagnostic system that provide fast and definite categorisation of lung nodules thereby early diagnosis of disease. For this purpose, 47 patients were included in the study. The amount of volatile organic compounds in the patients' breath was measured by capturing 27 VOCs in exhaled breath using a microreactor approach and quantifying them by mass spectrometry. Shape properties based on spherical harmonic, 7th-order Markov Gibbs Random Field (MGRF) based appearance model and volumetric properties (size) of pulmonary nodules were calculated from CT images. This data was inserted into the deep learning autoencoder classifier to classify the nodules. Retrospective CT scans from 467 patients with 727 pulmonary nodules and breath samples from 504 patients were also analyzed to increase the sample size and validate the methodology. In this way, the computer aided diagnostic system was developed successfully with 97.8%

accuracy, 97.3% sensitivity, 100% specificity and 99.1% area under the curve in classifying pulmonary nodules [35]. However, advances in standard clinical use and ultra-high sensitivity advanced mass spectrometry are critical to improve the effectiveness of these diagnostic methods based on VOC analysis in exhaled breath [31].

DNA methylation which is a DNA-based change, is an epigenetic modification of DNA that occurs commonly in various cancers such as ovarian, prostate, liver and cervical cancer [30, 31]. In most patients with cancer, tumoral DNA can be found both in exfoliative material and in the blood. Moreover, methylated DNA markers have been detected in many body fluids such as blood, serum, pleural effusion and ascites in lung cancer [31]. DNA-based diagnostics allows signal amplification by polymerase chain reaction (PCR) and can therefore provide improved sensitivity. Studies have shown that DNA methylation pattern analyses with high specificity and sensitivity can be a powerful tool for accurate and early diagnosis of lung cancer [30]. For example, Wielscher and colleagues were able to identify four methylated genes as markers for LC detection. These are homeobox D10, paired box 9, protein tyrosine phosphatase receptor type 2 and stromal antigen 3 [31, 36]. The commercially available test kit Epi proLung® (Epigenomics Inc.) based on methylation in the short stature homeobox 2 (SHOX2) gene, one of these genes, has been approved by the Chinese Food and Drug Administration (FDA) for use in LC screening. Analyses based on this method have high sensitivity and specificity. In fact, 70% sensitivity and 96% specificity were obtained in a meta-analysis to determine the sensitivity of the SHOX2 DNA methylation method. Thus, it was demonstrated that lung cancer can be effectively differentiated from other lung diseases and controls [31]. In another example, to determine the methylation pattern difference in cancerous tumor-benign lesions, DNA methylation profile of tissue samples (nodule size < 3 cm) was determined using DNA bisulfite sequencing. Afterwards, plasma sample classification was performed by eliminating methylation patterns displaying high background in circulating tumor DNA (ctDNA). In this way, 9 markers were selected. As a result of the studies, the sensitivity of the method in the differentiation of malignant and benign patients was 79.5% and the specificity was 85.2%. In addition, high specificity (93.2%) was found in the face of differences such as gender and age. It has been shown that the method is highly sensitive in detecting early-stage lung cancer, with a sensitivity of 75.0% in 20 stage Ia lung cancer patients and 85.7% in 7 stage Ib lung cancer [37]. Various methods such as sodium bisulfite conversion, restriction enzyme, specific antibodies, PCR, microarrays and next-generation sequencing (NGS) are used in the analysis of methylated DNA. However, random DNA fragments can occur in bisulfite conversion. In the restriction enzyme method, only certain patterns in the CpG region can be detected. The recovery rate of antibody-based methods is low [31].

MicroRNAs (miRNA) are small non-coding RNAs that can affect cancer metabolism. They exert their effects by modulating the tumor suppressor signaling pathways involved in glucose metabolism and the expression of glycolytic enzymes [31]. miRNA expression is also present in lung cancer and can be detected in various body fluids such as human serum/plasma and sputum. Therefore, miRNA expression patterns can be used as specific biomarkers for detection of lung cancer at all stages [31, 38, 39]. To demonstrate that 54 lung cancer-associated miRNAs, which they identified in a previous study, could be used as plasma biomarkers in the diagnosis of lung cancer, Leng *et al* quantified the expression of lung tumor-miRNAs in plasma using reverse transcription PCR in 180 subjects. When validation of miRNAs was performed in 64 of 180 subjects (34 lung cancer patients and 30 cancer-free smokers), 30 of 54 miRNAs were observed to have significantly different expression in lung cancer patients than in the other group. Of these 30 miRNAs, the best predictive results were obtained with miRNAs-126, -145, -210 and -205–5p (sensitivity 91.5% and specificity 96.2%). In addition, in this method, variables such as the stage and histological type of the lung tumor, age, gender and ethnicity of the patients did not affect the result [40]. Apart from this, plasma circulating miRNA-448, 506, 4316, and 4478 can also be used as biomarkers in the diagnosis of lung cancer. In a study to determine this, plasma samples from 90 lung cancer patients and 85 healthy individuals were taken and miRNA values were determined by quantitative reverse transcription polymerase chain reaction (qRTPCR) technique. Receiver operating curves (ROC) with area under the curve (AUC) were used to increase the discrimination of the method. Of these 4 microRNAs, miRNA-448 and 4478 were highly overexpressed in lung cancer patients in accordance with the healthy group, so further analyses were performed with these two molecules alone, and the sensitivity and specificity were found as 90% and 76.3%, respectively for patients with operable (stage Ia–IIb) non-small cell lung cancer [39]. Despite successful results, there are still several challenges for the clinical use of miRNAs as biomarkers. One of them is that miRNAs are only the visible part of non-coding genes in the entire genome. Therefore, more miRNA transcripts need to be uncovered. The other is that the roles of miRNAs in cancer biology should be determined in more detail. Others, the roles of miRNAs in cancer biology and the potential biological functions of circulating miRNAs containing multivesicular bodies (MVBs) in cell-cell communication, tumor immune evasion, and tumor microenvironment need to be determined in more detail, and the methods used in the detection and analysis of miRNAs—extraction and measurement methods—should be further optimized by comparing them with each other [41].

Finally, the discovery of activating mutations in genes such as epidermal growth factor receptor (EGFR) and anaplastic lymphoma kinase (ALK), which enables the clinical application of personalized medicine, can also be used in the detection of disease [42, 43]. In studies conducted in this context, as lung cancer biomarkers, Kang *et al* and other researchers have identified β-chain of human haptoglobin (HP), serum amyloid A (SAA), apolipoprotein A-1 (APOA1), annexin (ANXA), vimentin (VIM), non-muscle myosin (NM), calmodulin (CALM), cofilin (CFL), thymosin (TMS), and EGFR proteins [43]. To demonstrate the diagnostic significance of the EGFR mutation, a study of 1699 patients was conducted. While 750 of these patients were in the early stage of lung cancer, 949 were in its advanced stage. EGFR mutation rates measured by the amplification refractory mutation system (ARMS) method and EGFR mutation type were similar in the early stage and advanced stage groups. Direct DNA sequencing, COBAS, and droplet digital PCR methods can

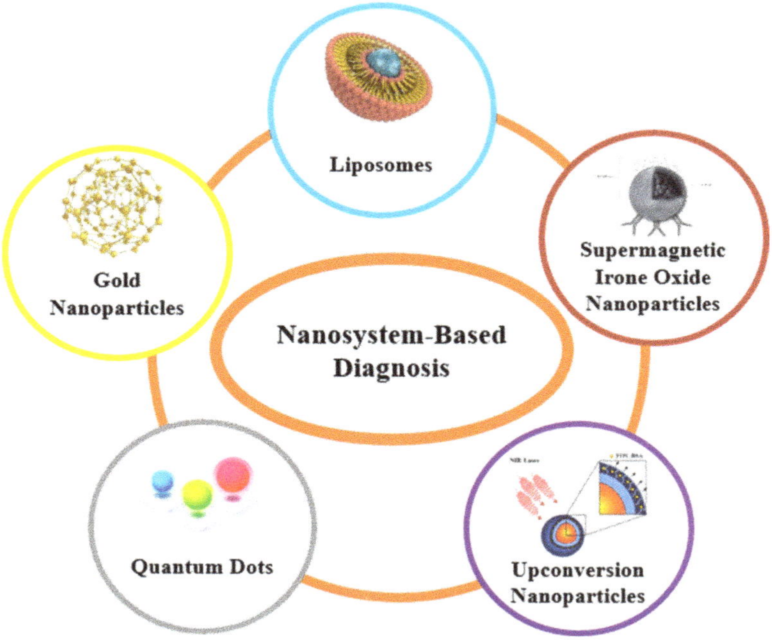

Figure 9.2. Schematic images of nanosystems used in lung diagnostics.

also be used to detect EGFR mutation [44]. In addition, mass spectrometry can be preferred to measure amounts of these proteomics in normal and tumor lung tissue [43].

9.2.2.2 Nanosystem-based diagnostic methods

Advances in nanotechnology have allowed imaging agents (contrast agents, radionuclide probes and fluorescent dyes)—as well as therapeutics—to be encapsulated or conjugated to nano-sized systems, enabling these systems to reach tumor tissue with a passive or active targeting approach and to mark tumor sites highly effectively. In this way, great advances have been achieved in the diagnosis and treatment of cancer. Various nanosystems have been developed for the imaging of lung cancer. The schematic visual of nanosystems designed for use in diagnostics is shown in figure 9.2. These are liposomes, nanostructured lipid carriers, gold and iron oxide nanoparticles (NPs) and quantum dots [45, 46]. Because cancerous tissue can be detected colorimetrically with gold and iron oxide nanoparticles, or quantum dots and nanosystems with upconversion properties can be used for *in vivo* imaging due to their fluorescent properties [46].

Substances used in the imaging and diagnosis of lung cancer and loaded into nanosystems could be gadolinium, fluorescent dye (DiD) and photosensitizers (PS) [45, 47]. Photosensitizer molecules are substances that can produce reactive oxygen species when exposed to light in the presence of molecular oxygen and emit fluorescent light. Therefore, they can be used in both tumor therapy (photodynamic therapy) and fluorescent imaging. For example, photodynamic therapy (PDT) and fluorescence diagnosis (FD) methods are very popular in Russia. Thus, even patients with central lung cancer (CLC) can be diagnosed earlier. Because, although at an early-stage computed tomography of the chest is useful in detecting peripheral NSCLC, it is unfortunately not sufficient for the diagnosis of CLC. For this reason, most patients cannot be diagnosed with CLC until signs and symptoms that indicate an advanced stage are observed, and the airway of these patients need to reopen palliatively via minimally invasive endobronchial techniques [47].

Fluorophore (indocyanine green (ICG) or cyanine 5.5 (Cy5.5)) conjugated glycol chitosan nanoparticles (CNPs) were prepared by On *et al.* Nanoparticles were prepared by chemical synthesis. For this purpose, glycol chitosan was solvated in a methanol/distilled water mixture and combined with N-hydroxysuccinimide (NHS) and 1-ethyl-3-(3-dimethyl laminopropyl)-carbodiimide hydrochloride (EDC). The methanolic solution of 5β-cholanic acid was added dropwise to this solution and stirred vigorously for 24 h. Dialysis method was used to remove unreacted 5β-cholanic acid, EDC and NHS. The remaining part was lyophilized to obtain nanoparticles. For use in imaging, CNPs obtained were dissolved in dimethyl sulfoxide (DMSO) and mixed with Cy5.5-NHS or ICG-NHS. Re-dialysis was performed to remove unreacted substances and followed by lyophilization. The lyophilized product was dispersed in sterile phosphate-buffered saline (PBS, pH 7.4) with a probe-type sonicator to generate Cy5.5-CNP or ICG-CNPs. These nanosystems were then applied to VX2 tumor-bearing mouse and rabbit models. According to their results, CNPs accumulated more in VX2 tumor cells in a dose-dependent manner without any cytotoxic effect. They also successfully visualized the distinction between tumor and normal tissue in mouse and rabbit VX2 tumor models [48].

Since visceral pleural invasion (PL) is a prognostic factor in lung cancer, a PL1 or higher level of pleural invasion is indicative of advanced lung cancer, even if the tumor diameter is the same. In order to make a definitive diagnosis according to the PL level, the specimens must be excised and pathologically examined. Only in this way can unnecessary surgeries for disseminated lesions be avoided. In cancer tissue 5-amino-levulinic acid (5-ALA) is metabolized to a photosensitive substance, or protoporphyrin IX (PPIX), and emits a red color in response to excitation light, thus it allows optical visualization of the region [49]. Since the inhaled administration of 5-ALA does not show any dose-related adverse effects, it is currently used clinically for the optical observation of bronchial malignancies. To demonstrate the ability of 5-ALA to detect lung cancer at an early stage, inhaled 5-ALA with a nebulizer was administered to seven patients who had positive or suspicious sputum cytology but negative for white light bronchoscopy. No adverse impacts were noticed in these patients. Fluorescence bronchoscopy was performed 3 h after inhalation. To convert 5-ALA to PPIX and thus fluoresce, patients were given violet light and an optical multichannel analyzer was used to image cancerous tissues. According to the results, since the emitted fluorescence was at high enough intensity for video imaging using the target-integrated color charge-coupled device (CCD) camera, fluorescent spectra were observed in the bronchial mucosa, thus enabling carcinoma and dysplasia to be visualized. Although with histological examinations after biopsy, the sensitivity of the method was found to be high, the specificity was found below 50%. This may be related to the light source and drug dose [50]. However, 5-ALA's ability to cross biological barriers and thus reach tumor tissue may be limited due to its charge and polarity. To overcome this situation, 5-ALA can be applied with drug delivery systems [51]. No 5-ALA-loaded nanosystem study has yet been found for the diagnosis of lung cancer. However, compared to free 5-ALA for glioma, periodic mesoporous organosilica coated Prussian blue nanoparticles containing 5-ALA provided more PPIX formation in tumor tissue [52]. From this point of view, 5-ALA-loaded nanosystems can increase the imaging sensitivity and contribute to the detection of lung cancer at an earlier stage.

Liposomes functionalized with gadodiamide (Gd) and loaded with paclitaxel-carboplatin with teratonistic (therapeutic and diagnostic) effect were prepared for imaging (Gd was used for imaging in MRI). The *in vivo* distribution of liposomes prepared in this way was observed by contrast-enhanced MRI. Thin film hydration method was used in the preparation of these liposomes. As lipids, distearoylphosphatidylcholine (DSPC), 1,2-distearoyl-sn-glycero-3-phosphoglycerol (DSPG), sodium;[(2R)-2,3-di(octadecanoyloxy)propyl] 2-(2-methoxyethoxycarbonylamino) ethyl phosphate (MPEG-2000-DSPE) and c(RGDyK)-PEG2000-DSPE were weighed in different ratios and dissolved in chloroform/methanol/water mixture and then paclitaxel was added into this solution. To form a thin film final solution was kept in a high vacuum overnight. Then, carboplatin and gadolinium-DTPA-BMA (Gd-DTPA-BMA is a contrast agent) solution was added to hydrate thin film, and liposome suspensions were obtained subject to sonication and extrusion. In terms of liposomal analyses, particle size and zeta potential with dynamic light scattering (DLS), particle imaging with transmission electron microscopy (TEM), and confirmation of peptide-lipid c(RGDyK)-PEG2000-DSPE conjugate was done by spectrophotometer and mass spectroscopy. Liposomes prepared in this way have been observed to effectively target non-small cell lung cancer cells in *in vitro* fluorescent microscopy and *in vivo* MRI studies. Tumor signals were greatly increased in a liposome loaded with Gd-DTPA-BMA according to the commercial contrast agent Omniscan® [53].

In cases of suspected lung cancer, although computed tomography (CT) is the standard imaging technique, it is not easy to distinguish between malignant and benign nodules. Therefore, to develop a procedure that is both non-invasive and has improved discrimination, researchers have prepared an actively targeted gold nanoparticle contrast agent. The epidermal growth factor receptor (EGFR) which is found on the cell surface of most lung adenocarcinomas was targeted with cetuximab. Gold nanoparticles (AuNPs) were obtained using the modified Friends method, which is based on the reduction of gold chloride salt with citrate. Tetrachloroauric acid ($HAuClR_4R$) was dissolved in water, after that the solution was heated to boiling point. A preheated solution of sodium citrate was speedily injected into this solution under strong stirring. At this stage, the color of the solution changes from yellow to dark red, indicating the formation of gold nanoparticles. The solution was stirred at 100 °C for an extra 15 min to complete the reaction and then its temperature was lowered to room temperature. The resulting solution was filtered through a 0.22 μm filter to remove aggregates with coarser particle size. The size and distribution of nanoparticles were measured by transmission electron microscopy. To conjugate antibodies to the gold NP surface a polyethylene glycol (PEG) linker, of which one of these contains a reactive NHS ester group to form covalent bonds with primary amines on the antibodies and the other contain a thiol group to bind to the gold nanoparticle surface, was used. The PEG-antibody conjugation reaction was carried out in HEPES-buffered saline (pH 8.6/4 °C overnight) and obtained PEG-antibodies were mixed with plain gold nanoparticles. For non-targeted nanoparticles, only PEGylation was performed on the NP surface. Three different formulations prepared in this way (non-targeted nanoparticles, nanoparticles conjugated with cetuximab, and the smaller single-domain llama-derived anti-EGFR antibody conjugated nanoparticles) were injected into the tail veins of animals *in vivo* and compared for their tumor-targeting efficacy. Although all of the nanoparticles accumulated in tumor tissue, cetuximab conjugated NPs showed higher accumulation than the other groups. This study demonstrates that targeted nanoparticles can be used to detect tumor receptor overexpression and have the potential to better distinguish malignant lung tumors from benign lesions, as they are combined with conventional imaging features [54]. It has been mentioned in the previous paragraph that volatile organic compound analysis is performed by GC–MS in the diagnosis of lung cancer. Similarly, VOCs can be measured with AuNP sensors and thus histological classification of lung cancer was also possible. In a study, after the prepared AuNPs (3–4 nm core diameter) were coated with organic ligands to create a large area where VOC would be adsorbed, the samples were analyzed using cross-reactive chemical resistances. When the signals come from AuNP was analyzed, an effective distinction could be made between LC and healthy cells, between SCLC and NSCLC, and between the two subtypes (adenocarcinoma and squamous cell carcinoma) of NSCLC [55]. Like Barash *et al*, Peng and coauthors tried to determine volatile organic substances in exhaled breath with gold nanoparticles. For this purpose, 42 volatile organic compounds were identified as lung cancer biomarkers by GC–MS. AuNP sensors have been optimized using only four of them. Within this scope, firstly AuNPs with a diameter of 5 nm coated with a monolayer were produced by a modified two-phase method. Dodecanethiol, decanethiol, 1-butanethiol, 2-ethylhexanethiol, hexanethiol, tert-dodecanethiol, 4-methoxy-toluenethiol, 2-mercaptobenzoxazole and 11-mercapto-1-undecanol were used as coating material. During preparation, $AuCl_4^-$ was transferred from the aqueous $HAuCl_4.xH_2O$ solution to a toluene solution, and the thiol required for coating was added in excess after the organic phase isolation. Sodium borohydride ($NaHB_4$) solution was added to the solution following it was vigorously stirred for 10 min, further stirred at room temperature for at least 3 h. Thus, it was observed that as the solution color turned brown, thiol-coated gold nanoparticles were formed. The solvent in the resulting solution was removed by rotary-evaporator, and the obtained nanoparticles were extracted several times to remove free thiols. The results showed that these developed sensors hold promise for rapid, easy and cost-effective diagnosis and screening of lung cancer [56]. In another study, to determine the sequence of heterogeneous nuclear ribonucleoprotein (hnRNP B1), a lung cancer biomarker, AuNPs were synthesized using citrate reduction technique and conjugated with single-stranded DNA. Size, morphology and shape analyses were performed on AuNPs by spectrophotometry and TEM to confirm their suitability for processing prior to conjugation. The results obtained from the study showed that the gold nanoprobe-based method is better than the PCR-based method since enzymatic amplification and gel electrophoresis are not required, and small amounts of sample are sufficient [57]. Similar to this study, Ho *et al* developed an electrochemical sandwich immunosensor using AuNPs that can detect α-enolase (ENO1) protein, which is one of the biomarkers of lung cancer (SCLC or NSCLC), and thus diagnose lung cancer. The method is based on measuring the protein that was physisorbed on the screen-printed carbon electrodes with PEG-coated, by contacting AuNPs modified with anti-ENO1 antibody. It has been shown in this study that the developed sensor can detect the biomarker even in trace amounts. These systems prepared using AuNPs are more advantageous than radioisotopic or enzymatic methods, as they have high chemical stability, low probability of hazard, simple and accurate production and improvement of biocompatibility with surface modification [58].

Although magnetic resonance guided focused ultrasound surgery (MRgFUS) is successful in non-invasive cancer treatment, its use is currently limited due to its inability to detect small tumors, insufficient accumulation of ultrasonic energy and damage to surrounding tissues. Therefore, researchers have developed an active targeted theranostic nano-sized superparamagnetic iron oxide (SPIO) system to improve imaging sensitivity and energy deposition efficiency. SPIOs synthesized and PEGylated for active targeting were modified with anti-EGFR antibodies (anti-EGFR mAb). For the production of iron oxide nanoparticles, ferric acetylacetonate ($Fe(acac)_3$), α,ω-dicarboxyl poly(ethylene glycol) (HOOC-PEG-COOH) and oleylamine were mixed in diphenyl oxide solution and the solution was heated under nitrogen. The iron solution was then stirred at 400 rpm. At this time, samples were taken intermittently and reacted at 37 °C by adding an ethanol/ether mixture. These reaction samples were pooled and isolated. After washing, the residue was dissolved in ethanol and precipitated by adding ether. The resulting SPIO-NPs were purified for use. Anti-EGFR-PEG-SPIOs are prepared by adding the solution of EDC and *N*-hydroxysulphosuccinimide sodium salt (sulfo-NHS) in PBS on PEGylated SPIO, followed by stirring for 15 min at room temperature, purification, and storage with cetuximab at 4 °C overnight, respectively. The results showed that non-targeting PEGylated SPIOs were more targeted to the human non-small cell lung carcinoma (NIC-H460) tumor cells than anti-EGFR mAb-targeted PEGylated SPIOs, greatly increasing MRI contrast and ultrasonic energy deposition at the tumor site [59]. Another SPIO nanoparticle production study based on surface modification was done by Huang *et al*. In this study, after the SPIO was synthesized, the surface modification was made by replacing the hydrophobic surfactants on its surface with the peptide containing PEG-linked cysteine. Similar to the previous method to prepare SPIO-NPs, $Fe(acac)_3$, oleic acid, oleylamine and 1,2-hexadecandiol were dissolved in phenyl ether. The mixture was heated under nitrogen at 200 °C and then refluxed at 300 °C. The SPIO particles formed were precipitated by adding ethanol and suspended in hexane. This process was repeated several times to obtain SPIO particles with homogeneous diameter (6.2±0.9 nm). Size and imaging analyses on the particles were performed by TEM. For surface modification, SPIO nanoparticles were dispersed in toluene and mixed with a solution of lung cancer-targeting and scrambled control peptide (LCP/SP-PEG-Cys) in DMSO. The mixture was held at 60 °C under nitrogen and then cooled to room temperature. Finally, the mix precipitated with an ethanol/chloroform/hexane mixture and redistributed in water to obtain peptide-coated SPIO. The size of the coated SPIO particles was measured by dynamic light scattering. Morphological analysis was performed using TEM. Apart from these analyses, the amount of protein bound to the particle surface, magnetic properties and T_2 relaxation times were also determined. In this way, biocompatible SPIO particles were obtained and it was observed that T_2 relaxation was high in the experiments. The system developed as a result of MR imaging and Prussian blue staining was found to be successful in targeting lung cancer cells expressing *αvβ6* [60]. Wan and colleagues synthesized immune superparamagnetic iron oxide nanoparticles that could be used in MR immunoimaging for sensitive detection of lung cancer metastasis. After production with SPOI-NP, their surfaces were covered with oleic acid and carboxymethyl dextran (CMD), and then conjugated with mouse anti-CD44v6 monoclonal antibody. The production phase is as follows: iron oxide (Fe_3O_4) nanoparticles were prepared by chemical co-precipitation method. According to this method, ferric chloride hexahydrate ($FeCl_3{\cdot}6H_2O$) and ferrous chloride tetrahydrate ($FeCl_2{\cdot}4H_2O$) were rapidly added to deoxygenated deionized water under nitrogen and the solution was heated to 80 ° C. Aqueous ammonium hydroxide (NH_4OH) solution was added dropwise under stirring at 800 rpm. At this stage, the color of the solution changes from brown to black, indicating that iron oxide particles are formed. For oleic acid coating, oleic acid was added to the black solution and stirred continuously under nitrogen. After the reaction was finished, the solutions were brought to room temperature and dialyzed for purification. For CMD coating, oleic acid coated SPIO-NPs and CMD solution were mixed and sonicated. NPs were removed from solution using magnets to remove free polymers. These SPIO-NPs were dispersed by sonication in distilled water. In order for the antibody to be conjugated to SPIO-NPs' surface, the carboxyl group on their surface must be activated. For this, SPIO-NPs were combined with EDC and NHS using mechanical shaker in HEPES medium. Then the pH of the medium was adjusted to 7.4 with sodium hydroxide (NaOH) and antibody was added to the medium. This system was incubated overnight. Dialysis was performed against HEPES to get rid of impurities. It was treated with fluorescein isothicynate (FITC) so that it could be visualized on MRI. The FITC solution in acetone was prepared and dried under nitrogen. The SPIO-NP solution was then added and sonicated. X-ray powder diffraction (XRD), thermogravimetric analysis (TGA), and Fourier transform infrared spectroscopy (FTIR) analyses were performed for the antibody unconjugated nanoparticles. In final NPs, size and imaging were performed by DLS and TEM, respectively. In conclusion, since SPIO-NPs have been shown to have relatively high saturation magnetization and can actively target human lung adenocarcinoma (A549) cells, it can be used as an effective contrast agent improving the detection limit by MRI [61]. Apart from the antibody, chemical ligands such as folate can also be used for surface modification of SPIO-NPs to enhance detection. Because there is overexpression of folate by cancerous tissue, such as lung adenosarcomas [62, 63]. In this case, the developed folate-conjugated nanosystems can also target tumor site and aid in diagnosis. In this context Yoo *et al* prepared folic acid-polyethylen glycol (FA-PEG) conjugated SPIO-NPs (FA-PEG-SPIO-NPs) by firstly synthesizing FA-PEG conjugate and then coating SPIO-NPs with FA-PEG similar to other studies. SPIO-NPs were treated with Cy5.5 for optical imaging of the prepared systems. The formulations (folic acid conjugated SPIO-NPs (FA-PEG-SPIO-NPs) and folic acid unconjugated SPIO-NPs (PEG-SPIO-NPs)) were injected into mice with lung cancer for determining targeting and imaging activity. In the folic acid pretreated group, cellular uptake of FA-PEG-SPIO-NPs was suppressed, suggesting their uptake by receptor-mediated endocytosis. In addition, PEG-SPIO-NPs conjugated with folic acid (FA-PEG-SPIO-NPs) had higher optical imaging signal than PEG-SPIO-NPs [64].

Another nanosystem used in the diagnosis of various types of lung cancer is quantum dots (QDs). Some researchers have prepared QDs with different properties using various methods. For instance, Kalkal *et al* have synthesized biofunctionalized graphene QDs that can quantify cancer biomarkers with higher accuracy and sensitivity, thus allowing for early diagnosis of the disease. Graphene QDs were obtained using the hydrothermal method. Briefly, citric acid was dissolved in distilled water, following diethylenetriamine (DETA) was added to this solution and stirred until a transparent solution was obtained. This solution was heated for a time at 170 °C and then cooled to room temperature. It was lyophilized after filtration and dialysis. Standard EDC-NHS coupling chemistry was used for antibody conjugation as described in other methods. The obtained nanoparticles were characterized by UV–vis, zeta potential and FTIR studies. The adhesion efficiency was found to be 88.13%. This indicates that amine-functionalized and nitrogen-doped graphene quantum dots (amine-N-GQDs) will be an effective fluorescent biosensor. In this study, QDs were used as the energy donor of the fluorescent open biosensor for the ultrasensitive detection of small cell lung cancer biomarkers. The energy acceptor of this system is gold nanoparticles (AuNPs). In a system developed in this way, the anti-NSE/amine-N GQDs@AuNPs nanoprobe gave a fast, wide and linear range and low level fluorescence response. In addition, the recovery value was obtained as approximately 94.69% [65]. Li *et al*, on the other hand, produced bicolor fluorescence quantum dots functionalized with two different biomarkers (carcinoembryonic antigen-CEA and neuron-specific enolase-NSE) that will enable the detection of lung cancer at an early stage. First, the researchers combined streptavidin-coated polystyrene beads with a solution containing two captured antibodies, two antigens, and two detection antibodies, allowing the beads to aggregate. In the second stage, dual color QDs with maximum emission at 525 and 655 nm washed, added to the above solution, and reacted with the antibodies it would identify. In the final step, the bead-QD conjugates were separated and the QDs were free for fluorescent detection of CEA and NSE. According to the results of the study, the system developed determined CEA and NSE precisely with fluorescent plate reader, and showed high precision for both targets. So much so that it showed comparable performance to the commercial single analyte ELISA. No cross-reactivity was observed during the experiments, and a good correlation was obtained for CEA and NSE in measurements made in 25 humans [66]. Since the efficiency of large-sized nanosystems in diagnosis and therapy is low, Shivaji *et al* synthesized cadmium sulfide quantum dots (CdS QDs) with a particle size of 2–5 nm for the production of low-size (<10 nm) nanoparticles such as semiconductor quantum dots. Tea leaf extract (*Camellia sinensis*) was used as a particle stabilizing agent during production. First, the plant extract to be used in QD synthesis was prepared. For this, *C. sinensis* was dried after washing in water and incubated in methanol for 24 h. The mixture was filtered through filter paper to get the fraction that passed into methanol. To prepare CdS QDs, cadmium sulfate ($CdSO_4$) was added to the *C. sinensis* extract and incubated in the dark. Afterwards, sodium sulfide (Na_2S) was added and incubated again to obtain CdS nanoparticles. The solid CdS QDs obtained after centrifugation of the final solution were lyophilized. According to the results of the study, high-contrast fluorescent images of A549 cells, a lung cancer cell line, were obtained by strong interaction of CdS QDs with cancer cell. It also has a cytotoxic effect on cells. Fluorescence emission and flow cytometry analyses showed that the fluorescent emission of CdS QDs is λexc=410 nm, and they inhibit further growth by arresting cell growth in the S phase of the cell cycle. Moreover, the results showed that CdS quantum dots prepared using *C. sinensis* was highly stable in the bio-environment [67]. Since the detection of micrometastases has an important role in the early diagnosis of cancers, Wang and collageous aimed to detect micrometastases of lung cancer in peripheral blood using magnetic nanoparticles (MNPs) and quantum dots (QDs). Iron oxide MNPs were prepared by Massart method that is co-precipitating ferrous chloride ($FeCl_2$) and ferric chloride ($FeCl_3$). Subsequently, oleic acid-modified MNPs were obtained by adding an excess of oleic acid was added to the dispersion of Fe_3O_4 MNP in water. This solution was washed and dried. To prepare Fe_3O_4/polystyrene MNPs, the oleic acid modified Fe_3O_4 MNPs obtained in the first stage were dispersed in styrene/cyclohexane (oil phase). Sodium dodecyl sulfate (SDS) and sodium bicarbonate ($NaHCO_3$) were dissolved in water (water phase). The oil phase and water phase were mixed in an ultrasonic bath in a cold environment. An aqueous solution of potassium persulfate on it to initiate the polymerization added at 70 °C. Fe_3O_4/polystyrene MNPs were obtained after a certain period of incubation. A carbodiimide-mediated condensation method was used to coat the surface of MNPs with pan-cytokeratin (pan-ck) antibody. For this, MNPs and coupling buffer were combined, and the activated MNPs were separated from the reaction medium. The MNPs were then suspended in coupling buffer and 1-ethyl-3-(3-dimethylaminopropyl)carbodiimide (EDAC) was added to the medium followed by pan-ck antibody. After stirring for a while, the resulting MNP-pan-ck was magnetically separated. For preparation of QDs, firstly, a solution of cadmium acetate dihydrate ($Cd(Ac)_2.2H_2O$) in water was prepared and thioglycolic acid was added. Its pH was adjusted to 9.5 with NaOH. The gas in the mixture was removed with nitrogen (N_2) and the oxygen-free sodium hydrogen telluride (NaHTe) solution was injected into the medium. The resulting mixture was refluxed until QDs of the desired size were obtained (determined by following ultraviolet-visible curves). Different lung antibodies were conjugated to different QDs: rabbit anti-human Lunx antibody for QD552 and rabbit anti-human SP-A antibody for QD625. After adding borate buffer (pH 7.5) to the QD solution, this solution was mixed with the aqueous solution of EDAC. After a sufficient period of incubation, the antibody was added to the mixture and dialysis was performed to purify. To determine the efficacy of the system, different epithelial tumor cells were first enriched with pan-ck antibody-MNPs (MNP-pan-ck) and then QDs with double-labeled antibodies were able to identify lung cancer cells A549 and SPC-A-1. Validation of the method was done with samples from 32 patients with non-small cell lung cancer (NSCLC). Of these, 26 had enriched circulating tumor cells (CTC), and QDs were able to identify 21 of them. Therefore, it has been shown that the developed system can be used simultaneously to identify CTCs from NSCLC patients [68]. Recent work on QDs concerns QDs synthesized by Fan *et al* to perform analysis of circulating microRNA in serum, which is itself a biomarker. To demonstrate that both the serum levels of miRNAs and the developed system can be used in the early diagnosis of the lung, serum samples from patients with NSCLC and healthy individuals were taken and miRNA quantities were appointed via quantitative reverse transcriptase polymerase chain reaction (qRTPCR). The presence of 12 miRNAs was detected in this analysis. Similarly, the same analysis was repeated, this time using a fluorescent quantum dot liquid bead array. As a result, it was observed that the amount of 5 serum miRNAs (miR-16–5p, miR-17b-5p, miR-19–3p, miR-20a-5p, and miR-92–3p) decreased significantly, whereas the amount of miR-15b-5p increased in patients, the expression of miR-15b-5p, miR-16–5p and miR-20a-5p could be a biomarker for NSCLC patients and serum miR-106–5p expression was higher in stage I. As summary, due to the size of miRNAs, RTPCR can lead to false positive results in the detection and quantification of miRNA. However, quantum dots increase the analysis sensitivity thanks to their high extinction coefficient and quantum efficiency. Fluorescent quantum dots liquid bead array method used in the detection and quantification analysis of miRNAs in this study showed high selectivity, sensitivity and reproducibility [69].

Upconversion nanoparticles (UCNPs) act as next-generation fluorophores. Because it can convert low-energy near-infrared radiations into high-energy visible radiations. In this respect, it can be used in both *in vitro* and *in vivo* applications for imaging and detection of biological materials [70]. Moreover, because UCNPs do not show autofluorescence, they can very precisely detect a small number of tumor cells to be collected for further analysis. In order to detect CTCs that indicate that cancer is metastatic and are used as biomarkers in cancer diagnosis, Wang *et al* developed a system in which a microfluidic silicon nanowire (SiNW) array is integrated with multifunctional magnetic upconversion nanoparticles (MUCNPs). This system ensures that CTCs are both captured and detected. To capture CTCs, MUCNPs were coated with anti-epithelial cell adhesion molecule (EpCAM) antibody. However, these NPs were integrated with the microfluidic SiNW array to increase the capture efficiency. Because UpNPs do not show autofluorescence, they can very precisely detect a small number of tumor cells to be collected for further analysis. Study results showed that this developed system can detect CTCs in blood samples from lung cancer patients, and consistent results are obtained when upconversion luminescence signals are compared with patient clinical results [71]. Near-infrared (NIR) fluorescence guided surgery has an important place in cancer treatment. However, conventional NIR fluorescent reagents have low sensitivity and specificity, do not have sufficient photostability, and cannot penetrate tissues sufficiently. In order to visualize lung cancer with fluorescence, NIR-visible upconversion nanoprobe with lanthanide nanoparticles that was targeted using RGD10 (ligand for integrin $\alpha v\beta 3/5$ receptor) and NGR9 (ligand for aminopeptidase N receptor) was developed. Dual-targeted UCNPs were synthesized in three steps. Firstly, UCNPs in core–shell structure were obtained because they abolished fluorescence quenching to improve upconversion luminescence. For this, the core ytterbium and thulium doped sodium yttrium fluoride ($NaYF_4$:Yb/Tm) particles and then the hexagonal sodium yttrium fluoride ($NaYF_4$) shell part were synthesized by solvothermal method. The surface of the obtained UCNPs was coated with polydopamine (PDA). The coating process was carried out by spontaneous polymerization of dopamine (DA) in alkaline solution. PDA-coated UCNPs were conjugated with the polypeptide chain RGD10 and NGR9 via Michael addition reaction. RGD and NGR were used for binding to integrin αvβ3/5 and aminopeptidase N, respectively. It has been determined that the obtained homogeneously distributed core–shell nanoprobes are biocompatible with cells and animals, can specifically target A549 cancer cells in analyses using cell binding and inductively coupled plasma-mass spectrometer (ICP-MS), and can separate tumor tissue from surrounding normal tissues in BALB/c nude mice carrying tumor xenografts [72]. To increase the imaging efficiency and safety of UCNPs in the biological environment, phosphate-coated UCNPs were synthesized by Li *et al.* Because UCNPs are produced using rare earth (RE) metals, however, intact RE nanoparticles (NPs) are not stable in an acidic physiological environment (e.g., lysosomes). With the disintegration of the lysosome, it can form a phosphate complex within the cell and lose its luminescence efficiency. In this study, polyethylene glycol-erbium and ytterbium doped sodium yttrium fluoride (PEG-NaYF4:Er/Yb) UCNPs were not synthesized and it was supplied from the market. UCNPs was dispersed in deionized water containing the coating phosphate material and reacted with these coating molecules at room temperature. N-(Phosphonomethyl)iminodiacetic acid hydrate, aminomethylphosphonic acid, (3-bromopropyl) phosphonic acid, or ethylenediamine tetra(methylenephosphonic acid) was used as phosphate resource. The solutions were centrifuged to obtained the coated particles. When the stability of commercially available and non-phosphate-coated UCNPs was evaluated in lysosomes and simulated lysosomal fluid, it was observed that they induced proinflammatory effects at the cellular level and intact lung, and decreased upconversion fluorescence efficiency. However, when coated with phosphate, it was found that especially EDTMP retained UCNPs' imaging intensity and did not cause proinflammatory effects *in vitro* and *in vivo* [73].

9.3 Conclusion

In conclusion, it is difficult to diagnose lung cancer at an early stage. Small lesions detected by various imaging methods require further examination like histological or cytological. For example, when using fine-needle aspirates (FNA) to remove these lesions, this procedure is often difficult as the reliability of the sample largely depends on the accurate finding of the biopsy site. Resection is an invasive method and is preferred only when the benefit to the patient is high. Although exfoliative materials (sputum, bronchoalveolar lavage and bronchial brushes) offer diagnostic possibilities as a non-invasive approach, the sensitivity of current cytological tests is not sufficient. However, significant progress has been made in non-invasive methods, especially with the detection of cancer cell-specific biomarkers. Today, studies continue on various analysis methods or analysis auxiliary components in order to detect these markers sensitively and accurately even at the lowest level. Nanosystems are also used to increase the sensitivity of the methods. Thanks to their nano size, these systems tend to passively go to tumor tissue rather than healthy tissues and show high accumulation there. However, in addition to passive targeting, active targeting is also used in order to distinguish between healthy tissue and tumor tissue more precisely. A tumor-specific ligand or antibody is conjugated to the surface of the nanosystem for active targeting. Usually, these ligands or antibodies are tumor-specific because they are overexpressed by tumor cells. In this way, nanosystems can go directly to the tumor site and this approach is often preferred in tumor treatment. As discussed in the chapter, the use of these systems for diagnosis is often supported by fluorescent or magnetic imaging. Nanosystems to be used in this way can be prepared to contain imaging concentrates or can be magnetically enhanced. Apart from this, there are also nanosystems that spontaneously luminescence depending on the particle size. The success of biomarkers or nanosystems in the diagnosis of lung cancer has been demonstrated by various clinical studies, and there are some diagnostic kits based on this approach in clinical use. However, there are still many steps to be taken to increase the diagnostic sensitivity, as well as to improve its properties such as biocompatibility and clinical use.

References

[1] Thai A A, Solomon B J, Sequist L V, Gainor J F and Heist R S 2021 Lung cancer *Lancet* **398** 535–54

[2] Sha X, Gong G, Qiu Q, Duan J, Li D and Yin Y 2019 Identifying pathological subtypes of non-small-cell lung cancer by using the radiomic features of ^{18}F-fluorodeoxyglucose positron emission computed tomography *Transl. Cancer Res.* **8** 1741–9

[3] Zappa C and Mousa S A 2016 Non-small cell lung cancer: current treatment and future advances *Transl. Lung Cancer Res.* **5** 288–300

[4] Sita T L, Iyengar P, Abazeed M E and Kruser T J 2021 Radiotherapy for metastatic non–small cell lung cancer: an emerging tool for systemic control *Adv. Oncol.* **1** 15–28

[5] Rudin C M *et al* 2019 Molecular subtypes of small cell lung cancer: a synthesis of human and mouse model data *Nat. Rev. Cancer* **19** 289–97

[6] Raso M G, Bota-Rabassedas N and Wistuba I I 2021 Pathology and classification of SCLC *Cancers* **13** 820
[7] Akhtar N and Bansal J G 2017 Risk factors of lung cancer in nonsmoker *Curr. Probl. Cancer* **41** 328–39
[8] Bade B C and Cruz C S D 2020 Lung cancer 2020: epidemiology, etiology, and prevention *Clin. Chest Med.* **41** 1–24
[9] Corrales L, Rosell R, Cardona A F, Martin C, Zatarain-Barrón Z L and Arrieta O 2020 Lung cancer in never smokers: the role of different risk factors other than tobacco smoking *Crit. Rev. Oncol./Hematol.* **148** 102895
[10] de Groot P and Munden R F 2012 Lung cancer epidemiology, risk factors, and prevention *Radiol. Clin.* **50** 863–76
[11] Himbert C, Klossner N, Coletta A M, Barnes C A, Wiskemann J, LaStayo P C, Varghese T K Jr and Ulrich C M 2020 Exercise and lung cancer surgery: a systematic review of randomized-controlled trials *Crit. Rev. Oncol./Hematol.* **156** 103086
[12] Pêgo-Fernandes P M, Haddad F J, Imaeda C J and Sandrini M 2021 The role of the surgeon in treating patients with lung cancer. An updating article *Sao Paulo Med. J.;* **139** 293–300
[13] Li Z, Feiyue Z and Gaofeng L 2021 Traditional Chinese medicine and lung cancer-from theory to practice *Biomed. Pharmacother.* **137** 111381
[14] Reuss J E, Gosa L and Liu S V 2021 Antibody drug conjugates in lung cancer: state of the current therapeutic landscape and future developments *Clin. Lung Cancer* **22** 483–99
[15] Shao W, Zhou Q and Tang X 2020 Current and emerging treatment options for lung cancer in patients with pre-existing connective tissue disease *Pulm. Pharmacol. Ther.* **63** 101937
[16] Wulf J, Haedinger U, Oppitz U, Thiele W, Mueller G and Flentje M 2004 Stereotactic radiotherapy for primary lung cancer and pulmonary metastases: a noninvasive treatment approach in medically inoperable patients *Int. J. Radiat. Oncol. Biol. Phys.* **60** 186–96
[17] Ferrell B, Koczywas M, Grannis F and Harrington A 2011 Palliative care in lung cancer *Surg. Clin.* **91** 403–17
[18] Lee S H 2019 Chemotherapy for lung cancer in the era of personalized medicine *Tuberc. Respir. Dis.* **82** 179–89
[19] Choi H K and Mazzone P J 2020 Lung cancer screening *Surg. Oncol. Clin. N Am.* **29** 509–24
[20] Toumazis I, Bastani M, Han S S and Plevritis S K 2020 Risk-based lung cancer screening: a systematic review *Lung Cancer* **147** 154–86
[21] Sim A J, Kaza E, Singer L and Rosenberg S A 2020 A review of the role of MRI in diagnosis and treatment of early stage lung cancer *Clin. Transl. Radiat. Oncol.* **24** 16–22
[22] Rivera M P, Detterbeck F and Mehta A C 2003 Diagnosis of lung cancer: the guidelines *Chest* **123** 129S–36S
[23] Ho H, Williamson C, Regis S M, Stock C T, Quadri S M, McKee B J, McKee A B and Servais E L 2021 Surgery and invasive diagnostic procedures for benign disease are rare in a large low-dose computed tomography lung cancer screening program *J. Thorac. Cardiovasc. Surg.* **161** 790–802
[24] Yasufuku K and Fujisawa T 2007 Staging and diagnosis of non-small cell lung cancer: invasive modalities *Respirology* **12** 173–83
[25] Kulkarni A and Panditrao A 2014 Classification of lung cancer stages on CT scan images using image processing *IEEE Int. Conf. on Advanced Communications, Control and Computing Technologies* 1384–88

[26] He T, Xue Z, Lu K, y Alvarado M V, Wong K K, Xie W and Wong S T 2012 A minimally invasive multimodality image-guided (MIMIG) system for peripheral lung cancer intervention and diagnosis *Comput. Med. Imag. Graph.* **36** 345–55
[27] Hirsch F R, Scagliotti G V, Mulshine J L, Kwon R, Curran W J, Wu Y L and Paz-Ares L 2017 Lung cancer: current therapies and new targeted treatments *Lancet* **389** 299–311
[28] Jonas D E *et al* 2021 Screening for lung cancer with low-dose computed tomography: updated evidence report and systematic review for the US Preventive Services Task Force *JAMA* **325** 971–87
[29] Veronesi G *et al* 2008 Lung cancer screening with low-dose computed tomography: a non-invasive diagnostic protocol for baseline lung nodules *Lung Cancer* **61** 340–49
[30] Tsou J A, Hagen J A, Carpenter C L and Laird-Offringa I A 2002 DNA methylation analysis: a powerful new tool for lung cancer diagnosis *Oncogene* **21** 5450–61
[31] Li Z, Shu J, Yang B, Zhang Z, Huang J and Chen Y 2020 Emerging non-invasive detection methodologies for lung cancer *Oncol. Lett.* **19** 3389–99
[32] Ye M *et al* 2021 Circulating genetically abnormal cells add non-invasive diagnosis value to discriminate lung cancer in patients with pulmonary nodules ⩽ 10 mm *Front. Oncol.* **11** 638223
[33] Bajtarevic A *et al* 2009 Noninvasive detection of lung cancer by analysis of exhaled breath *BMC Cancer* **9** 348
[34] Jia Z, Zhang H, Ong C N, Patra A, Lu Y, Lim C T and Venkatesan T 2018 Detection of lung cancer: concomitant volatile organic compounds and metabolomic profiling of six cancer cell lines of different histological origins *ACS Omega* **3** 5131–40
[35] Shaffie A, Soliman A, Fu X A, Nantz M, Giridharan G, van Berkel V, Khalifeh H A, Ghazal M, Elmaghraby A and El-Baz A 2021 A novel technology to integrate imaging and clinical markers for non-invasive diagnosis of lung cancer *Sci. Rep.* **11** 1–10
[36] Wielscher M, Vierlinger K, Kegler U, Ziesche R, Gsur A and Weinhäusel A 2015 Diagnostic performance of plasma DNA methylation profiles in lung cancer, pulmonary fibrosis and COPD *EBioMedicine* **2** 929–36
[37] Liang W *et al* 2019 Non-invasive diagnosis of early-stage lung cancer using high-throughput targeted DNA methylation sequencing of circulating tumor DNA (ctDNA) *Theranostics* **9** 2056–70
[38] Ulivi P and Zoli W 2014 miRNAs as non-invasive biomarkers for lung cancer diagnosis *Molecules* **19** 8220–37
[39] Powrózek T, Krawczyk P, Kowalski D M, Kuźnar-Kamińska B, Winiarczyk K, Olszyna-Serementa M, Batura-Gabryel H and Milanowski J 2016 Application of plasma circulating microRNA-448, 506, 4316, and 4478 analysis for non-invasive diagnosis of lung cancer *Tumor Biol.* **37** 2049–55
[40] Leng Q, Lin Y, Jiang F, Lee C J, Zhan M, Fang H, Wang Y and Jiang F 2017 A plasma miRNA signature for lung cancer early detection *Oncotarget* **8** 111902–11
[41] Lan H, Lu H, Wang X and Jin H 2015 MicroRNAs as potential biomarkers in cancer: opportunities and challenges *BioMed Res. Int.* **2015** 125094
[42] Cryer A M and Thorley A J 2019 Nanotechnology in the diagnosis and treatment of lung cancer *Pharmacol. Ther.* **198** 189–205
[43] Zamay T N, Zamay G S, Kolovskaya O S, Zukov R A, Petrova M M, Gargaun A, Berezovski M V and Kichkailo A S 2017 Current and prospective protein biomarkers of lung cancer *Cancers* **9** 155

[44] Pi C, Xu C R, Zhang M F, Peng X X, Wei X W, Gao X, Yan H H and Zhou Q 2018 EGFR mutations in early-stage and advanced-stage lung adenocarcinoma: analysis based on large-scale data from China *Thoracic Cancer* **9** 814–9

[45] Haider N, Fatima S, Taha M, Rizwanullah M, Firdous J, Ahmad R, Mazhar F and Khan M A 2020 Nanomedicines in diagnosis and treatment of cancer: an update *Curr. Pharm. Des.* **26** 1216–31

[46] Kumar K and Chawla R 2021 Nanocarriers-mediated therapeutics as a promising approach for treatment and diagnosis of lung cancer *J. Drug Delivery Sci. Technol.* **65** 102677

[47] Akopov A and Papayan G 2021 Photodynamic theranostics of central lung cancer: present state and future prospects *Photodiagn. Photodyn. Ther.* **33** 102203

[48] On K C, Rho J, Yoon H Y, Chang H, Yhee J Y, Yoon J S, Jeong S Y, Kim H K and Kim K 2020 Tumor-targeting glycol chitosan nanoparticles for image-guided surgery of rabbit orthotopic VX2 lung cancer *Pharmaceutics* **12** 621

[49] Kitada M, Ohsaki Y, Yasuda S, Abe M, Takahashi N, Okazaki S, Ishibashi K and Hayashi S 2017 Photodynamic diagnosis of visceral pleural invasion of lung cancer with a combination of 5-aminolevulinic acid and autofluorescence observation systems *Photodiagn. Photodyn. Ther.* **20** 10–5

[50] Baumgartner R, Huber R M, Schulz H, Stepp H, Rick K, Gamarra F, Leberig A and Roth C 1996 Inhalation of 5-aminolevulinic acid: a new technique for fluorescence detection of early stage lung cancer *J. Photochem. Photobiol.,* B **36** 169–74

[51] Babič A, Herceg V, Bastien E, Lassalle H P, Bezdetnaya L and Lange N 2018 5-Aminolevulinic acid-squalene nanoassemblies for tumor photodetection and therapy: *in vitro* studies *Nanoscale Res. Lett.* **13** 1–9

[52] Wang X, Tian Y, Liao X, Tang Y, Ni Q, Sun J, Zhao Y, Zhang J, Teng Z and Lu G 2020 Enhancing selective photosensitizer accumulation and oxygen supply for high-efficacy photodynamic therapy toward glioma by 5-aminolevulinic acid loaded nanoplatform *J. Colloid Interface Sci.* **565** 483–93

[53] Ren L, Chen S, Li H, Zhang Z, Zhong J, Liu M and Zhou X 2016 MRI-guided liposomes for targeted tandem chemotherapy and therapeutic response prediction *Acta Biomater.* **35** 260–8

[54] Ashton J R, Gottlin E B, Patz E F Jr, West J L and Badea C T 2018 A comparative analysis of EGFR-targeting antibodies for gold nanoparticle CT imaging of lung cancer *PLoS One* **13** e0206950

[55] Barash O, Peled N, Tisch U, Bunn P A Jr, Hirsch F R and Haick H 2012 Classification of lung cancer histology by gold nanoparticle sensors *Nanomed. Nanotechnol. Biol. Med.* **8** 580–9

[56] Peng G, Tisch U, Adams O, Hakim M, Shehada N, Broza Y Y, Billan S, Abdah-Bortnyak R, Kuten A and Haick H 2009 Diagnosing lung cancer in exhaled breath using gold nanoparticles *Nat. Nanotechnol.* **4** 669–73

[57] Daraee H, Pourhassanmoghadam M, Akbarzadeh A, Zarghami N and Rahmati-Yamchi M 2016 Gold nanoparticle–oligonucleotide conjugate to detect the sequence of lung cancer biomarker *Artif. Cells Nanomed. Biotechnol.* **44** 1417–23

[58] Ho J A A, Chang H C, Shih N Y, Wu L C, Chang Y F, Chen C C and Chou C 2010 Diagnostic detection of human lung cancer-associated antigen using a gold nanoparticle-based electrochemical immunosensor *Anal. Chem.* **82** 5944–50

[59] Wang Z *et al* 2017 Active targeting theranostic iron oxide nanoparticles for MRI and magnetic resonance-guided focused ultrasound ablation of lung cancer *Biomaterials* **127** 25–35

[60] Huang G, Zhang C, Li S, Khemtong C, Yang S G, Tian R, Minna J D, Brown K C and Gao J 2009 A novel strategy for surface modification of superparamagnetic iron oxide nanoparticles for lung cancer imaging *J. Mater. Chem.* **19** 6367–72
[61] Wan X, Song Y, Song N, Li J, Yang L, Li Y and Tan H 2016 The preliminary study of immune superparamagnetic iron oxide nanoparticles for the detection of lung cancer in magnetic resonance imaging *Carbohydr. Res.* **419** 33–40
[62] O'Shannessy D J, Yu G, Smale R, Fu Y S, Singhal S, Thiel R P, Somers E B and Vachani A 2012 Folate receptor alpha expression in lung cancer: diagnostic and prognostic significance *Oncotarget* **3** 414–25
[63] Kato T *et al* 2017 Nanoparticle targeted folate receptor 1-enhanced photodynamic therapy for lung cancer *Lung Cancer* **113** 59–68
[64] Yoo M K, Park I K, Lim H T, Lee S J, Jiang H L, Kim Y K, Choi Y J, Cho M H and Cho C S 2012 Folate–PEG–superparamagnetic iron oxide nanoparticles for lung cancer imaging *Acta Biomater.* **8** 3005–13
[65] Kalkal A, Pradhan R, Kadian S, Manik G and Packirisamy G 2020 Biofunctionalized graphene quantum dots based fluorescent biosensor toward efficient detection of small cell lung cancer *ACS Appl. Bio. Mater.* **3** 4922–32
[66] Li H, Cao Z, Zhang Y, Lau C and Lu J 2011 Simultaneous detection of two lung cancer biomarkers using dual-color fluorescence quantum dots *Analyst* **136** 1399–405
[67] Shivaji K, Mani S, Ponmurugan P, De Castro C S, Lloyd Davies M, Balasubramanian M G and Pitchaimuthu S 2018 Green-synthesis-derived CdS quantum dots using tea leaf extract: antimicrobial, bioimaging, and therapeutic applications in lung cancer cells *ACS Appl. Nano Mater.* **1** 1683–93
[68] Wang Y, Zhang Y, Du Z, Wu M and Zhang G 2012 Detection of micrometastases in lung cancer with magnetic nanoparticles and quantum dots *Int. J. Nanomed.* **7** 2315–24
[69] Fan L, Qi H, Teng J, Su B, Chen H, Wang C and Xia Q 2016 Identification of serum miRNAs by nano-quantum dots microarray as diagnostic biomarkers for early detection of non-small cell lung cancer *Tumor Biol.* **37** 7777–84
[70] Wang M, Abbineni G, Clevenger A, Mao C and Xu S 2011 Upconversion nanoparticles: synthesis, surface modification and biological applications *Nanomed. Nanotechnol. Biol. Med.* **7** 710–29
[71] Wang C, Ye M, Cheng L, Li R, Zhu W, Shi Z, Fan C, He J, Liu J and Liu Z 2015 Simultaneous isolation and detection of circulating tumor cells with a microfluidic silicon-nanowire-array integrated with magnetic upconversion nanoprobes *Biomaterials* **54** 55–62
[72] Cao J, Zhang L, Ding X, Liu D, Su B and Shi J 2020 Dual-targeting peptides RGD10-NGR9-conjugated lanthanide nanoparticle@ polydopamine as upconversion nanoprobes for *in vivo* imaging of lung cancer *Small Methods* **4** 2000648
[73] Li R *et al* 2015 Enhancing the imaging and biosafety of upconversion nanoparticles through phosphonate coating *ACS Nano* **9** 3293–306

IOP Publishing

Detection Systems in Lung Cancer and Imaging, Volume 1

Ayman El-Baz and Jasjit S Suri

Chapter 10

Heat shock proteins as biomarkers for early-stage diagnosis of lung cancer

Adria Hasan, Suroor Fatima Rizvi, Sana Parveen and Snober S Mir

Cancer cells have high expression of heat shock proteins (HSPs). Moreover, their expression can also define the level of aggressiveness in certain cancers and are generally linked with poor prognosis. As HSPs can stabilize several mutated cancer genes or oncogenic kinases, overexpression of HSPs is usually linked with apoptosis evasion, metastasis, and drug resistance in cancers. Thus, assessing the levels of HSPs in cancer patients may help in the early detection of the carcinogenesis process. Although several diagnostic methods such as MRI, CT scan and PET scan are used, early detection of cancers is still an issue. HSPs are highly upregulated in lung cancer and can be used as biomarkers for its early diagnosis. This chapter discusses the conventional methods of cancer diagnosis followed by elaborating the role of HSPs in the diagnosis and prognosis of lung cancer.

10.1 Introduction

Cancer is the second major cause of mortality worldwide where lung, stomach, prostate, liver and colorectal are most common in men, while breast, lung, colorectal and thyroid cancers commonly occur in women [1]. However, in terms of metastasis, lung cancer has a high metastatic rate and is the most common metastatic site (49.1%) [2]. Lung cancer is divided into two histological subtypes: small cell lung carcinoma (SCLC; 15% caseload) and non-small cell lung carcinoma (NSCLC; 85% caseload). In NSCLC, lung adenocarcinoma (LUAD) and lung squamous cell carcinoma (LUSC) are the most common subtypes [3]. In India, lung cancer accounts for 5.5% of total cancer cases [1]. In recent years, adenocarcinoma has taken over squamous cell carcinoma as the leading type of NSCLC (figure 10.1a, 10.1b). According to WHO, lung cancer deaths will keep on increasing due to a large amount of tobacco consumption. In lung cancer, tobacco is the most common associated risk factor while smoking being the second most common cause of it [4].

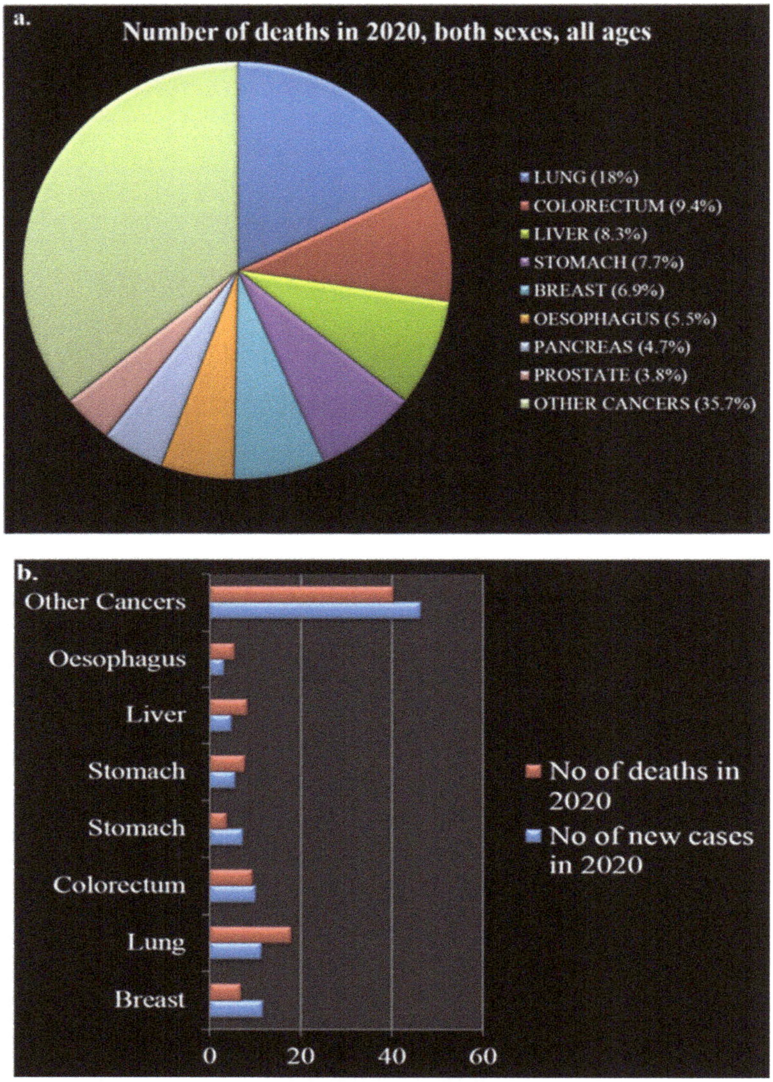

Figure 10.1. Lung cancer accounts for maximum number of cancer related deaths worldwide. Source: GLOBOCAN 2020.

However, passive smoking, pollution, or inherited genetic susceptibility are also common causes of lung cancer, especially in women [5, 6].

10.1.1 Risk factors and symptoms associated with lung cancer

Tobacco smokers alone account for nearly 80% of lung cancer cases [7]. Apart from tobacco, factors such as arsenic, asbestos, emphysema, chronic bronchitis, tuberculosis, and asthma are other causes of lung cancer development. Further, any

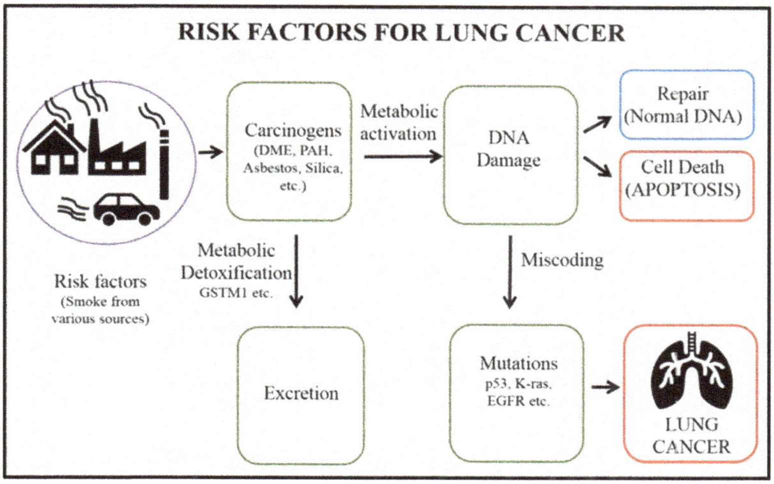

Figure 10.2. Major risk factors associated with lung cancer. Carcinogens such as DME (diesel motor exhaust), PAH (polycyclic aromatic hydrocarbons) may cause DNA damage, which, if not repaired may lead to mutations in either tumor suppressor genes (TP53) or the oncogenic genes (EGFR, K-RAS) leading to lung cancer progression.

mutations in tumor suppressor genes or DNA damage may also promote lung cancer progression. Moreover, human immunodeficiency virus (HIV), human papillomavirus (HPV), and Epstein–Barr virus (EBV) infections have been observed in association with lung cancer [8].

Further, primary symptoms of lung cancer include weakness, weight loss, bone pain, chest pain, cough, shortness of breath, hemoptysis, and swallowing discomfort. Small pulmonary nodules are usually asymptomatic. However, tumors with an endobronchial component, central tumors or large pulmonary lesions result in symptoms such as cough and chest pain [9]. Symptoms usually appear based on tumor location and metastasis site, while three-fourths of lung cancer cases are detected in advanced cancer cases [10]. A study reported that approximately 50% of cases reported non-massive hemoptysis (42.45%), chronic cough (44.1%), asymptomatic (35.65%), significant weight loss (27.9%), dyspnea (18.35%), poor appetite (13.75%) and chest pain (8.8%) [11] (figure 10.2).

10.2 Conventional diagnostic methods of lung cancer

10.2.1 Chest radiography

Chest radiography (CXR) is an imaging technique used to detect lung cancer [12]. However, if any abnormalities are detected in CXRs, computed tomography is subsequently performed. It is an easy to perform technique, and has very low levels of radiation exposure, making it a standard diagnostic tool for detecting respiratory diseases [12]. During imaging, lung cancer may be seen as a speculated mass or lobar collapse. In cases of bulky or obvious contralateral mediastinal adenopathy, no further imaging is required. However, a CT (computerized tomography) scan may further be used as chest radiographs are less sensitive in the detection of mediastinal lymph node metastases and mediastinal and chest wall invasion [13].

Moreover, CXRs are more likely to have misinterpretation where, of all misdiagnosed lung cancer cases, 10% used CT scans and other diagnostic methods while 90% of cases were diagnosed by CXRs [14]. Early identification of lesions is the key to a better prognosis of lung cancer, a delay in diagnosis due to misinterpretation of results in more negative clinical outcomes [14, 15]. Yet, studies have demonstrated that using CXRs for the early diagnosis of lung cancer may improve survival chances [15, 16]. Another study reported a reduction of 18% in lung cancer mortality with CXR screening in the population at-risk. Moreover, it was shown in a case control study that more than 20% of lung cancer mortality was reduced when it was screened at early stages by CXR [17]. Thus, CXRs may significantly help in the screening of lung cancer.

10.2.2 CT scan

Computed tomography (CT) is used as a detection tool for the diagnosis of early stages of lung cancer [18, 19]. A CT scan can detect specific features in lung nodules, such as fungus balls, arteriovenous fistulae, mucoid impaction, rounded atelectasis, and infarcts [20]. As CT scans can evaluate the entire thorax at the time of nodule assessment, it is beneficial at the initial diagnostic stages. Further, spiral or helical CT is efficient in the detection of small nodules between slices [21, 22]. Non-enhanced CT through thorax and adrenals can stage patients with newly diagnosed NSCLC as it was reported by Patz *et al* that there was no difference in the radiological stage of non-contrast-enhanced scans and contrast-enhanced scans in 84 patients [23]. However, another study comprising 50 patients reported an 11% higher detection rate of enlarged mediastinal nodes after contrast enhancement than unenhanced CT [24].

Further, when high-risk populations were screened using CT scans, chest radiography, and sputum analysis in large screening programs conducted in the United States of America and Czechoslovakia, an increase in the diagnosis of early-stage lung cancer was observed along with improved 5-year survival rates in the screened versus control groups. However, no significant difference was observed in the overall mortality rate [25–29]. These trials indicate that CT scans may detect more lung nodules than chest radiography. Although, only a small fraction of these nodules can lead to lung cancer.

In a trial conducted in the Mayo Clinic for early detection of lung cancer, approximately 50% patients had at least one nodule. However, by assessing calcification patterns at low-dose and high-resolution CT (HRCT) and repeating the scans after an interval, the Early Lung Cancer Action Project (ELCAP) group had performed only one biopsy for a benign, non-calcified nodule. It is a matter of concern to perform a number of biopsies to distinguish between benign and malignant nodules [26, 28]. Although low-dose CT can detect early-stage lung cancer 6–10 times more frequently than chest radiography, there has not been a similar fall in the occurrence of the advanced stage of lung cancer [28, 30, 31].

10.2.3 MRI (magnetic resonance imaging)

MRIs are more sensitive than CT scans in detecting stage IIIa (resectable) from IIIb (generally unresectable) tumors as they can identify invasion of major mediastinal structures [32]. Other advantages that MRIs have over CT scans include better soft-tissue contrast, multiplanar imaging capability [33, 34]. MRI can also assess mediastinal and chest wall invasion to determine fat-stripe invasion and involvement of the diaphragm and spinal canal. Further, MRIs can differentiate lymph nodes from hila vessels due to the 'flow void' phenomenon [35].

Although MRIs are majorly used in cancer detection, they are scarcely used in early detection of lung cancer due to physical properties such as low tissue density. Further, the high air content of the lung drastically reduces the signal-to-noise ratio (SNR) as the MR signal is directly proportional to proton density [36]. However, a higher magnetic field can improve SNR theoretically. Still, it would also aggravate susceptibility artifacts due to magnetic field inhomogeneities caused by omnipresent microscopic tissue–air interfaces smaller than standard voxel sizes [36]. Additionally, motion caused via cardiac and respiratory cycles may cause ghosting artifacts on the MR images [37].

The major disadvantage associated with MRI for lung cancer detection is its high cost, poor spatial resolution, and limited lung parenchyma information. MRIs may overestimate lymph node size due to respiratory movements, leading to the blurring together of discrete nodes into a larger, conglomerate mass. Moreover, MRIs are also difficult for patients suffering from claustrophobia. [38].

10.2.4 PET (positron emission tomography) scan

PET scanning is a rather sensitive imaging modality that can accurately detect malignancies in the entire body in one examination. PET scan uses a radiopharmaceutical that generally labels metabolic markers such as amino acids or glucose with positron-emitting radionuclides like fluorine-18. The radiomarker is then imaged by coincidence detection of two 511 KeV photons produced by annihilating the emitted positrons. The radiopharmaceutical 18F-2-deoxy-D-glucose (FDG) is generally used for PET scans. Scans performed with this agent exploit the differences in glucose metabolism between normal versus neoplastic cells, along with precise identification between benign and malignant abnormalities [39]. FDG uptake is proportional to tumor aggressiveness and growth rates [40]. Generally, an uptake ratio of v2.5 indicates a benign lesion [41, 42]. PET scans can detect malignancy in focal pulmonary opacities with a sensitivity of 96%, specificity of 88%, and an accuracy of 94% in lesions of 10 mm [43, 44].

However, PET has a poor spatial resolution, which prevents it from accurately assessing anatomical assessment of primary tumors [45]. Moreover, lungs with tuberculous infection or histoplasmosis also give a false-positive PET [45, 46]. Compared to CT scans, PET can detect mediastinal nodal metastases with a sensitivity ranging from 67%–100% [47, 48]. They can also detect recurrent lung cancers and distinguish persistent or recurrent tumors from fibrotic scars [45, 49].

However, the major disadvantage for PET is the lack of availability and relatively high cost [50].

Despite tremendous advances in diagnostics and therapeutics, early detection of cancer is still difficult. There is an increasing interest in using molecular markers as tools for cancer detection and prognosis. Thus, these biomarkers can be used either as stand-alone tests or combined with existing imaging methods to aid in early detection, diagnosis, prognosis, and monitoring the patient's response towards the cancer treatment.

10.3 Biomarkers as tools for early cancer detection

Biomarkers are the molecular markers that could be assessed for early diagnosis, prognosis, and monitoring of cancer progression. Advancement in molecular diagnostics such as epigenomics, genomics, and proteomics, has enabled the monitoring of genome changes easily. Changes in the genetic markers refer to any modifications in the structure or sequence of the genetic material. These changes have a major role in the pathogenesis of lung cancer and can be checked for early detection of cancer development. Hence, genome testing can be done to detect genomic changes as potential lung cancer biomarkers [51]. The primary feature of genetic markers is their polymorphic status. Polymorphism refers to the presence of multiple forms of a gene or genetic phenotypes. Thus, genetically based diseases can be detected by analyzing the polymorphic markers specific to that disease [52]. Further, epigenetic markers such as DNA methylation that play an essential role in the cell cycle can be checked for early cancer diagnosis [53, 54].

Lung cancer is generally detected in advanced stages, making the treatment options limited. In patients with clinical stage IA in the classification of tumor-lymph nodes-metastasis, 5-year survival rate is nearly 60%, indicating that majority of lung cancer cases either go undetected or are detected at the advanced metastatic stage [55–57]. Lung cancer usually results from the last stage of multistage carcinogenesis with gradual genetic and epigenetic changes and not from any sudden transformations in bronchia epithelioma with gradually increasing genetic and epigenetic changes [57, 58]. The primary cause of lung cancer is the activation of oncogenes that results in uncontrolled cell proliferation. Frequently mutated proto-oncogenes in lung cancer include RAS, MYC, and HER family of genes. Moreover, lung cancers also harbor mutations in the tumor suppressor genes such as TP53, RB, and p16 [59–61]. In NSCLC, 56% of patients harbor mutations in p53, 27% of patients harbor mutations in KRAS (Kirsten rat sarcoma viral oncogene), and p16 methylation was observed in 38% of patients NSCLC. KRAS mutation was the first identified mutations in NSCLC. However, mutations in the RAS family of genes such as KRAS, HRAS, NRA, and EGFR were observed in only 3% of SCCs cases [62].

Thus, the need of the hour is the identification of such biomarkers that are expressed in nearly all types of lung cancer. Heat shock proteins (HSPs) may play a significant role in this regard as their high expression has been reported in approximately all types of cancers. HSPs help in cancer cell proliferation by providing cytoprotection to cells undergoing extreme stress due to chemotherapy. Therefore, analyzing the levels of HSPs in cancer patients may serve as a tool for early cancer diagnosis.

HSPs were initially identified almost four decades ago in Drosophila melanogaster as proteins expressed due to chemical and physical stress or heat shock [63–65]. Over the years, many studies have identified that HSPs take part in a plethora of cellular functions. HSPs can be induced by several stressors, including the increase in the levels of reactive oxygen species and cytotoxicity induced due to any known toxic compound, including chemotherapeutics [63]. HSPs are named according to their molecular weight, and the major classes of HSPs include HSPB (small HSPs), DnaJ (Hsp40), HSPA (Hsp70), HSPC (Hsp90), and HSPH (Hsp110) [66].

HSPs are transcriptionally controlled by the heat shock factor-1 (HSF1). The HSF gene family includes HSF1 that is the primary regulator of the heat shock response, HSF2 (heat shock transcription factor 2), and HSF4 (heat shock transcription factor 4) [67–69]. HSF1 and HSF2 are hyperphosphorylated during stress by mitogen-activated protein (MAP) kinases in a ras-dependent manner followed by binding of phosphorylated HSF1 to heat shock elements present in the promoter region of all stress-inducible genes. This leads to an increase in the induction of Hsp proteins due to the transcription of HSP genes [70]. Primarily, all HSPs are molecular chaperones as they assist in the proper folding of non-native proteins.

10.3.1 The chaperoning activity of HSPs

Proteins are synthesized on the ribosome and should fold correctly to attain their functional conformations. However, unfolded or aggregated proteins should be refolded to maintain their functional activity [71]. HSPs help a protein achieve its correct structural conformation by identifying the changes in structural characteristics of incorrectly folded proteins. Hydrophobic residues which are present in the protein core get exposed on the outer surface due to misfolding and thus can cause aggregation of non-native proteins. HSPs detect and bind with hydrophobic regions of the clients to halt their aggregation [72]. Hsp27, an ATP-independent HSP, can switch between shorter and larger oligomeric forms to bind and hold unfolded proteins so as to prevent their aggregation with other native proteins [73–75]. Hsp27 may play a crucial role in preventing protein aggregation in an ATP-independent manner, especially during heat shock, where ATP production is disturbed, and other ATP-dependent HSPs may not function properly [76]. A model has been proposed for cellular conditions where the need for refolding exceeds the ATP-dependent chaperones' capacity. In this case, Hsp27 may harbor non-native intermediates in a 'folding-permissive' state, which protects against the formation of insoluble protein aggregates until Hsp70 and Hsp90 progressively process them throughout the recovery phase [77]. Hsp70 binds with unfolded or partially folded polypeptides associated with Hsp27. Hsp70 transitions between ATP-bound, polypeptide-free, and ADP-polypeptide-bound states, in which the client proteins are reorganized and folded to their native conformation. Several co-chaperones help Hsp70 properly fold

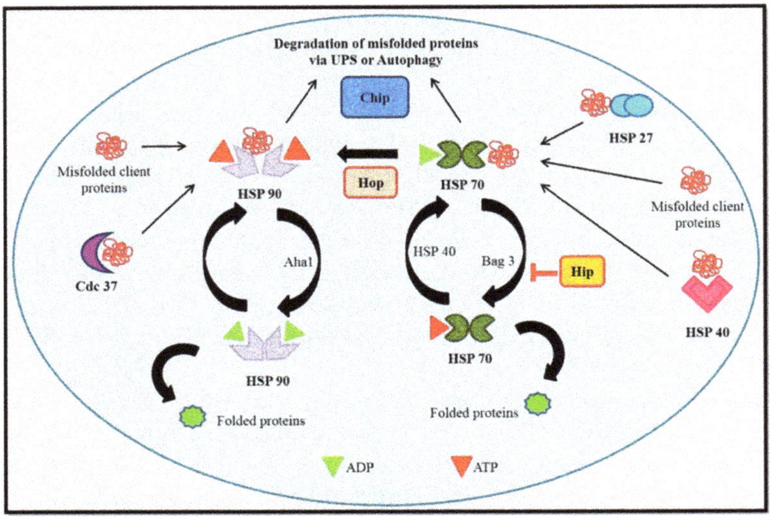

Figure 10.3. Hsp27, Hsp70, and Hsp90 maintain the cellular proteostasis. Substrates are either bound directly to Hsp70 and Hsp90 or are recruited by Hsp27, Hsp70 co-chaperones (Hsp40 family members), and Hsp90 co-chaperones (Cdc37) for proper folding. Unfolded client proteins are transferred from Hsp27 or Hsp40 to the ATP-bound Hsp70 for proper folding. The folded client proteins are released in the cell in their native form, degraded by autophagy pathway, or transferred to Hsp90 for further folding, where Hsp90 and its co-chaperones further fold the client proteins to their native form.

the client proteins, including detecting potential clients (J domain proteins such as Hsp40) and nucleotide exchange (Hspbp1, Bag1, and Bag3). However, these co-chaperone proteins, which help the HSPs in their chaperoning activity, may also participate in tumorigenesis [78]. If Hsp70-client proteins are not folded completely, they may either undergo autophagic degradation or be transferred to Hsp90 for further folding [79, 80]. The co-chaperone HOP facilitates the transfer of Hsp70 clients to Hsp90. HOP binds to the C-terminal TPR binding domains found in Hsp70 and Hsp90 and forms a transient Hsp70-client protein-Hsp90 co-chaperone complex [81]. Hsp70 dissociates from this complex, and Hsp90 and its co-chaperones carry out the folding of client proteins to their native, functional form. The co-chaperone Cdc37 is the crucial player that helps Hsp90 conduct its chaperoning activity [82–84]. The client proteins dissociate from the Hsp90 chaperoning complex after attaining their proper structural and functional form to perform their cellular functions. However, if oncogenic kinases are chaperoned, they may help in the process of malignant transformation [85] (figure 10.3).

10.3.2 Role of HSPs in cancer

HSPs are highly expressed in cancers and associated with cancer cell growth, survival, metastasis, and chemoresistance. They interact with and stabilize several oncogenic molecules known as the client proteins to form a fostering environment that is crucial for the development of tumors [86, 87]. Furthermore, cells with high expression of HSPs have been observed to be resistant for radiation-induced cell death [88]. Thus, it could be implied that cancer cells may depend on HSPs for survival and growth.

In lung cancer, studies have shown that HSPs such as Hsp90 is overexpressed and provide protection against chemotherapeutics [89]. Thus, the HSPs can serve as potential biomarkers for the early detection of lung cancer [90]. Moreover, high expression of HSPs is associated with poor prognosis of lung cancer, thus, making these proteins a therapeutic target and biomarkers in lung cancer detection and treatment strategies.

10.3.3 HSPs as biomarkers for lung cancer

10.3.3.1 Hsp27

Hsp27 is an ATP-independent HSP which belongs to the family of small HSPs. Hsp27 functions through phosphorylation, a post-translational modification, and abnormal phosphorylation of Hsp27 is related to the progression of cancer [91]. High expression of Hsp27 is associated with poor prognosis in lung cancer and promotes chemoresistance in NSCLC, lung cancer stem-like cells, and laryngeal cancers [92–94]. Lelj-Garolla *et al* reported that inhibiting Hsp27 with OGX-427 sensitizes NSCLC tumors to chemotherapy in highly metastatic NSCLC [95]. Hsp27 interacts with and inhibits various apoptotic proteins such as Bax, cytochrome c, and pro-caspase 3 through the activation of the oncogenic PI3K/Akt pathway [96–98].

Furthermore, overexpression of Hsp27 has also been observed in the serum samples of NSCLC patients compared to the serum samples of normal control patients even at early stages of cancer [99]. Furthermore, a single nucleotide polymorphism (SNP; 1271 G > C) in the HSP27 gene was observed to be associated with poor survival and an increased risk of lung cancer development in NSCLC patients [100]. In contrast, another study reported that this mutation contributed to the survival of patients with advanced stage NSCLC [101]. Thus, screening the samples of NSCLC patients for an SNP in the Hsp27 gene could serve as a biomarker, predict the disease outcome, and help determine the treatment regimens.

Hsp27 also acts as a biomarker to diagnose determine TNM (tumor (T), nodes (N), and metastases (M)) staging of NSCLC, where low expression of Hsp27 is associated with a better prognosis. Moreover, a meta-analysis revealed that Hsp27 expression could be a strong biomarker to predict the poor clinicopathological and prognostic characteristics in lung cancer [102]. Thus, determining the expression levels of Hsp27 may serve as an important tool for the early diagnosis of lung cancer and may help design better treatment modalities.

10.3.3.2 Hsp60

HSPD1 gene encodes Hsp60 which belongs to a family of chaperonins localized in the mitochondrial matrix. It works as an anti-aggregative protein by ensuring correct folding of mitochondrial proteins [103]. Hsp60 works in concert with Hsp10 which serves as a co-factor for its catalytic activity. The involvement of Hsp60 has been reported in cancer progression. In fact, overexpression of Hsp60 was also correlated with poor prognosis [104].

In tissue samples from patients suffering from lung adenocarcinoma, 68% of samples tested positive for Hsp60. Overexpression of Hsp60 and annexin 2 was also observed in adeno or squamous cell carcinoma suggesting that these two proteins can be used as biomarkers for diagnosis of lung cancer [105]. However, no difference in the expression of Hsp60 was observed in early and advanced stage lung cancers.

Nevertheless, Hsp60 expression can be used as a biomarker for lung adenocarcinoma diagnosis, but its expression in other lung cancer types is still ambiguous. Therefore, studies based on screening of lung cancer patients with diverse tumor histotypes may substantiate its use in diagnosis and prognosis (table 10.1).

10.3.3.3 Hsp70

Hsp70 is an ATP-dependent chaperone which includes two major isoforms, the constitutively expressed Hsc70, and inducible Hsp70. Hsp70 family also includes endoplasmic reticulum and mitochondria localized forms namely Grp78 (glucose-regulated protein 78) and Grp75 (glucose-regulated protein 75). The primary function of Hsp70 is to ensure error free folding of native proteins [106]. However, Hsp70 gets highly upregulated and protects the cells against stress conditions such as low oxygen (hypoxia), stress induced by ROS, changes in pH, and DNA damage response [107]. Several studies have suggested that Hsp70 phosphorylation plays a significant role in regulating cell survival and death, protein degradation, and resistance to anticancer compounds. Overexpression of Hsp70 has been observed in different cancer types, including lungs, and is correlated with poor prognosis [108, 109]. A study related to the Japanese population revealed that Hsp70 expression was higher among male lung cancer patients than females [109].

Moreover, high serum Hsp70 levels were observed in patients suffering from lung adeno and squamous cell carcinoma as compared to normal healthy controls. Thus, it was proposed that serum Hsp70 levels can be used as a tool for early detection of lung cancer [110]. However, another study reported high levels of carcinoembryonic antigen (CEA) and low levels of circulating Hsp70 in the plasma of NSCLC patients compared to healthy individuals [111]. Hence, the ratio of circulating Hsp70 along with CEA can be used as a biomarker for the early detection of NSCLC. Apart from Hsp70, high levels of Grp78 and Grp75 have also been observed in lung cancer patients and may serve as biomarkers for lung cancer detection [112].

Grp78 is highly expressed in poorly differentiated lung tumors than moderately or well-differentiated tumors [112]. Grp78 contributes towards the metastasis of the advanced stage of NSCLC, specifically in patients with lymph node metastasis [113]. Furthermore, NSCLC patients with a polymorphism in the intronic region (rs430397 G > A) in Grp78 respond better to platinum-based chemotherapy [114]. However, Grp78 overexpression was observed in patients with A/A genotype and they responded poorly towards platinum-based agents. Thus, identifying any polymorphism in Grp78 may play an essential role in lung cancer management, and give us an insight towards response to therapy.

Table 10.1. Role of different HSPs in lung cancer.

S.no.	HSP	Expression level	Effect	References
1.	Hsp27	overexpressed	• poor prognosis • promotes chemoresistance in NSCLC • induces lung cancer stem like cells • inhibits apoptosis	[92, 96, 98, 128]
2.	Hsp60	loss or downregulated	• low expression of Hsp60/Hsp10 causes defective mitochondrial internalization of FHIT leading to loss of apoptotic function • promotes cancer cell survival	[129, 130, 131, 132]
3.	Hsp70	overexpressed	• poor prognosis and low survival rates	[108, 109, 110, 133, 134
4.	Grp78	overexpressed	• used as a biomarker to correlate with the stage and grade of lung cancer. • responsible for tumor progression and metastasis.	[113]
5.	Hsp90	overexpressed	• maintains the stability of oncogenic kinases • poor prognosis, low survival rates • inhibits apoptosis • promotes angiogenesis and metastasis	[116, 117]
6.	Grp94	overexpressed	• overexpressed in lung cancer stage I, II & III and • may act as independent prognostic factor for NSCLC patients.	[121]

10.3.3.4 Hsp90

Hsp90 is a molecular chaperone which is conserved across kingdoms. Hps90 has two isoforms, namely the inducible Hsp90α and constitutive Hsp90β. Grp94 (glucose-regulated protein 94) and TRAP1/Hsp75 (TNF receptor-associated protein1) are resident Hsp90 homologs localized in the endoplasmic reticulum and mitochondrial matrix, respectively [115]. Hsp90 is highly upregulated in cancer. Hsp90 and other co-chaperones maintain the structure and stability of several oncogenic kinases implicated in lung cancer progression [116, 117]. Hsp90 overexpression has been correlated with shorter survival of NSCLC patients [118]. High levels of Hsp90α were reported in the plasma of lung cancer patients with advanced stage of lung cancer and were correlated with poor prognosis [119, 120]. Further, high expression of Hsp90β and Grp94 has been correlated with poor survival of NSCLC patients [121, 122]. An increase in the expression of serum Hsp90β correlates with the differentiated grade and advanced clinical stage of patients with lung cancer [123]. In one comparative study, Hsp90β presents a higher expression in lung adenocarcinoma (LAC) tissues than in laryngeal squamous cell carcinoma (LSCC). It correlates with the poor survival of LAC patients [124]. Moreover, approximately 10% of NSCLC patients harbor EGFR mutations, and Hsp90 stabilizes mutant EGFR leading to lung cancer progression [125]. The T2821 and T2851 lung cancer cells harbor high expression of Hsp90 and promote radio-resistance in them [126]. Increased expression of Hsp90 was also observed in SPCA-1 and H446 lung cancer cell lines that led to cisplatin resistance [127]. Thus, monitoring Hsp90 levels can serve as a biomarker for the early detection and prognosis of lung cancer (figure 10.4).

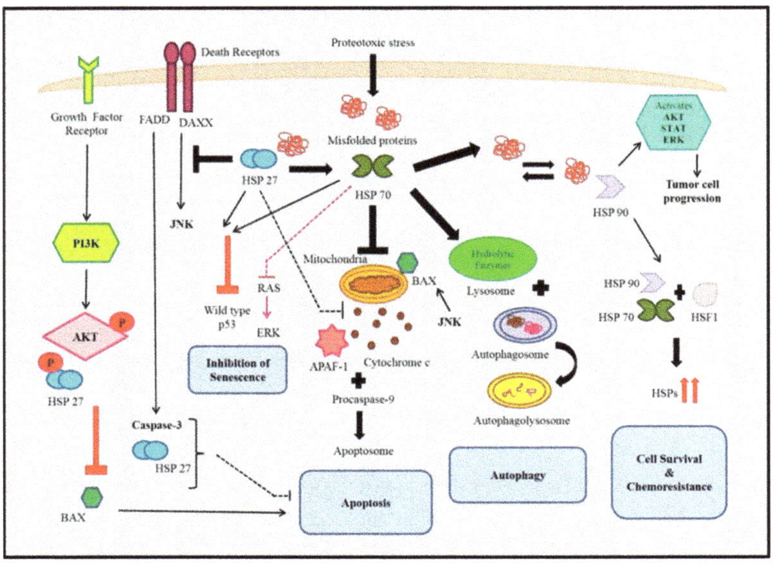

Figure 10.4. Heat shock proteins mediate lung cancer proliferation by interacting with several apoptotic molecules. Hsp27 interacts with and inhibits various apoptotic proteins, including cytochrome c, caspase 3, BAX, to promote cancer cell survival. Hsp70 inhibits apoptosis and promotes cell survival by interacting with pro-apoptotic molecules. Hsp90 inhibits the pro-apoptotic BAX, cytochrome c, caspase 9 and stabilizes the oncogenic PI3K and AKT to promote cancer cell survival.

10.4 Conclusion

Multiple studies have reported the role of HSPs in cancer progression. The expression of HSPs may be correlated to the degree of differentiation and aggressiveness of certain cancers. Serum levels of Hsp and anti-Hsp antibodies in cancer patients can be used in tumor diagnosis. HSP may also predict the response to some anticancer treatments. Pharmacological inhibition of HSPs or using them as adjuvant therapy can be used as a successful target for cancer treatment. Even though more studies are required to authenticate the molecular chaperone expression as diagnostic or prognostic markers or as drug targets in lung cancer patient management, there is a hope that the HSPs may serve as potential biomarkers and drug targets against lung cancer.

Declarations of interest: none

Acknowledgments

The authors are thankful to Hon'ble Vice-Chancellor, Integral University, Lucknow for providing infrastructural support and Dean Office, R&D, Integral University for providing manuscript communication number (IU/R&D/2021-MCN0001202).

References

[1] Sung H, Ferlay J, Siegel R L, Laversanne M, Soerjomataram I, Jemal A and Bray F 2021 Global cancer statistics 2020: GLOBOCAN estimates of incidence and mortality worldwide for 36 cancers in 185 countries *CA Cancer J. Clin.* **71** 209–49

[2] Tantraworasin A, Saeteng S, Lertprasertsuke N, Arreyakajohn N, Kasemsarn C and Patumanond J 2013 Prognostic factors of tumor recurrence in completely resected non-small cell lung cancer *Cancer Manag. Res.* **5** 77

[3] Molina J R, Yang P, Cassivi S D, Schild S E and Adjei A A 2008 Non-small cell lung cancer: epidemiology, risk factors, treatment, and survivorship *Mayo Clin. Proc* **83** 584–94

[4] Alberg A J, Brock M V, Ford J G, Samet J M and Spivack S D 2013 Epidemiology of lung cancer: diagnosis and management of lung cancer: American College of Chest Physicians evidence-based clinical practice guidelines *Chest* **143** e1S–29S

[5] Hackshaw A K, Law M R and Wald N J 1997 The accumulated evidence on lung cancer and environmental tobacco smoke *Brit. Med. J.* **315** 980–8

[6] Vineis P *et al* 2005 Environmental tobacco smoke and risk of respiratory cancer and chronic obstructive pulmonary disease in former smokers and never smokers in the EPIC prospective study *Brit. Med. J.* **330** 277

[7] Minna J D, Roth J A and Gazdar A F 2002 Focus on lung cancer *Cancer Cell* **1** 49–52

[8] Akhtar N and Bansal J G 2017 Risk factors of lung cancer in nonsmoker *Curr. Probl. Cancer* **41** 328–39

[9] Ost D E, Yeung S C, Tanoue L T and Gould M K 2013 Clinical and organizational factors in the initial evaluation of patients with lung cancer: diagnosis and management of lung cancer: American College of Chest Physicians evidence-based clinical practice guidelines *Chest* **143** e121S–41S

[10] Tantraworasin A, Suksomboonchroen T, Wannasopha Y, Kongkarnka S, Saeteng S, Lertprasertsuke N, Euathrongchit J and Chewaskulyong B 2015 Lung cancer: diagnosis and treatment approach *Int. Manual of Oncology Practice (iMOP)* (Cham: Springer) pp 97–144
[11] Paesmans M 2012 Prognostic and predictive factors for lung cancer *Breathe.* **9** 112–21
[12] Kim J and Kim K H 2020 Role of chest radiographs in early lung cancer detection *Transl. Lung Cancer Res.* **9** 522–31
[13] Hollings N and Shaw P 2002 Diagnostic imaging of lung cancer *Eur. Respir. J.* **19** 722–42
[14] White C S, Salis A I and Meyer C A 1999 Missed lung cancer on chest radiography and computed tomography: imaging and medicolegal issues *J. Thorac Imag.* **14** 63–8
[15] Strauss G M and Dominioni L 2013 Chest x-ray screening for lung cancer: overdiagnosis, endpoints, and randomized population trials *J. Surg. Oncol.* **108** 294–300
[16] Strauss G M, Gleason R E and Sugarbaker D J 1995 Chest x-ray screening improves outcome in lung cancer: a reappraisal of randomized trials on lung cancer screening *Chest* **107** 270S–9S
[17] Nakayama T, Baba T, Suzuki T, Sagawa M and Kaneko M 2002 An evaluation of chest X-ray screening for lung cancer in Gunma Prefecture, Japan: a population-based case–control study *Eur. J. Cancer* **38** 1380–7
[18] Bach P B *et al* 2012 Benefits and harms of CT screening for lung cancer: a systematic review *JAMA* **307** 2418–29
[19] National Lung Screening Trial Research Team 2011 Reduced lung-cancer mortality with low-dose computed tomographic screening *N. Engl. J. Med.* **365** 395–409
[20] Webb W R 1990 Radiologic evaluation of the solitary pulmonary nodule *AJR Am. J. Roentgenol.* **154** 701–8
[21] Remy-Jardin M, Remy J, Giraud F and Marquette C H 1993 Pulmonary nodules: detection with thick-section spiral CT versus conventional CT *Radiology* **187** 513–20
[22] Tillich M, Kammerhuber F, Reittner P, Riepl T, Stoeffler G and Szolar D H 1997 Detection of pulmonary nodules with helical CT: comparison of cine and film-based viewing *AJR Am. J. Roentgenol.* **169** 1611–4
[23] Patz E F Jr, Erasmus J J, McAdams H P, Connolly J E, Marom E M, Goodman P C, Leder R A, Keogan M T and Herndon J E 1999 Lung cancer staging and management: comparison of contrast-enhanced and nonenhanced helical CT of the thorax *Radiology* **212** 56–60
[24] Cascade P N, Gross B H, Kazerooni E A, Quint L E, Francis I R, Strawderman M and Korobkin M 1998 Variability in the detection of enlarged mediastinal lymph nodes in staging lung cancer: a comparison of contrast-enhanced and unenhanced CT *AJR Am. J. Roentgenol.* **170** 927–31
[25] Tockman M S 1986 Survival and mortality from lung cancer in a screened population: the Johns Hopkins study *Chest* **89** 324S–5S
[26] Fontana R S, Sanderson D R, Woolner L B, Taylor W F, Miller W E and Muhm J 1986 Lung cancer screening: the Mayo program *J. Occup. Med.* **28** 746–50
[27] Kubik A, Parkin D M, Khlat M, Erban J, Polak J and Adamec M 1990 Lack of benefit from semi-annual screening for cancer of the lung: follow-up report of a randomized controlled trial on a population of high-risk males in Czechoslovakia *Int. J. Cancer* **45** 26–33

[28] Henschke C I *et al* 1999 Early Lung Cancer Action Project: overall design and findings from baseline screening *Lancet* **354** 99–105
[29] Kaneko M, Eguchi K, Ohmatsu H, Kakinuma R, Naruke T, Suemasu K and Moriyama N 1996 Peripheral lung cancer: screening and detection with low-dose spiral CT versus radiography *Radiology* **201** 798–802
[30] Patz E F Jr, Goodman P C and Bepler G 2000 Screening for lung cancer *N. Engl. J. Med.* **343** 1627–33
[31] Sone S *et al* 2001 Results of three-year mass screening programme for lung cancer using mobile low-dose spiral computed tomography scanner *Br. J. Cancer* **84** 25–32
[32] Gefter W B 1990 Magnetic resonance imaging in the evaluation of lung cancer *Semin. Roentgen.* **25** 73–84
[33] Hatabu H, Stock K W, Sher S, Edinburgh K J, Levin D L, Garpestad E, Albert M S, Mai V M, Chen Q and Edelman R R 1999 Magnetic resonance imaging of the thorax: past, present, and future *Clin. Chest Med.* **20** 775–803
[34] Batra P, Brown K, Steckel R J, Collins J D, Ovenfors C O and Aberle D 1988 MR imaging of the thorax: a comparison of axial, coronal, and sagittal imaging planes *J. Comp. Assist. Tomogr.* **12** 75–81
[35] Aitken K and Armstrong P 1992 Clinical imaging for staging lung cancer *Imaging* **4** 15–22
[36] Wild J M, Marshall H, Bock M, Schad L R, Jakob P M, Puderbach M, Molinari F, Van Beek E J and Biederer J 2012 MRI of the lung (1/3): methods *Insights Imag.* **3** 345–53
[37] Boiselle P M, Biederer J, Gefter W B and Lee E Y 2013 Expert opinion: why is MRI still an under-utilized modality for evaluating thoracic disorders? *J. Thorac. Imag.* **28** 137
[38] Wang Y X, Lo G G, Yuan J, Larson P E and Zhang X 2014 Magnetic resonance imaging for lung cancer screen *J. Thorac. Dis.* **6** 1340
[39] Erasmus J J and Patz E F Jr 1999 Positron emission tomography imaging in the thorax *Clin. Chest Med.* **20** 715–24
[40] Duhaylongsod F G, Lowe V J, Patz E F Jr, Vaughn A L, Coleman R E and Wolfe W G 1995 Lung tumor growth correlates with glucose metabolism measured by fluoride-18 fluorodeoxyglucose positron emission tomography *Ann. Thorac. Surg.* **60** 1348–52
[41] Lowe V J *et al* 1998 Prospective investigation of positron emission tomography in lung nodules *J. Clin. Oncol.* **16** 1075–84
[42] Lowe V J, Duhaylongsod F G, Patz E F, Delong D M, Hoffman J M, Wolfe W G and Coleman R E 1997 Pulmonary abnormalities and PET data analysis: a retrospective study *Radiology* **202** 435–9
[43] Conti P S, Lilien D L, Hawley K, Keppler J, Grafton S T and Bading J 1996 PET and [18F]-FDG in oncology: a clinical update *Nucl. Med. Biol.* **23** 717–35
[44] Gupta N C, Maloof J and Gunel E 1996 Probability of malignancy in solitary pulmonary nodules using fluorine-18-FDG and PET *J. Nucl. Med.* **37** 943–48
[45] Erasmus J J, McAdams H P and Patz E F Jr 1999 Non-small cell lung cancer: FDG-PET imaging *J Thorac. Imag.* **14** 247–56
[46] Scott W J, Schwabe J L, Gupta N C, Dewan N A, Reeb S D and Sugimoto J T 1994 Positron emission tomography of lung tumors and mediastinal lymph nodes using [18F] fluorodeoxyglucose *Ann. Thorac. Surg.* **58** 698–703
[47] Steinert H C, Hauser M, Allemann F, Engel H, Berthold T, Von Schulthess G K and Weder W 1997 Non-small cell lung cancer: nodal staging with FDG PET versus CT with correlative lymph node mapping and sampling *Radiology* **202** 441–6

[48] Guhlmann A, Storck M, Kotzerke J, Moog F, Sunder-Plassmann L and Reske S N 1997 Lymph node staging in non-small cell lung cancer: evaluation by [18F] FDG positron emission tomography (PET) *Thorax* **52** 438–41

[49] Bury T, Corhay J L, Duysinx B, Daenen F, Ghaye B, Barthelemy N, Rigo P and Bartsch P 1999 Value of FDG-PET in detecting residual or recurrent non-small cell lung cancer *Eur. Respir. J.* **14** 1376–80

[50] Gambhir S S, Shepherd J E, Shah B D, Hart E, Hoh C K, Valk P E, Emi T and Phelps M E 1998 Analytical decision model for the cost-effective management of solitary pulmonary nodules *J. Clin. Oncol.* **16** 2113–25

[51] Garcia-Gimenez J L, Seco-Cervera M, Tollefsbol T O, Roma-Mateo C, Peiro-Chova L, Lapunzina P and Pallardo F V 2017 Epigenetic biomarkers: current strategies and future challenges for their use in the clinical laboratory *Crit. Rev. Clin. Lab. Sci.* **54** 529–50

[52] Pass H I, Beer D G, Joseph S and Massion P 2013 Biomarkers and molecular testing for early detection, diagnosis, and therapeutic prediction of lung cancer *Thorac. Surg. Clin.* **23** 211–24

[53] Calabrese F, Lunardi F, Pezzuto F, Fortarezza F, Vuljan S E, Marquette C and Hofman P 2019 Are there new biomarkers in tissue and liquid biopsies for the early detection of non-small cell lung cancer? *J. Clin. Med.* **8** 414

[54] Wadowska K, Bil-Lula I, Trembecki Ł and Śliwińska-Mossoń M 2020 Genetic markers in lung cancer diagnosis: a review *Int. J. Mol. Sci.* **21** 4569

[55] Lu S *et al* 2018 Two plasma microRNA panels for diagnosis and subtype discrimination of lung cancer *Lung Cancer* **123** 44–51

[56] Jakubek Y *et al* 2016 Genomic landscape established by allelic imbalance in the cancerization field of a normal appearing airway *Cancer Res.* **76** 3676–83

[57] Hirsch F R, Franklin W A, Gazdar A F and Bunn P A 2001 Early detection of lung cancer: clinical perspectives of recent advances in biology and radiology *Clin. Cancer Res.* **7** 5–22

[58] Gazdar A F and Brambilla E 2010 Preneoplasia of lung cancer *Cancer Biomark.* **9** 385–96

[59] Hubers A J, Prinsen C F, Sozzi G, Witte B I and Thunnissen E 2013 Molecular sputum analysis for the diagnosis of lung cancer *Br. J. Cancer* **109** 530–7

[60] Ahrendt S A, Chow J T and Xu L H *et al* 1999 Molecular detection of tumor cells in bronchoalveolar lavage fluid from patients with early stage lung cancer *J. Natl. Cancer Inst.* **91** 332–9

[61] Kopczynski P and Krawczynski M 2012 The role of oncogenes and tumor suppressor genes in oncogenesis *Now Lekarskie* **81** 679–81

[62] Chakravarthi S and Karikalan B 2021 Molecular biomarkers for lung adenocarcinoma: a short review *Curr. Cancer Ther. Rev.* **17** 97–106

[63] Shankar K and Mehendale H M 2014 Heat-shock proteins *Encyclopedia of Toxicology* 3rd edn (Amsterdam: Elsevier) pp 830–1

[64] Lindquist S and Craig E A 1988 The heat shock proteins *Ann. Rev. Genet.* **22** 631–37

[65] Georgopolis C and Welch W J 1993 Role of the major heat shock proteins as molecular chaperones *Ann. Rev. Cell Biol.* **9** 601–34

[66] Kampinga H H, Hageman J, Vos M J, Kubota H, Tanguay R M, Bruford E A, Cheetham M E, Chen B and Hightower L E 2009 Guidelines for the nomenclature of the human heat shock proteins *Cell Stress Chaperones* **14** 105–11

[67] Rabindran S K, Giorgi G, Clos J and Wu C 1991 Molecular cloning and expression of a human heat shock factor, HSF1 *Proc. Natl. Acad. Sci. U. S. A.* **88** 6906–10

[68] Schuetz T J, Gallo G J, Sheldon L, Tempst P and Kingston R E 1991 Isolation of a cDNA for HSF2: evidence for two heat shock factor genes in humans *Proc. Natl. Acad. Sci. U. S. A.* **88** 6911–5
[69] Nakai A, Tanabe M, Kawazoe Y, Inazawa J, Morimoto R I and Nagata K 1997 HSF4, a new member of the human heat shock factor family which lacks properties of a transcriptional activator *Mol. Cell. Biol.* **17** 469–81
[70] Cadenas C, Marchan R and Bolt H M 2013 Role of heat shock proteins in stress response and carcinogenesis *Arch. Toxicol.* **87** 1–2
[71] Lang B J, Guerrero-Giménez M E, Prince T L, Ackerman A, Bonorino C and Calderwood S K 2019 Heat shock proteins are essential components in transformation and tumor progression: Cancer cell intrinsic pathways and beyond *Int. J. Mol. Sci.* **20** 4507
[72] Rudiger S, Buchberger A and Bukau B 1997 Interaction of Hsp70 chaperones with substrates *Nat. Struct. Biol.* **4** 342–9
[73] Lelj-Garolla B and Mauk A G 2006 Self-association and chaperone activity of Hsp27 are thermally activated *J. Biol. Chem.* **281** 8169–74
[74] Hayes D, Napoli V, Mazurkie A, Stafford W F and Graceffa P 2009 Phosphorylation dependence of hsp27 multimeric size and molecular chaperone function *J. Biol. Chem.* **284** 18801–7
[75] Cox D, Whiten D R, Brown J, Horrocks M H, San Gil R, Dobson C M, Klenerman D, van Oijen A M and Ecroyd H 2018 The small heat shock protein Hsp27 binds α-synuclein fibrils, preventing elongation and cytotoxicity *J. Biol. Chem.* **293** 4486–497
[76] Patriarca E J and Maresca B 1990 Acquired thermotolerance following heat shock protein synthesis prevents impairment of mitochondrial ATPase activity at elevated temperatures in Saccharomyces cerevisiae *Exp. Cell. Res.* **190** 57–64
[77] Ehrnsperger M, Graber S, Gaestel M and Buchner J 1997 Binding of non-native protein to Hsp25 during heat shock creates a reservoir of folding intermediates for reactivation *EMBO J.* **16** 221–9
[78] Calderwood S K and Murshid A 2017 Molecular chaperone accumulation in cancer and decrease in Alzheimer's disease: the potential roles of HSF1 *Front. Neurosci.* **11** 192
[79] Workman P 2004 Altered states: selectively drugging the Hsp90 cancer chaperone *Trends Mol. Med.* **10** 47–51
[80] Cuellar J, Martin-Benito J, Scheres S H, Sousa R, Moro F, Lopez-Vinas E, Gomez-Puertas P, Muga A, Carrascosa J L and Valpuesta J M 2008 The structure of CCT-Hsc70 NBD suggests a mechanism for Hsp70 delivery of substrates to the chaperonin *Nat. Struct. Mol. Biol.* **15** 858–64
[81] Kamal A, Thao L, Sensintaffar J, Zhang L, Boehm M F, Fritz L C and Burrows F J 2003 A high-affinity conformation of Hsp90 confers tumour selectivity on Hsp90 inhibitors *Nature* **425** 407–10
[82] Gray P J, Prince T, Cheng J, Stevenson M A and Calderwood S K 2008 Targeting the oncogene and kinome chaperone CDC37 *Nat. Rev. Cancer* **8** 491–5
[83] Gray P J, Stevenson M A and Calderwood S K 2007 Targeting Cdc37 inhibits multiple signaling pathways and induces growth arrest in prostate cancer cells *Cancer Res.* **67** 11942–50
[84] Eguchi T, Prince T L, Tran M T, Sogawa C, Lang B J and Calderwood S K 2019 MZF1 and SCAND1 reciprocally regulate CDC37 gene expression in prostate cancer *Cancers* **11** 792

[85] Miyata Y, Nakamoto H and Neckers L 2013 The therapeutic target Hsp90 and cancer hallmarks *Curr. Pharm. Des.* **19** 347–65

[86] Calderwood S K and Gong J 2016 Heat shock proteins promote cancer: it's a protection racket *Trends Biochem. Sci.* **41** 311–23

[87] Kirschke E, Goswami D, Southworth D, Griffin P R and Agard D A 2014 Glucocorticoid receptor function regulated by coordinated action of the Hsp90 and Hsp70 chaperone cycles *Cell* **157** 1685–97

[88] Calderwood S K, Khaleque M A, Sawyer D B and Ciocca D 2018 Heat shock proteins in cancer: chaperones of tumorigenesis *Trends Biochem. Sci.* **31** 164–72

[89] Hasan A, Haque E, Hameed R, Maier P N, Irfan S, Kamil M, Nazir A and Mir S S 2020 Hsp90 inhibitor gedunin causes apoptosis in A549 lung cancer cells by disrupting Hsp90: Beclin-1: Bcl-2 interaction and downregulating autophagy *Life Sci.* **256** 118000

[90] Ciocca D R and Calderwood S K 2005 Heat shock proteins in cancer: diagnostic, prognostic, predictive, and treatment implications *Cell Stress Chaperones* **10** 86–103

[91] Katsogiannou M, Andrieu C and Rocchi P 2014 Heat shock protein 27 phosphorylation state is associated with cancer progression *Front. Genet.* **5** 346

[92] Berrieman H K, Cawkwell L, O'Kane S L, Smith L and Lind M J 2006 Hsp27 may allow prediction of the response to single-agent vinorelbine chemotherapy in non-small cell lung cancer *Oncol. Rep.* **15** 283–6

[93] Han-Shui H, Jiun-Han L, Wen-Chien H, Tien-Wei H, Kelly S, Shih-Hwa C, Yo-Ting T and Shih-Chieh H 2010 Chemoresistance of lung cancer stem-like cells depends on activation of Hsp27 *Cancer* **117** 1516–28

[94] Lee J-H, Sun D, Cho K-J, Kim M-S, Hong M-H, Kim I-K, Lee J-S and Lee J-H 2007 Overexpression of human 27 kDa heat shock protein in laryngeal cancer cells confers chemoresistance associated with cell growth delay *J. Cancer Res. Clin. Oncol.* **133** 37–46

[95] Lelj-Garolla B, Kumano M, Beraldi E, Nappi L, Rocchi P, Ionescu D N, Fazli L, Zoubeidi A and Gleave M E 2015 Hsp27 Inhibition with OGX-427 sensitizes non–small cell lung cancer cells to erlotinib and chemotherapy *Mol. Cancer Ther.* **14** 1107–16

[96] Concannon C G, Gorman A M and Samali A 2003 On the role of Hsp27 in regulating apoptosis *Apoptosis* **8** 61–70

[97] Havasi A, Li Z, Wang Z, Martin J L, Botla V, Ruchalski K, Schwartz J H and Borkan S C 2008 Hsp27 inhibits bax activation and apoptosis via a phosphatidylinositol 3-kinase-dependent mechanism *J. Biol. Chem.* **283** 12305–313

[98] Zhang S A I, HU Y, Huang Y, Xu H, WU G and Dai H 2015 Heat shock protein 27 promotes cell proliferation through activator protein-1 in lung cancer *Oncol. Lett.* **9** 2572–6

[99] Zimmermann M, Nickl S, Lambers C, Hacker S, Mitterbauer A, Hoetzenecker K, Rozsas A, Ostoros G, Laszlo V and Hofbauer H *et al* 2012 Discrimination of clinical stages in non-small cell lung cancer patients by serum HSP27 and HSP70: a multiinstitutional case–control study *Clin. Chim. Acta* **413** 1115–20

[100] Xu T, Wei Q, Guerra J L L, Wang L-E, Liu Z, Gomez D, O'Reilly M, Lin S H, Zhuang Y and Levy L B *et al* 2012 HSPB1 gene polymorphisms predict risk of mortality for US patients after radio(chemo)therapy for non-small-cell lung cancer *Int. J. Radiat. Oncol. Biol. Phys.* **84** e229–35

[101] Guo H, Bai Y, Xu P, Hu Z, Liu L, Wang F, Jin G, Wang F, Deng Q and Tu Y *et al* 2010 Functional promoter −1271G>C variant of HSPB1 predicts lung cancer risk and survival *J. Clin. Oncol.* **28** 1928–35

[102] Li S, Zhang W, Fan J, Lai Y and Che G 2016 Clinicopathological and prognostic significance of heat shock protein 27 (HSP27) expression in non-small cell lung cancer: a systematic review and meta-analysis *Springerplus* **5** 1165

[103] Oba M, Yano S, Shuto T, Suico M A, Eguma A and Kai H 2008 IFN-gamma down-regulates Hsp27 and enhances hyperthermia-induced tumor cell death *in vitro* and tumor suppression *in vivo Int. J. Oncol.* **32** 1317–24

[104] Xu X, Wang W, Shao W, Yin W, Chen H, Qiu Y, Mo M, Zhao J, Deng Q and He J 2011 Heat shock protein-60 expression was significantly correlated with the prognosis of lung adenocarcinoma *J. Surg. Oncol.* **104** 598–603

[105] Agababaoglu I, Onen A, Demir A B, Aktaş S, Altun Z, Ersoz H, Şanlı A, Ozdemir N and Akkoçlu A 2017 Chaperonin (HSP60) and annexin-2 are candidate biomarkers for non-small cell lung carcinoma *Medicine (Baltimore)* **96** e5903

[106] Rosenzweig R, Nillegoda N B, Mayer M P and Bukau B 2019 The Hsp70 chaperone network *Nat. Rev. Mol. Cell Biol.* **20** 665–80

[107] Knighton L E, Delgado L E and Truman A W 2019 Novel insights into molecular chaperone regulation of ribonucleotide reductase *Curr. Genet.* **65** 477–82

[108] Nitika T A W 2017 Cracking the chaperone code: cellular roles for Hsp70 phosphorylation *Trends Biochem. Sci.* **42** 932–5

[109] Suzuki K, Ito Y, Wakai K, Kawado M, Hashimoto S, Seki N, Ando M, Nishino Y, Kondo T and Watanabe Y *et al* 2006 Serum heat shock protein 70 levels and lung cancer risk: a case-control study nested in a large Cohort study *Cancer Epidemiol. Biomarkers Prev.* **15** 1733–7

[110] Gunther S, Ostheimer C, Stangl S, Specht H M, Mozes P, Jesinghaus M, Vordermark D, Combs S E, Peltz F and Jung M P *et al* 2015 Correlation of Hsp70 Serum levels with gross tumor volume and composition of lymphocyte subpopulations in patients with squamous cell and adeno non-small cell lung cancer *Front. Immunol.* **6** 556

[111] Tang T, Yang C, Brown H E and Huang J 2018 Circulating heat shock protein 70 is a novel biomarker for early diagnosis of lung cancer *Dis. Markers* **2018** 6184162

[112] Wang Q, He Z, Zhang J, Wang Y, Wang T, Tong S, Wang L, Wang S and Chen Y 2005 Overexpression of endoplasmic reticulum molecular chaperone GRP94 and GRP78 in human lung cancer tissues and its significance *Cancer Detect. Prev.* **29** 544–51

[113] Sun Q, Hua J, Wang Q, Xu W, Zhang J, Zhang J, Kang J and Li M 2012 Expressions of GRP78 and Bax associate with differentiation, metastasis, and apoptosis in non-small cell lung cancer *Mol. Biol. Rep.* **39** 6753–61

[114] Zhu X, Lin M C M, Fan W, Tian L, Wang J, Ng S S, Wang M, Kung H and Li D 2018 An intronic polymorphism in GRP78 improves chemotherapeutic prediction in non-small cell lung cancer *Chest* **141** 1466–72

[115] Subbarao Sreedhar A, Kalmar E, Csermely P and Shen Y-F 2004 Hsp90 isoforms: functions, expression and clinical importance *FEBS Lett.* **562** 11–5

[116] Whitesell L and Lindquist S L 2005 HSP90 and the chaperoning of cancer *Nat. Rev. Cancer* **5** 761

[117] Khalil A A, Kabapy N F, Deraz S F and Smith C 2011 Heat shock proteins in oncology: diagnostic biomarkers or therapeutic targets? *Biochim. Biophys. Acta* **1816** 89–104

[118] Gallegos Ruiz M I *et al* 2008 Integration of gene dosage and gene expression in non-small cell lung cancer, identification of HSP90 as potential target *PLoS One* **3** e0001722
[119] Wang X, Song X, Zhuo W, Fu Y, Shi H, Liang Y, Tong M, Chang G and Luo Y 2009 The regulatory mechanism of Hsp90α secretion and its function in tumor malignancy *Proc. Natl Acad. Sci.* **106** 21288–93
[120] Shi Y, Liu X, Lou J, Han X, Zhang L, Wang Q, Li B, Dong M and Zhang Y 2014 Plasma levels of heat shock protein 90 alpha associated with lung cancer development and treatment responses *Clin. Cancer Res.* **20** 6016–22
[121] Kim S-H, Lee G, Lee J-S, Cho Y J, Jeong Y Y, Kim H-C, Lee J D, Lee J H, Lee E H and Lee H W 2014 Association of high expression of Hsp90-beta and GRP 94 with poor survival in resected non-small cell lung cancer patients *J. Clin. Oncol.* **32** e22183–2183
[122] Kim S H *et al* 2015 High-level expression of Hsp90β is associated with poor survival in resectable non-small-cell lung cancer patients *Histopathology* **67** 509–19
[123] Rong B, Zhao C, Liu H, Ming Z, Cai X, Gao W and Yang S 2014 Identification and verification of Hsp90-beta as a potential serum biomarker for lung cancer *Am. J. Cancer Res.* **4** 874
[124] Minghui W A, Lin F E, Ping L I, Naijun H A, Yanning G A and Ting X I 2016 Hsp90AB1 protein is overexpressed in non-small cell lung cancer tissues and associated with poor prognosis in lung adenocarcinoma patients *Zhongguo Fei Ai Za Zhi.* **19**
[125] Ahsan A *et al* 2012 Wild-type EGFR is stabilized by direct interaction with HSP90 in cancer cells and tumors *Neoplasia* **14** 670–7
[126] Gomez-Casal R, Epperly M W, Wang H, Proia D A, Greenberger J S and Levina V 2015 Radioresistant human lung adenocarcinoma cells that survived multiple fractions of ionizing radiation are sensitive to HSP90 inhibition *Oncotarget* **6** 44306
[127] Ting L I, Xiaokun W A and Zhang L 2011 The correlation between the up-regulation of Hsp90 and drug resistance to cisplatin in lung cancer cell line *Zhongguo Fei Ai Za Zhi* **14**
[128] Hsu H S, Lin J H, Huang W C, Hsu T W, Su K, Chiou S H, Tsai Y T and Hung S C 2011 Chemoresistance of lung cancer stem-like cells depends on activation of Hsp27 *Cancer.* **117** 1516–28
[129] Cappello F, Di Stefano A, D'Anna S E, Donner C F and Zummo G 2005 Immunopositivity of heat shock protein 60 as a biomarker of bronchial carcinogenesis *Lancet Oncol.* **6** 816
[130] Clare D K and Saibil H R 2013 ATP-driven molecular chaperone machines *Biopolymers* **99** 846–59
[131] Corrao S *et al* 2014 Hsp10 nuclear localization and changes in lung cells response to cigarette smoke suggest novel roles for this chaperonin *Open Biol.* **4** 140125
[132] Fucarino A and Pitruzzella A 2020 Role of HSP60/HSP10 in lung cancer: simple biomarkers or leading actors? *J. Oncol.*
[133] Volm M, Koomägi R, Mattern J and Stammler G 1995 Heat shock (hsp70) and resistance proteins in non-small cell lung carcinomas *Cancer Lett.* **95** 195–200
[134] Michils A, Redivo M, de Beyl V Z, De Maertelaer V, Jacobovitz D, Rocmans P and Duchateau J 2001 Increased expression of high but not low molecular weight heat shock proteins in resectable lung carcinoma *Lung Cancer* **33** 59–67

www.ingramcontent.com/pod-product-compliance
Ingram Content Group UK Ltd.
Pitfield, Milton Keynes, MK11 3LW, UK
UKHW051356100926
8556IPUK00005B/656

9 780750 33353